DBT® Skills Manual for Adolescents

Jill H. Rathus
Alec L. Miller

Foreword by Marsha M. Linehan

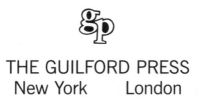

THE GUILFORD PRESS
New York   London

© 2015 The Guilford Press
A Division of Guilford Publications, Inc.
370 Seventh Avenue, Suite 1200, New York, NY 10001
www.guilford.com

Printed in the United States of America

This book is printed on acid-free paper.

Last digit is print number: 9   8   7   6   5   4   3   2

The authors have checked with sources believed to be reliable in their efforts to provide information that is
complete and generally in accord with the standards of practice that are accepted at the time of publication.
However, in view of the possibility of human error or changes in behavioral, mental health, or medical
sciences, neither the authors, nor the editors and publisher, nor any other party who has been involved
in the preparation or publication of this work warrants that the information contained herein is in every
respect accurate or complete, and they are not responsible for any errors or omissions or the results obtained
from the use of such information. Readers are encouraged to confirm the information contained in this
book with other sources.

Library of Congress Cataloging-in-Publication Data

Rathus, Jill H.
  DBT skills manual for adolescents / Jill H. Rathus, Alec L. Miller.
     pages cm
  Includes bibliographical references and index.
  ISBN 978-1-4625-1535-6 (pbk. : acid-free paper)
  1. Dialectical behavior therapy.   2. Adolescent psychotherapy.   3. Adolescent psychology.   I. Miller,
Alec L.   II. Title.   III. Title: Dialectical behavior therapy skills manual for adolescents.
  RC489.B4R36 2015
  616.89′142—dc23

                                                                                      2013043128

Illustrations by Sam Miller

DBT is a registered trademark of Marsha M. Linehan.

DBT® SKILLS MANUAL FOR ADOLESCENTS

Also from Jill H. Rathus and Alec L. Miller

Dialectical Behavior Therapy with Suicidal Adolescents
Alec L. Miller, Jill H. Rathus, and Marsha M. Linehan

About the Authors

Jill H. Rathus, PhD, is Professor of Psychology at Long Island University—C. W. Post Campus, where she directs the DBT scientist-practitioner training program within the clinical psychology doctoral program. She is also Co-Director and Co-Founder of Cognitive Behavioral Associates, a group private practice in Great Neck, New York, specializing in dialectical behavior therapy (DBT) and cognitive-behavioral therapy (CBT). Her clinical and research interests include DBT, CBT, adolescent suicidality, marital distress, intimate partner violence, anxiety disorders, and assessment, and she publishes widely in these areas. Dr. Rathus is coauthor (with Alec L. Miller and Marsha M. Linehan) of *Dialectical Behavior Therapy with Suicidal Adolescents*, and she trains mental health professionals internationally.

Alec L. Miller, PsyD, is Professor of Clinical Psychiatry and Behavioral Sciences, Chief of Child and Adolescent Psychology, and Director of the Adolescent Depression and Suicide Program at Montefiore Medical Center of the Albert Einstein College of Medicine. He is also Co-Founder of Cognitive and Behavioral Consultants of Westchester and Manhattan. Dr. Miller has published widely on DBT, adolescent suicide, childhood maltreatment, and borderline personality disorder, and has trained thousands of mental health professionals in DBT. A Fellow of Divisions 12 (Clinical Psychology) and 53 (Clinical Child and Adolescent Psychology) of the American Psychological Association, he is coauthor (with Jill H. Rathus and Marsha M. Linehan) of *Dialectical Behavior Therapy with Suicidal Adolescents*.

Foreword

Jill Rathus and Alec Miller attended one of my first dialectical behavior therapy (DBT®) intensive trainings. They were working on learning DBT and applying it to an urban, multiproblem, suicidal adolescent population at Montefiore Medical Center, Bronx, New York. When they returned for Part II of the intensive training, during which teams present their programs, I was struck by their passion and compassion, by how deeply they grasped the treatment, and by how thoughtfully they applied it to adolescents. I realized then how fabulous their work was for DBT and for teens in need of DBT.

Rathus and Miller infused their version of DBT with original, creative, and developmentally appropriate elements. They included family members in the treatment through skills training, family sessions, and parent coaching modalities, to directly address adolescents' environments; this helps not only adolescents, but also their parents, who are often despondent and don't know what to do. They identified new dialectical dilemmas that they observed in the struggles between parents and teens, parents and parents, and teens and therapists. They developed a new skills module that addresses family conflict by explicitly teaching dialectics as a skill set not only for DBT therapists, but also for teens and their parents; validation, which families desperately need; and behavior change, which families often attempt ineffectively and also desperately need. They devised a sensitive way to teach the biosocial theory to parents, developed teaching points for the DBT assumptions that address the negative attributions parents and teens often make for one another's behavior, figured out how to handle matters of confidentiality, and devised mindfulness exercises that appeal to teens—to name just a few of their creative ideas. They thoughtfully explicated these innovations and more in an earlier book, *Dialectical Behavior Therapy with Suicidal Adolescents*. Rathus and Miller developed the teen-based treatment and wrote the 2007 book; I was simply a coauthor, serving as consultant and confidant on DBT when needed. That work has become the primary text on applying DBT with adolescents, and as such is a companion volume to the present book.

Throughout the nearly two decades I have known them, Jill Rathus and Alec Miller have also published research, expanded their clinical practices, and trained professionals around the world to conduct DBT with adolescents. They have been a driving force behind the international proliferation of adolescent DBT programs, and in disseminating this treatment to youth and families who in the past were often rejected from treatment settings and clinical research trials.

The current volume presents their latest contribution to adolescent DBT, and is certain to be as influential as their 2007 book. It is written for clinicians in various settings to use with adolescents coping with a broad array of emotional and behavioral difficulties. The book presents 10 chapters on conducting skills training with adolescents and their caregivers. The first four chapters contain everything practitioners need to know about setting up and structuring an adolescent DBT skills training program. This section includes solutions to problems and questions regarding such topics as whom to include in skills training; group management strategies; skills training challenges; variations on the basic skills training format; therapy-interfering behaviors of teens *and* parents; dialectical tensions that arise in skills training; and dialectical dilemmas and their related treatment targets, not only in the context of individual and family therapy with adolescents, but also within the modality of skills training. The next six chapters provide the teaching notes corresponding to each adolescent skills training module: Mindfulness, Distress Tolerance, Walking the Middle Path, Emotion Regulation, and Interpersonal Effectiveness. These notes contain not only the basic "how-to" of teaching each skill group, but also the authors' collective clinical wisdom regarding teen- and family-based teaching stories, examples, exercises, role plays, and possible responses to likely questions/challenges by parents or teens.

Finally, the volume contains a set of skills handouts and practice worksheets. Whereas we at the University of Washington have used the adult versions of handouts and worksheets with our adolescent clients at high risk for suicide (and teens seems to understand them better than their parents), many clinicians and treatment programs are more comfortable with skills designed specifically for adolescents. These skills handouts and worksheets are wonderfully done. While keeping to the essence of the skills content from standard DBT, Rathus and Miller have added several new versions of skills tailored to teen and family work, such as the Parent–Teen Shared Pleasant Activities List, a Pleasant Activities List for teens, and the Crisis Survival Kit for school.

Make no mistake: Jill Rathus and Alec Miller are the experts on adolescent DBT. No clinicians in this rapidly expanding field better know the ins and outs of working with teens. This volume reveals in fine detail how to deliver this treatment to teens and their families in a way that will engage them, reach them, and offer them hope. This skills manual is an essential addition to their body of work, likely to make clinicians' jobs easier while enhancing outcomes, and sure to touch many lives.

MARSHA M. LINEHAN, PhD, ABPP
University of Washington

Preface

Marsha M. Linehan's dialectical behavior therapy (DBT®; Linehan, Armstrong, Suarez, Allmon, & Heard, 1991; Linehan, 1993a, 1993b) has revolutionized cognitive-behavioral therapies, with constructs such as mindfulness and acceptance now permeating behavioral approaches. Her technology for treating complex problems of emotional and behavioral dysregulation has brought compassionate treatment to clients who had been previously rejected by many therapists.

Linehan originally developed her treatment for clients with suicidal or self-injurious behaviors who were at high risk of suicide. Her work evolved using an iterative approach, systematically developing solutions for each problem that arose. To address the problem that patients receiving DBT lack certain capabilities, Linehan developed a set of standardized skills to teach clients how to regulate emotions, recognize internal states, focus attention, tolerate distress, and develop and sustain satisfying interpersonal relationships. To address the problem that therapists cannot teach new skillful behaviors while managing crises, Linehan determined that it is necessary to have skills training delivered as a separate modality. Linehan designed DBT as a comprehensive treatment package, including not only skills training, but also individual therapy, between-session telephone coaching, and therapist peer consultation (Linehan, 1993a, 1993b).

In the 1990s, we began applying DBT to suicidal multiproblem adolescents and families in an inner-city outpatient clinic and used the original Linehan (1993b) skills training manual. We recognized that many of the youth and their parents had difficulty reading and comprehending the material. However, we were reluctant to adapt the protocol before we had used it in its entirety. We piloted the adult manual as written with cohorts of adolescent patients and their caregivers in order to gain clinical information before making any modifications.

ADAPTING THE ADULT SKILLS TRAINING MANUAL FOR ADOLESCENTS

Direct participant feedback coupled with our clinical observations informed our initial alterations to the adult manual (Miller, Rathus, Linehan, Wetzler, & Leigh, 1997), and we have continued to make minor modifications as reflected in our 2007 book, *Dialectical Behavior Therapy with Suicidal Adolescents* (Miller, Rathus, & Linehan, 2007), and in the present manual.

We have modified only where necessary while maintaining the essential elements of DBT, such as its dialectical underpinnings; its biosocial theory of disorder; its functions; its assumptions; its targets; its change procedures; its treatment strategies (i.e., core, dialectical, stylistic, case management); and its skills. We have retained virtually all of Linehan's original DBT skills because (1) we have no basis for determining which, if any, are nonessential; (2) clients are idiosyncratic with regard to which skills they find most helpful, so we believe exposure to all skills is helpful; (3) while we do not expect clients to master the skills during skills training group, they have opportunities for mastery through the take-home practice exercises, practice exercise review, application in problem solving during individual therapy, and phone coaching; and (4) clients have an opportunity to relearn the skills by repeating the cycle through the skills modules or in a graduate group, described in Chapter 2.

This fidelity requires, of course, that clinicians conducting DBT with adolescents know DBT, and do not mistake DBT with adolescents for a treatment other than DBT. We based our 2007 book, written with Linehan (Miller et al., 2007), on our research and clinical work with this population and followed the treatment as it had been originally developed by Linehan.

We based modifications to the treatment on characteristics inherent to adolescents—they differ from adult clients with regard to emotional and cognitive developmental level—and context—they overwhelmingly attend school, and reside with their families and depend on them for daily functioning, including for getting to therapy. Thus, we considered developmentally relevant as well as family-based targets, cognitive processing and capability differences, distinct liability issues, and interventions with their environments, that is, their caregivers. We identified adolescent-quality-of-life treatment targets (e.g., skipping school) and adolescent–family secondary treatment targets, emphasized adolescent-appropriate therapeutic interactions, and increased the use of environmental intervention. The latter meant including parents in treatment by offering as-needed family or parenting sessions as well as including parents in skills training. With parents participating in skills training, we added a family-based module called Walking the Middle Path Skills. In addition, we modified the language and look of the original skills materials to enhance accessibility for adolescents, given their cognitive processing and capability differences. Additional changes included (1) slightly reducing the amount of content; (2) limiting the amount of information presented on a single handout; (3) simplifying language on handouts given that many patients and parents had reading levels at or below a middle school level, due to learning disabilities or speaking English as a second language; (4) adjusting the teaching stories, exercises, and examples on handouts and in the teaching notes to be developmentally relevant for an adolescent population (in both language and content); (5) adding graphics, pictures, and varied fonts to make handouts more visually and emotionally accessible to distractable and dysregulated teens; and (6) adding a fifth module, called Walking the Middle Path Skills, to target prominent issues that arose when working with teens and families, such as polarizing conflict, behavioral extremes, invalidation, and ineffective behavior change strategies. To counter these problems, the module teaches (1) principles of dialectics and adolescent–family dialectical dilemmas to reduce extreme thinking and behavior and enhance perspective taking, (2) validation skills, and (3) behavior change/learning principles and strategies for obtaining changes in one's own or others' behaviors. We believed that through such modifications, we could more effectively deliver Linehan's DBT skills to a teen population.

ADDITIONAL SKILLS IN THIS MANUAL

Along with the original set of DBT skills (Linehan, 1993a) and those from the Walking the Middle Path Skills module introduced in our 2007 book (Miller et al., 2007), we have included several additional skills. The following handouts are based on Linehan's recently revised skills manual (Linehan, 2015a; Linehan, 2015b): "Crisis Survival Skills: TIPP Skills for Managing Extreme Emotions" (Distress Tolerance Handout 11), "Building Mastery and Coping Ahead" (Emotion Regulation Handout 15), and "Check the Facts and Problem Solving" (Emotion Regulation Handout 19). The "Wise Mind Values and Priorities List" (Emotion Regulation Handout 13) is also based on Linehan's revised skills manual. To date, with the exception of Cope Ahead, these skills have not been included in adolescent research trials.

Original to this manual is the "Parent–Teen Shared Pleasant Activities List" (Emotion Regulation Handout 11). This handout expands the emotion regulation skill of Accumulating Positives in the short term to address the deficit in positive interactions that we have noted within many families seeking DBT. We also include two supplemental handouts to the emotion regulation PLEASE skill, for those who need more in-depth information on managing eating ("FOOD and Your MOOD," Emotion Regulation Handout 16a) and sleep ("BEST Ways to Get REST: 12 Tips for Better Sleep," Emotion Regulation Handout 16b). We have also expanded the validation skill in the Walking the Middle Path Skills module to formally include self-validation (see "How Can We Validate Ourselves?," Walking the Middle Path Handout 10). This is a secondary treatment target in DBT and a skill often lacking in teens. Finally, in the Interpersonal Effectiveness Skills module, we include the optional THINK skill. We developed this skill based on Crick and Dodge's (1994) social information-processing model after noticing that teens and families often assumed the worst about others' intentions and needed more help with perspective taking. THINK skills are not part of standard DBT and have not been used in any clinical trials to date.

Our skills adaptations for adolescents were designed as part of a comprehensive DBT treatment package, which is fully described in *Dialectical Behavior Therapy with Suicidal Adolescents* (Miller et al., 2007). This skills manual can serve as a companion to that 2007 book. Since then, however, clinicians and researchers have found DBT treatment and skills applicable to a much broader range of adolescents, many of whom have never been suicidal (see Groves, Backer, van den Bosch, & Miller, 2012, for review). Clinicians can, therefore, use this manual in the treatment of adolescents across diagnoses and behavioral problems who present with emotional and behavioral dysregulation.

Our adapted adolescent skills handouts are being used in multiple research settings; many clinical settings around the world employ some version of our materials. The publication of this manual makes them more widely available, along with group management strategies and skills teaching notes to assist the DBT skills trainer working with adolescents. We also believe in the importance of establishing a standardized and replicable set of materials to enhance research and clinical applications with materials faithful to DBT, and to reduce piecemeal application or continued reinvention of the adolescent materials.

Throughout this book, we use the terms "family member," "parent," or "caregiver" interchangeably. Our adolescent clients come from various backgrounds and settings. Some youth live with their parents or stepparents, some with a grandparent or other relative, and others in foster care or group home settings. Thus, some youth will invite nontraditional caregivers to participate in their treatment.

We hope this in-depth presentation of skills training for teens and families will help clinicians and researchers as they work toward improving the lives of adolescents who suffer from and struggle with emotional and behavioral dysregulation.

Acknowledgments

Both of us are deeply indebted to Marsha Linehan for her friendship, collaboration, and mentoring over the past two decades. We thank her for supporting this work and sharing her insights and materials with us.

We especially want to acknowledge our illustrator, Sam Miller (MFA, Columbia University), whose creativity, artistry, and sensitivity enhanced the communication of our words.

Our wonderful and talented team at The Guilford Press deserves so much credit for helping to usher this book through to completion: Bob Matloff, President; Seymour Weingarten, Editor-in-Chief; Kitty Moore, our acquisitions editor; Barbara Watkins, our developmental editor; Laura Specht Patchkofsky, our production editor; Judith Grauman, Managing Editor; and many other Guilford staff. We are grateful for their influence in the shaping of this volume, their patient and thorough work, and their investment in this project.

We also wish to mention some of our current and former colleagues at Montefiore Medical Center who helped encourage us when we first endeavored to adapt DBT for teens and families. These colleagues include Scott Wetzler, Bill Sanderson, and especially the late Marcia Landsman, who joined us during the first 4 years of our journey, helping us adapt these skills for teens.

Finally, we would like to thank so many of our DBT colleagues for their friendship, wisdom, and support of our work over the years. While we cannot recognize the entire DBT community by name, we want to extend a special thank you to Charlie Swenson, Larry Katz, Michael Hollander, Lizz Dexter-Mazza, Jim Mazza, Blaise Aguirre, Tony DuBose, Linda Dimeff, Helen Best, Alan Fruzzetti, Christine Foertsch, Kelly Koerner, Adam Payne, Lars Mehlum, Emily Cooney, Seth Axelrod, Gwen Abney-Cunningham, Perry Hoffman, Matthew Nock, and the late Cindy Sanderson.

I want to thank my dear coauthor, Alec Miller, for 20-plus years of friendship and collaboration. We've spent countless hours together discussing, researching, and writing. We've inspired each other and remoralized each other when needed, and it never fails to be a delight to work together.

I'd like to thank my family for their love, encouragement, and unwavering support. Now that my children are solidly into their teen years, they keep me on my toes, teach me every day about my work, and keep me smiling.

In addition, I am extremely grateful to my colleagues and friends at Long Island University–C. W. Post Campus (LIU Post) for being a long-standing source of support, personally and professionally: Bob Keisner, Eva Feindler, David Roll, Camilo Ortiz, Danielle Knafo, Geoff Goodman, Hilary Vidair, Marc Deiner, Cathy Kudlak, and Katherine Hill Miller. I also want to thank my assistant program director, Pam Gustafson, for always looking out for me and anticipating program and faculty needs. I also want to acknowledge the wonderful graduate students at LIU Post for participating in my DBT Clinical Research Lab, filling my DBT electives and workshops, sharing their enthusiasm with me, and keeping me fresh. For their help at various stages with research for this book and with running my DBT Lab, I would like to thank Erika Rooney, Melody Wysocki, Neal Bauer, Shannon York, Rivka Halpert, and Rebecca Kason.

I want to express special appreciation to my wonderful friend, codirector, and cofounder of Cognitive Behavioral Associates, LLP (CBA), Ruth DeRosa. Ruth anchors our practice and our team, and infuses our work with thoughfulness, positivity, creativity, clarity, and clinical acumen. I also want to extend a thank you to my other fabulous and talented DBT team members—Michelle Chung, Nira Nafisi, Shamshy Schlager, Hilary Vidair, and Vince Passarrelli—and our current and recent psychology externs—Gus Cutz, Kristin Wyatt, Lisa Shull Gettings, Avigail Margolis, Steve Mazza, and Esther Pearl. Hilary has been my longest-running skills group coleader at CBA and brings great skill and precision to skills training.

My friend, colleague, and fellow Guilford author, Valerie Gaus, provided helpful tips for the book, and I am grateful to her. I also thank Martha Guerra for all of her help and dedication. In addition, I thank Rahsaan Robinson for being a well of optimism and encouragement.

I also thank those who provided mentoring and modeling at Stony Brook, particularly Daniel O'Leary. I also thank Dina Vivian, Marv Goldfried, Dan Klein, Everett Waters, and the late Ted Carr. And I'd like to acknowledge the late Stephen Parrish—a Romantic Poetry scholar and my caring and dedicated English mentor at Cornell. His voice remains with me as I write.

I am deeply grateful to my clients, the teens, adults, parents, and families who work so hard to accept—and change—their problems. They show tremendous courage, honesty, perseverance, and good humor; they teach and inspire me each week. This work is for them.

—J. H. R.

I feel deep gratitude for my colleagues and trainees at Montefiore Medical Center's Department of Psychiatry and Behavioral Sciences who have supported my DBT treatment and training program for the past 20 years. Specifically, within Montefiore's Adolescent Depression and Suicide Program (ADSP), many have helped contribute to the development and refinement of my thinking about skills training with adolescents and families. I want to give a special thanks to Heather Smith, who has served as my Associate Director over the past 10 years and is ceaselessly committed to teaching DBT skills to Bronx youth and their caregivers. My research director, Miguelina German, and dozens of research assistants have helped enhance our understanding and application of DBT with Hispanic families. Jenny Seham and Michelle Lupkin are talented attending psychologists in the ADSP and continue to provide support to me at Montefiore and within our DBT program. None of this would be possible without Madelyn Garcia, my administrative assistant for the past 18 years, who continues to smile while seamlessly doing much of the heavy lifting to support our team.

My DBT team at Cognitive and Behavioral Consultants, LLP (CBC), has helped me grow as a DBT team leader, individual therapist, and skills trainer. Lata McGinn, my cofounder, has continued to be a great support to me over the past 24 years and to our DBT treatment and training program. At CBC, I continue to learn from and feel supported by many exceptional DBT clinicians, including Sara Steinberg, Jennifer Steinberg, Michelle Greenberg, Colleen Lang, Courtney Berry, Johanna Wekar, Amanda Edwards, Suzanne Davino, Yeraz Meschian, Liz Courtney-Seidler, Karen Burns, Irene Zilber, Arva Bensaheb, and Chad Brice. Dena Klein and Becky Hashim, two former students and now talented therapist colleagues with whom I have had the pleasure of working both at Montefiore Medical Center and CBC, continue to provide ongoing encouragement and creative thinking as it applies to DBT for specialized populations.

Many clients and their families in the Bronx and Westchester County, New York, have enhanced my skills as a DBT therapist and skills trainer. This book and my career would not have been possible without this group of remarkable people. Every day they teach me more about humility, compassion, curiosity, flexibility, commonalities, resilience, dialetics, the power of behavioral principles and validation, and the ultimate wisdom that comes from decades of experience.

I am forever grateful to my wife and children for their love, support, and patience during the writing of this book. They helped me become a better husband, father, and skills trainer, in fact, by providing me with opportunities to practice my DBT skills in daily life. Every life hiccup and hardship provides me with a new teaching example and an opportunity to practice DBT skills.

Finally, I want to thank Jill Rathus, my dear friend, cotreatment developer, coauthor, and former co-intern; together we have spent thousands of hours developing and challenging one another's thinking about how to adapt and improve DBT for adolescents and families. Thank you for sharing this journey with me.

—A. L. M.

Contents

PART III. Skills Training Handouts

Purchasers can download copies of the handouts
from *www.guilford.com/rathus-forms*.

PART I

Dialectical Behavior Therapy Skills Training Structure and Strategies

CHAPTER 1

An Introduction to Dialectical Behavior Therapy and Skills Training

DBT® Skills Manual for Adolescents offers a guide for mental health practitioners working with adolescents who struggle to control their emotions and behaviors. Emotional and behavioral dysregulation often contribute to an adolescent's difficulties in establishing a stable sense of self and forming fulfilling and stable relationships with peers and family members. Furthermore, problematic impulsive or avoidant behavior is often a consequence of emotion dysregulation or an effort to re-regulate. The five sets of skills in this book directly correspond to the five major problems that are associated with emotional dysregulation in adolescents. Mindfulness skills help adolescents increase their self-awareness and attentional control while reducing suffering and increasing pleasure; distress tolerance skills offer tools to reduce impulsivity and accept reality as it is; emotion regulation skills help increase positive emotions and reduce negative emotions; interpersonal effectiveness skills help adolescents improve and maintain peer and family relationships and build self-respect; and walking the middle path skills teach methods for reducing family conflict by teaching validation, behavior change principles, and dialectical thinking and acting.

We divide this book into three sections. The first section (Chapters 1–4) contains information for understanding dialectical behavior therapy (DBT) and its skills training mode, and for setting up and running a DBT skills training program. It explains the structure of skills training programs, describes the running and management of DBT multifamily groups and other skills training formats, and highlights the art and style of conducting DBT skills training. The second section (Chapters 5–10) contains the teaching notes, lecture points, examples, and strategies for orienting clients and teaching the specific DBT skills. The third section contains the skills training handouts for teens and families in the Orientation, Mindfulness, Distress Tolerance, Walking the Middle Path, Emotion Regulation, and Interpersonal Effectiveness Skills modules.

Parts of this chapter are adapted from Miller, Rathus, and Linehan (2007) and Linehan, Cochran, and Kehrer (2001). Copyright 2007 and 2001 by The Guilford Press. Adapted by permission.

ADOLESCENTS WHO CAN BENEFIT FROM DBT SKILLS TRAINING

Adolescents can be categorized along a continuum from typical, relatively asymptomatic adolescents to severely emotionally and behaviorally dysregulated teens who may require a restrictive setting (i.e., inpatient or residential treatment). We believe that DBT skills can be beneficial to all these populations, applied within a primary, secondary, or tertiary prevention framework. Primary prevention programs are intended to ward off future problems for a general population who are not presently at risk or seeking mental health services. From this vantage point, DBT skills can be applied broadly to middle school, high school, and early college-age youth with normal moodiness, occasional relational difficulties, and perhaps experimentation with risk behaviors. Many normal adolescents exhibit some degree of emotional dysregulation, and training in DBT skills, by itself, may benefit these teens. Secondary prevention programs are intended to protect against the full blossoming of mental health disorders for at-risk individuals characterized by mild or early indicators of mental health needs (e.g., school difficulties, attentional problems, sad or anxious mood, family conflict). DBT skills can be applied to these individuals in schools or clinical settings.

Tertiary preventions target individuals with significant emotional and behavioral disorders in order to actively treat the disorders while improving functioning. For this population, practitioners often apply DBT skills as part of a comprehensive DBT treatment program in outpatient, inpatient, residential, and juvenile justice settings. Linehan (1993a, 1993b) designed DBT as a comprehensive treatment program for high-risk clients diagnosed with borderline personality disorder (BPD). Comprehensive DBT with severely dysregulated adolescents follows Linehan's original model, with multiple treatment modalities. Many of the youth treated with comprehensive DBT typically carry two to four DSM-5 disorders as well as many other life problems not captured by these diagnoses. Such severely dysregulated teens are typically not able to fully benefit from skills training without a more comprehensive DBT program that usually includes individual therapy, telephone coaching of skills, and a consultation team of therapists working together, in addition to skills training. For example, individual therapy in DBT requires adolescents to intensively self-monitor their behavioral urges, actions, and skills on a diary card as well as to practice using skills in place of problem behaviors. When problem behaviors show up on a teen's diary card, the individual DBT therapist conducts what we term *behavioral chain* and *solution analyses* with the teen. This process identifies places in the behavioral sequence where skills can be used to replace the problem behaviors. Teens are encouraged to call their individual DBT therapists for intersession telephone coaching of skills to interrupt their impulse to engage in problem behaviors. At a minimum, severely emotionally dysregulated teens at risk for suicidal behavior need a practitioner other than the skills trainers to intensively oversee their treatment, remain available to them when needed, assess for suicidal behavior, and manage risk. This person, ideally, would be trained in an empirically validated suicide risk management protocol such as the Linehan Risk Assessment and Management Protocol (LRAMP; Linehan, Comtois, & Ward-Ciesielski, 2012).

HOW DBT CONCEPTUALIZES THE EMOTIONALLY DYSREGULATED ADOLESCENT

DBT can be applied to youth presenting with multiple, serious problems that may include suicidal behaviors, nonsuicidal self-injury, high-risk sexual behaviors, disordered eating, illicit drug use, binge drinking, and other harmful behaviors. Youth may also have less severe problems such as light social drinking; first signs of nonsuicidal and nonsevere self-harm behavior; anger dyscontrol; school avoidance; impaired self-awareness of emotions, goals, and values; and frequent relationship breakups. DBT views all these problems as consequences of emotional dysregulation or as attempts to cope with emotional dysregulation. In other words, emotional dysregulation can lead to interpersonal, behavioral, cognitive, and self-dysregulation.

From a DBT perspective, many problematic adolescent behaviors, including suicidal behaviors, are influenced by two significant factors: (1) the lack of important interpersonal, self-regulation, and distress tolerance capabilities; and (2) personal and environmental factors that inhibit the use of those skills teens may already have. These personal and environmental factors also interfere with the development of new skills and capacities, in addition to reinforcing inappropriate, dysregulated, and dysfunctional behaviors.

Comprehensive DBT directly addresses these factors by:

1. Increasing teens' (and families') capabilities by teaching specific skills for self-regulation (including emotion regulation and mindfulness), interpersonal effectiveness, distress tolerance, and balanced thinking and acting ("Walking the Middle Path"), as shown in Table 1.1.
2. Structuring the environment to motivate, reinforce, and individualize appropriate use of the skills.

TABLE 1.1. Characteristics of Dysregulation and Corresponding DBT Skills Modules

Some characteristics of dysregulation	DBT skills modules
Emotion dysregulation	
Emotional vulnerability; emotional reactivity; emotional lability; angry outbursts; steady negative emotional states such as depression, anger, shame, anxiety, and guilt; deficits in positive emotions and difficulty in modulating emotions.	Emotion Regulation
Interpersonal dysregulation	
Unstable relationships, interpersonal conflicts, chronic family disturbance, social isolation, efforts to avoid abandonment, and difficulties getting wants and needs met in relationships and maintaining one's self-respect in relationships.	Interpersonal Effectiveness
Behavioral dysregulation	
Impulsive behaviors such as cutting classes, blurting out in class, spending money, risky sexual behavior, risky online behaviors, bingeing and/or purging, drug and alcohol abuse, aggressive behaviors, suicidal and nonsuicidal self-injurious behavior.	Distress Tolerance
Cognitive dysregulation and family conflict	
Nondialectical thinking and acting (i.e., extreme, polarized, or black-or-white), poor perspective taking and conflict resolution, invalidation of self and other, difficulty effectively influencing own and others' behaviors (i.e., obtaining desired changes).	Walking the Middle Path
Self-dysregulation	
Lacking awareness of emotions, thoughts, action urges; poor attentional control; unable to reduce one's suffering while also having difficulty accessing pleasure; identity confusion, sense of emptiness, and dissociation.	Core Mindfulness

Note. From Miller, Rathus, and Linehan (2007, Table 2.1, p. 36). Copyright 2007 by The Guilford Press. Adapted by permission.

3. Improving teens' motivation to increase the use of new skills, reduce the use of prior dysfunctional behaviors, and identify the factors (e.g., thoughts, feelings, behaviors, contextual variables) that maintain problematic behavioral patterns and inhibit more skillful ways of responding.
4. Providing methods to encourage the generalization of new skill capabilities from therapy to the life situations where they are needed.
5. Providing support for therapists treating multiproblem adolescents.

To fulfill the above functions, Linehan (1993a) developed treatment modes that may vary across treatment settings. Comprehensive DBT for pervasive emotional dysregulation typically includes four modes: individual therapy, group skills training, between-session telephone coaching, and a therapist consultation team. Comprehensive adolescent outpatient DBT slightly modifies these modes by conducting skills training groups with both adolescents and parents present in a multifamily skills group, providing phone coaching not only for adolescents but also for parents, offering family therapy sessions as needed, and offering parenting sessions as needed (Miller, Rathus, & Linehan, 2007). See Table 1.2 for a summary.

Other core elements of DBT include a biosocial theory of emotion dysregulation; an overall dialectical stance that emphasizes the transactional nature of the therapeutic relationship; a framework of treatment stages and, within each stage, a hierarchical prioritizing of behavioral treatment targets; and sets of acceptance, change, communication, structural, and dialectical strategies to achieve the behavioral targets. In the sections below, we briefly describe these elements and then review the skills modules taught. The chapter concludes with a brief summary of the outcome literature on DBT with an emphasis on DBT with adolescents.

DBT'S BIOSOCIAL THEORY

DBT (Linehan, 1993a) theorizes that the problem behaviors of emotionally dysregulated individuals stem from a combination of biological and environmental factors. Specifically, these factors are a biological vulnerability to emotional dysregulation and an invalidating social environment (an environment where coaching in emotion regulation is inadequate and dysfunctional learning takes place)—hence the term *biosocial* theory.

TABLE 1.2. Modes in Comprehensive Outpatient DBT with Multiproblem Adolescents

- Multifamily skills training group
- Individual DBT therapy
- Telephone coaching for teens *and* family members
- Family sessions (as needed)
- Parenting sessions (as needed)
- Therapist consultation team meeting
- Possible ancillary treatments
    o Pharmacotherapy
    o Therapeutic/residential schools

Biological Vulnerability

Linehan (1993a) theorized that biological factors play a primary role in the initial vulnerability to emotional dysregulation. Emotional vulnerability is defined as a high sensitivity to emotional stimuli, high reactivity (i.e., intense emotional responses), and a slow return to emotional baseline. A person may be vulnerable to intense emotion across several (perhaps all) emotions, positive and negative, combined with difficulties in modulating emotional reactions. However, most individuals with an initial biological vulnerability do not develop persistent emotional dysregulation. According to the theory, persistent emotional dysregulation occurs when an emotionally vulnerable individual is exposed to a pervasively invalidating environment.

Invalidating Environment

The invalidating environment is defined by the tendency of (often well-meaning) others (typically family members, but also teachers and other school personnel, peers, health professionals, etc.) to negate and/or respond erratically and inappropriately to private experiences, particularly private experiences not accompanied by public signs (e.g., feeling sick without having a high temperature). Private experiences, especially emotional experiences, are often not taken as valid responses to events. The person's experiences are punished, trivialized, ignored, dismissed, and/or attributed to socially unacceptable characteristics such as overreactivity, inability to see things realistically, lack of motivation, or failure to adopt a positive (or discriminating) attitude. Yet at times, the environment may reinforce escalating communications of distress, such as by attending to a family member lovingly and removing demands after a suicidal communication. In this regard, the invalidating environment also intermittently reinforces escalated emotional displays. Invalidating environments emphasize the need to control emotional expressiveness, oversimplify the ease of solving problems, and are generally intolerant of displays of negative affect.

The transactional nature of biosocial theory implies that individuals may develop patterns of dysregulation via somewhat different routes. A person with extreme emotional vulnerability may develop patterns of dysregulation in a family with a "normal" level of invalidation, and may even inadvertently elicit invalidation from the environment. Conversely, a highly invalidating environment might transact with a moderate to low level of emotional vulnerability to yield persistent emotional dysregulation. A different scenario might involve an anxious, school-refusing adolescent who finally musters the nerve to go to school and shows up late. When he arrives late to class, the teacher scoffs at him, telling him he failed to get a late pass and needs to check in with the assistant principal. The assistant principal berates the student for having missed days of school and speculates judgmentally that he has been out due to drug use. The student feels increasingly ashamed and walks back to class with his head down, only to be bullied by a group of teenagers who call him a loser. Too upset to return to class now, the security guard catches him "cutting class" and reports him to the principal for detention. When this type of school scenario repeats itself, it becomes an independent, pervasively invalidating environment. It is important to recognize the manifold potential sources of invalidation in an adolescent's life, while also remembering the transactional nature of this invalidation with the adolescent's biological emotional vulnerability. From this perspective, we aim to increase validation from the teen's environment (as well as toward the environment from the teen), and at the same time we aim to increase the teen's capacity for emotion regulation. Although all DBT skills are relevant when addressing these goals, we emphasize validation skills and emotion regulation skills to target invalidation and emotional vulnerability, respectively.

Regardless of its source, a transactional pattern between emotion dysregulation and invalidating environments results in an individual who has never learned how to label and regulate emotional arousal, how to tolerate emotional distress, or when to trust his or her own emotional responses as reflections of valid interpretations of events (Linehan, 1993a). The individual learns to mistrust his or her internal states and instead scans the environment for cues about how to act, think, or feel. This general reliance on others results in the individual's tendency to self-invalidate, which is often depressogenic and may contribute to confusion about self—that is, about one's goals, values, interests, and emotions. Emotion dysregulation also interferes with the development and maintenance of stable interpersonal relationships, which depend on both a stable sense of self and a capacity to regulate emotions. Moreover, the tendency of the invalidating environment to punish or ignore the expression of negative emotion, while reinforcing negative expression at others, shapes an expressive style later seen in individuals who vacillate between suppression of emotional experience and extreme behavioral displays. Behaviors such as not showing up for a test, drug use, running away, and self-injury may have important affect-regulating properties and are sometimes quite effective in eliciting helping behaviors from an environment that otherwise may ignore expressions of emotional pain.

DIALECTICS AND A DIALECTICAL STANCE

A dialectical worldview considers reality as continuous, dynamic, and holistic. Reality from this perspective is simultaneously whole and consisting of bipolar opposites (e.g., an atom consisting of opposing positive and negative charges). Dialectical truth emerges through the combination (or "synthesis") of elements from both opposing positions (the "thesis" and "antithesis"). The tension between the thesis and antithesis within each system—positive and negative, good and bad, children and parents, client and therapist, person and environment, and so forth—and their subsequent integration, produce change. Following change through synthesis, the new state also consists of polar forces. Thus change is continuous, and contradictory truths do not necessarily cancel each other out.

From the point of view of therapeutic dialogue and relationship, "dialectics" refers to change by persuasion and by making use of the oppositions inherent in one's thinking and behaviors and within the therapeutic relationship. Through the therapeutic opposition of contradictory positions, both client and therapist can arrive at new meanings within old meanings, moving closer to the essence of the subject under consideration. The spirit of a dialectical point of view is never to accept a proposition as a final truth or an undisputable fact. Thus the question addressed by both client and therapist is, "What is being left out of our understanding?" Related to this question is the holistic consideration of a patient's environmental context and the disordered behavior occurring transactionally in relation to that context.

A dialectical therapeutic position is one of constantly combining acceptance with change, flexibility with stability, nurturing with challenging, and a focus on capabilities with a focus on deficits. The goal is to highlight the opposites, both in therapy and in clients' lives, and to provide conditions for syntheses. The presumption is that we can facilitate change by emphasizing acceptance, and acceptance by emphasizing change.

DBT TREATMENT STAGES AND PRIMARY TREATMENT TARGETS

DBT conceptualizes treatment in stages that correspond to the severity and complexity of the client's problems. As Table 1.3 shows, each stage has its own hierarchy of treatment priorities or targets.

In comprehensive DBT, the pretreatment stage is typically several weeks long and involves assessing the client, orienting the client to DBT, and securing commitment to treatment and to the treatment goals for each individual teen. Clients in Stage 1 are severely and pervasively

TABLE 1.3. Standard DBT Stages and Their Hierarchies of Primary Treatment Targets

Pretreatment stage: Orientation and commitment to treatment, agreement on goals

Targets: 1. Inform adolescent about, and orienting adolescent to, DBT.
2. Inform adolescent's family about, and orienting family to, DBT.
3. Secure adolescent's commitment to treatment.
4. Secure adolescent's family's commitment to treatment.
5. Secure therapist's commitment to treatment.

Stage 1: Attaining basic capacities, increasing safety, reducing behavioral dyscontrol

Primary targets in individual DBT:
1. Decrease life-threatening behaviors.
2. Decrease therapy-interfering behaviors.
3. Decrease quality-of-life-interfering behaviors.
4. Increase behavioral skills.

Primary targets in DBT skills training:
1. Decrease behaviors likely to destroy therapy.
2. Increase skill acquisition, strengthening, and generalization.
   a. Core mindfulness
   b. Interpersonal effectiveness
   c. Emotion regulation
   d. Distress tolerance
   e. Walking the middle path
3. Decrease therapy-interfering behaviors.

Stage 2: Increasing nonanguished emotional experiencing, reducing traumatic stress

Primary target in individual DBT:
1. Decrease avoidance of emotional experience and posttraumatic stress.

Stage 3: Increasing self-respect and achieving individual goals, addressing normal problems in living

Primary targets in individual DBT:
1. Increase respect for self.
2. Achieve individual goals.

Stage 4: Finding joy, meaning, connection, and self-actualization

Primary targets in individual DBT:
1. Resolve a sense of incompleteness.
2. Find freedom and joy.

Note. From Linehan (1993a, Table 6.1, p. 167). Copyright 1993 and 2007 by The Guilford Press. Adapted by permission.

dysregulated and are at high risk for self-harm or suicide. Therefore, the main task with Stage 1 clients is to help them attain basic capacities that establish safety and behavioral control. This is the stage that comprises comprehensive, "standard DBT" and the vast majority of outcome data.

In Stage 1, skills training is typically separated from individual therapy, and each mode has somewhat different treatment priorities, as shown in Table 1.3. Aided by the client-completed diary card (Figure 1.1), Stage 1 individual therapy in DBT is structured to focus on its hierarchy of primary treatment targets: decreasing life-threatening behaviors, therapy-interfering behaviors, and quality-of-life-interfering behaviors and increasing behavioral skills. Each teen also works on specific, individualized treatment targets. Although increasing behavioral skills is a primary treatment target for the individual DBT therapist in Stage 1, it takes the lowest priority. The necessity of attending to crises, maintaining the patient in therapy, and reducing the severe behaviors that interfere with life quality make skills acquisition within individual psychotherapy nearly impossible. Trying to increase capabilities while addressing ongoing risky behaviors is like trying to build a shelter in the midst of a storm. One cannot address crises without skills; one cannot learn skills while responding to crisis. Thus, a separate component of treatment directly targets the acquisition of behavioral skills, and this component typically occurs in a group format. In DBT with adolescents, we recommend a multifamily skills group format, when possible.

Stage 2 of DBT involves emotionally processing past trauma and grief, and typically denotes a departure from Stage 1 skills acquisition and the highly structured individual sessions. However, skills are to be used and strengthened throughout Stage 2 and all later stages of DBT. Stage 3 addresses ordinary happiness and unhappiness and problems in living. Stage 4 addresses the attainment of transcendence and joy, and making meaning. Linehan (1993a) fully explicates each treatment stage and its goals.

Stage 1 Secondary Treatment Targets: Dialectical Dilemmas

Individuals with pervasive emotional dysregulation learn to alternate between behavioral extremes that either underregulate or overregulate emotion. DBT views these patterns as dialectical dilemmas for the client: The client alternately tries each extreme approach to emotion regulation but is unable to make either work. The first three Stage 1 primary treatment targets (life-threatening behaviors, therapy-interfering behaviors, quality-of-life-interfering behaviors) are themselves expressions of these dialectical extremes. Because these behaviors endanger the client's life, the therapy itself, or the quality of the client's life, they must be immediately addressed. But the overall patterns help sustain the dysfunctional behaviors, and they can also derail the skills acquisition process. Therefore, the patterns themselves need to be targeted by treatment if there is to be long-term change. The standard DBT dialectical dilemmas are:

- Emotional vulnerability versus self-invalidation.
- Active passivity versus apparent competence.
- Unrelenting crises versus inhibited experiencing.

Emotional vulnerability refers to the experience of high emotional arousal, a central experience for people entering DBT. *Self-invalidation* refers to dismissal of one's own emotions, perceptions, and problem-solving approaches. *Apparent competence* refers to the tendency of clients with chronic emotional dysregulation to appear at times more competent and in control than they actually are. *Active passivity* refers to being passive and helpless in the face of

Dialectical Behavior Therapy Adolescent Diary Card

First Name: _____

Filled out in session? Y/N

How often did you fill out this section? ___ Daily ___ 2–3x ___ Once
How often did you use phone consult? ___

Date started ___/___/___

Date	Self-Harm Urge	Self-Harm Actions	Suicidal Thoughts	Suicidal Actions	Alcohol Urge	Alcohol Use amount/type	Drugs Urge	Drugs Use amount/type	Meds Taken as prescribed?	Cut class/ school?	Risky sex?	What time did you go to sleep?	What time did you wake?	Anger	Fear	Happy	Anxious	Sad	Shame	Misery	Skills	Notes/DBT homework:
	0–5	Yes/No	0–5	Yes/No	0–5		0–5		Yes/No	Yes/No	Yes/No	Ex: 10:00 P.M.	Ex: 6:00 A.M.	0–5	0–5	0–5	0–5	0–5	0–5	0–5	0–7	
___/___																						
___/___																						
___/___																						
___/___																						
___/___																						
___/___																						
___/___																						

(columns grouped under: Self-Harm | Suicidal | Alcohol | Drugs | Meds | Other | Emotions)

*USED SKILLS
0 = Not thought about or used
1 = Thought about, not used, didn't want to
2 = Thought about, not used, wanted to
3 = Tried, but couldn't use them
4 = Tried, could do them but they didn't help
5 = Tried, could use them, helped
6 = Didn't try, used them, didn't help
7 = Didn't try, used them, helped

Rating Scale for Emotions and Urges (above):
0 = Not at all; 1 = A bit; 2 = Somewhat; 3 = Rather strong; 4 = Very strong; 5 = Extremely strong

Urge to quit therapy: _____   Misery Index: _____

Instructions: Circle the days you worked on each skill

	Skill							
Core Mindfulness	1. Wise mind	Mon	Tues	Wed	Thur	Fri	Sat	Sun
	2. Observe (Just notice what's going on inside)	Mon	Tues	Wed	Thur	Fri	Sat	Sun
	3. Describe: (Put words on the experience)	Mon	Tues	Wed	Thur	Fri	Sat	Sun
	4. Participate (Enter into the experience)	Mon	Tues	Wed	Thur	Fri	Sat	Sun
	5. Don't judge (Nonjudgmental stance)	Mon	Tues	Wed	Thur	Fri	Sat	Sun
	6. Stay focused (One-mindfully, in-the-moment)	Mon	Tues	Wed	Thur	Fri	Sat	Sun
	7. Do what works (Effectiveness)	Mon	Tues	Wed	Thur	Fri	Sat	Sun
Distress Tolerance	8. Accepts (Distract)	Mon	Tues	Wed	Thur	Fri	Sat	Sun
	9. Self-soothe (Five senses)	Mon	Tues	Wed	Thur	Fri	Sat	Sun
	10. Improve the moment	Mon	Tues	Wed	Thur	Fri	Sat	Sun
	11. Pros and cons	Mon	Tues	Wed	Thur	Fri	Sat	Sun
	12. TIPP	Mon	Tues	Wed	Thur	Fri	Sat	Sun
	13. Radical acceptance	Mon	Tues	Wed	Thur	Fri	Sat	Sun
Walking the Middle Path	14. Positive reinforcement	Mon	Tues	Wed	Thur	Fri	Sat	Sun
	15. Validate self	Mon	Tues	Wed	Thur	Fri	Sat	Sun
	16. Validate someone else	Mon	Tues	Wed	Thur	Fri	Sat	Sun
	17. Think dialectically (non–black and white)	Mon	Tues	Wed	Thur	Fri	Sat	Sun
	18. Act dialectically (walk the middle path)	Mon	Tues	Wed	Thur	Fri	Sat	Sun
Emotion Regulation	19. Identify and label emotions	Mon	Tues	Wed	Thur	Fri	Sat	Sun
	20. Engage in pleasant activities	Mon	Tues	Wed	Thur	Fri	Sat	Sun
	21. Values and priorities	Mon	Tues	Wed	Thur	Fri	Sat	Sun
	22. Work toward long-term goals	Mon	Tues	Wed	Thur	Fri	Sat	Sun
	23. Build mastery	Mon	Tues	Wed	Thur	Fri	Sat	Sun
	24. Cope ahead	Mon	Tues	Wed	Thur	Fri	Sat	Sun
	25. PLEASE	Mon	Tues	Wed	Thur	Fri	Sat	Sun
	26. Opposite ACTION to current emotion	Mon	Tues	Wed	Thur	Fri	Sat	Sun
	27. Check the facts	Mon	Tues	Wed	Thur	Fri	Sat	Sun
	28. Do problem solving	Mon	Tues	Wed	Thur	Fri	Sat	Sun
Interpersonal Effectiveness	29. DEAR MAN (Getting what you want)	Mon	Tues	Wed	Thur	Fri	Sat	Sun
	30. GIVE (Improving the relationship)	Mon	Tues	Wed	Thur	Fri	Sat	Sun
	31. FAST (Feeling effective and keeping your self-respect)	Mon	Tues	Wed	Thur	Fri	Sat	Sun
	32. Cheerleading statements for worry thoughts	Mon	Tues	Wed	Thur	Fri	Sat	Sun
	33. THINK	Mon	Tues	Wed	Thur	Fri	Sat	Sun

FIGURE 1.1. Diary card.

11

problems while actively eliciting the help of others to solve one's problems. *Unrelenting crisis* refers to the immediate and impulsive escape from emotional pain, a "crisis-of-the-week" syndrome. *Inhibited experiencing* refers to involuntary, automatic avoidance of cues that evoke past losses, trauma, or painful emotional states. It involves a shutting down of the normal processing of grief or the experiencing of other difficult emotions.

In addition, we developed three additional dialectical dilemmas, specific to adolescent–family interactions (Rathus & Miller, 2000):

- Excessive leniency versus authoritarian control.
- Normalizing pathological behaviors versus pathologizing normative behaviors.
- Forcing autonomy versus fostering dependence.

The Walking the Middle Path Skills module directly addresses these adolescent-specific dilemmas. Parents, therapists, and adolescents can all vacillate between being too loose or too strict, making too light of serious problem behaviors or making too much of normal, typical teen behavior, and forcing independence too soon or fostering dependence.

At each of the polar extremes above, there are two secondary treatment targets: one aimed at decreasing the maladaptive behavior, the other aimed at increasing a more adaptive response. Table 1.4 lists the dialectical dilemmas and corresponding secondary treatment targets in standard DBT, and Table 1.5 lists those developed for an adolescent population and their families. We say more about dialectical dilemmas in skills training in Chapters 4 and 8.

DBT TREATMENT STRATEGIES

DBT uses five sets of treatment strategies to address the specific treatment targets described above: (1) dialectical strategies, (2) validation strategies, (3) problem-solving strategies, (4) stylistic (communication) strategies, and (5) case management or structural strategies. Validation and problem-solving strategies, together with dialectical strategies, constitute the core strategies in DBT. Validation strategies focus on acceptance. Problem-solving strategies focus on change, and traditional behavioral therapy strategies fall under this set. Dialectical strategies primarily concern how the therapist structures interactions and defines skillful behaviors. As discussed

TABLE 1.4. Standard DBT Dialectical Dilemmas with Corresponding Secondary Treatment Targets

Dilemma	Targets
Emotional vulnerability versus self-invalidation	Increasing emotion modulation; decreasing emotional reactivity
Active passivity versus apparent competence	Increasing active problem solving; decreasing active passivity
Unrelenting crises versus inhibited experiencing	Increasing realistic decision making and judgment; decreasing crisis-generating behaviors

Note. From Miller, Rathus, and Linehan (2007, Table 5.1, p. 97). Copyright 2007 by The Guilford Press. Adapted by permission.

TABLE 1.5. Adolescent Dialectical Dilemmas, with Corresponding Secondary Treatment Targets

Dilemma	Targets
Excessive leniency versus authoritarian control	Increasing authoritative discipline; decreasing excessive leniency
	Increasing adolescent self-determination; decreasing authoritarian control
Normalizing pathological behaviors versus pathologizing normative behaviors	Increasing recognition of normative behaviors; decreasing pathologizing of normative behaviors
	Increasing identification of pathological behaviors; decreasing normalization of pathological behaviors
Forcing autonomy versus fostering dependence	Increasing individuation; decreasing excessive dependence
	Increasing effective reliance on others; decreasing excessive autonomy

Note. From Miller, Rathus, and Linehan (2007, Table 5.2, p. 98). Copyright 2007 by The Guilford Press. Reprinted by permission.

earlier, a dialectical therapeutic position is one of constantly combining acceptance of what *is* with a push toward change. Note that these strategies do not apply only to individual DBT therapy; group leaders employ them during skills training as well. Falling within change-oriented, problem-solving strategies are techniques based on traditional behavioral principles: positive and negative reinforcement, shaping, extinction, and punishment. These behavioral strategies permeate DBT along with acceptance-oriented ones such as validation. In Chapter 3 we say more about orienting and commitment strategies, which are types of change-oriented problem solving. In Chapter 4 we discuss other core strategies and their application to skills training.

MULTIFAMILY SKILLS GROUPS FOR ADOLESCENTS AND THEIR FAMILIES

For skills training with adolescents, we recommend a multifamily group format when possible. In this format, parents learn the same didactic content side by side with their adolescents. The group provides a forum that can improve interactions and enhance closeness. Including multiple families also helps maintain the didactic agenda, as opposed to drifting into a single family's problem of the week. Having multiple families in the room offers a built-in support network; provides powerful coping models, motivation, and hope; and tends to expand group members' repertoires of skill use. For example, when review of homework exposes each member to 10 other examples of a skill's application, members can develop a more thorough and flexible understanding of the skill's use. A multifamily format also allows for feedback and practice across families, such as a teen practicing a skill with another teen's parent, or a parent gently providing input to another parent's teen. In such interactions, clients' emotions tend to remain better regulated, and thus new learning can be enhanced (the goal would then be to work toward direct interactions with one's own family members, to enhance generalization). Additionally, individual members often benefit from feelings of mastery when they can explain a concept to a newer member. Teens and parents alike report feeling validated to hear of the similar struggles of others, especially after a period of feeling very much alone. Finally, at the graduation ceremony (see Chapter 2), teens and parents offer their parting constructive feedback and encouragement to one another, which powerfully affects the graduates themselves and the remaining group members. Receiving the repeated supportive comments crystallizes family members' newly formed self-constructs as capable, effective, functional, goal-oriented, and hopeful about their progress, both individually and collectively. Most graduating members also report dramatic improvement in the relationships with their participating family members. These public expressions capturing the progress within each individual and family demonstrate to other members how life can be improved, and models the need for perseverance and commitment to the DBT skills training group. This experience validates the challenges and pain the remaining families are enduring while also inspiring them to work harder and remain hopeful.

DBT Skills

The skills taught are grouped within five modules: Mindfulness Skills, Emotion Regulation Skills, Interpersonal Effectiveness Skills, Distress Tolerance Skills, and Walking the Middle Path Skills. This fifth module was specifically developed for adolescents and their families (Miller et al., 2007), and it is generally not taught in DBT skills training for adults. One complete course through all the skills modules typically takes 6 months (24 weeks), the same time frame as standard DBT. However, the adolescent skills program has five skills modules rather than four and so less time is devoted to each module than in standard DBT. Table 1.6 lists the skills taught in our adolescent DBT program.

As the list in Table 1.6 shows, a number of specific skills are referred to by acronyms or other mnemonics. For example, DEAR MAN, an interpersonal effectiveness skill, is an acronym for the steps to follow in effectively asking for something or saying no (Describe, Express, Assert, Reinforce; stay Mindful, Appear confident, Negotiate). The word *improve* in the distress tolerance skill of "IMPROVE the Moment" is an acronym for a set of various ways that distress might be made more tolerable. Group members are taught all the strategies and encouraged to try them out in order to find some that prove helpful.

TELEPHONE CONSULTATION TO FAMILY MEMBERS

In running multifamily skills groups, we have observed that family members benefit from telephone coaching of skills as much as their adolescents. This creates a dilemma: Adolescents call their individual therapist for coaching, but parents in skills training do not have an individual therapist to call. Phoning their teen's therapist poses obvious problems involving privacy and trust. We thus offer parents the opportunity to call the skills group leaders or their parenting therapist (see the next section on parent training sessions), and to limit these contacts to as-needed phone coaching for skills generalization (as opposed to other purposes, such as repairing the relationship or sharing good news). In cases where one of the skills group leaders is the primary therapist for their child, the parents may call only the other group leader. In settings in which the primary therapist is also the sole skills trainer and there is no separate therapist for the parents, allowing the parents to call the adolescent's therapist puts the teen's trust at risk. In such situations, the parent and adolescent need to agree to clear guidelines on what can be discussed in the therapist–parent skills coaching call. The parent and therapist should routinely disclose to the teen any calls made. Alternatively, skills coaching for parents may need to be restricted to the context of skills training or family sessions. Even if the parent's phone coach is someone other than the adolescent's primary therapist, we encourage parents to tell their adolescent when such a phone contact has been made so the adolescent remains confident that the treatment team is not operating in a deceptive manner.

TABLE 1.6. Overview of DBT Skills by Module

Core mindfulness skills
  "Wise Mind" (States of Mind)
  "What Skills" (Observe, Describe, Participate)
  "How Skills" (Don't Judge, Stay Focused, Do What Works)

Distress tolerance skills
  Crisis Survival Skills
    Distract with "Wise Mind ACCEPTS"
      (<u>A</u>ctivities, <u>C</u>ontributing, <u>C</u>omparisons, <u>E</u>motions, <u>P</u>ushing away, <u>T</u>houghts, <u>S</u>ensations)
    Self-soothe with six senses
      (vision, hearing, touch, smell, taste, movement)
    IMPROVE the Moment
      (<u>I</u>magery, <u>M</u>eaning, <u>P</u>rayer, <u>R</u>elaxing, <u>O</u>ne thing in the moment, <u>V</u>acation, <u>E</u>ncouragement)
    Pros and cons
    TIPP Skills (<u>T</u>emperature, <u>I</u>ntense exercise, <u>P</u>aced breathing, <u>P</u>rogressive relaxation)

  Reality Acceptance Skills
    Half-Smile
    Radical Acceptance
    Turning the Mind
    Willingness

Walking the middle path skills
  Dialectics
    Dialectical Thinking and Acting
    Dialectical Dilemmas
  Validation
    Validation of Others
    Self-Validation
  Behavior Change
    Positive Reinforcement
    Negative Reinforcement
    Shaping
    Extinction
    Punishment

Emotion regulation skills
  Understanding Emotions
    Observing and Describing Emotions
    What Emotions Do for You
  Reducing Emotional Vulnerability
    ABC (<u>A</u>ccumulate positives, long and short term; <u>B</u>uild mastery; <u>C</u>ope ahead)
    PLEASE (treat <u>P</u>hysica<u>L</u> illness, balance <u>E</u>ating, avoid mood-<u>A</u>ltering drugs; balance <u>S</u>leep,
      get <u>E</u>xercise)
  Changing Unwanted Emotions
    Check the Facts
    Problem Solving
    Opposite Action (to the current emotion)
  Reduce Emotional Suffering
    The Wave: Mindfulness of Current Emotion

(continued)

TABLE 1.6. *(continued)*

Interpersonal effectiveness skills
    Goals and priorities
    Maintaining relationships and reducing conflict: GIVE
      (be <u>G</u>entle, act <u>I</u>nterested, <u>V</u>alidate, use an <u>E</u>asy manner)
    Getting what you want or saying no: DEAR MAN
      (<u>D</u>escribe, <u>E</u>xpress, <u>A</u>ssert, <u>R</u>einforce, be <u>M</u>indful, <u>A</u>ppear confident, <u>N</u>egotiate)
    Keeping your self-respect: FAST
      (be <u>F</u>air, no <u>A</u>pologies, <u>S</u>tick to your values, be <u>T</u>ruthful)
    Wise Mind self-statements to combat worry thoughts
    Factors to Consider in Asking or Saying No
    Optional: Reducing conflict and negative emotion: THINK
      (<u>T</u>hink from the other's perspective, <u>H</u>ave empathy, other <u>I</u>nterpretations, <u>N</u>otice the other,
        be <u>K</u>ind)

Note. From Miller, Rathus, and Linehan (2007, Table 4.2, p. 74). Copyright 2007 by The Guilford Press. Adapted by permission.

PARENT TRAINING SESSIONS

Over the years many parents have told us they needed more guidance with the parenting skills we introduce in the Walking the Middle Path Skills module. They feel they need help not only with dialectics and validation but also with the behavior change skills of reinforcement, shaping, extinction/ignoring, and consequences. Many parents feel that their parenting is erratic, reactive, and extreme toward their emotionally dysregulated teens, and the parents often struggle with emotional dysregulation themselves while trying to implement parenting skills. We have thus made available optional, separate sessions for parents with a therapist on the treatment team who is not the adolescent's primary therapist. The therapist works with the teen's parent(s) to implement more consistent and effective parenting strategies, while bringing in other DBT skills as needed (e.g., mindfulness, distress tolerance). We offer this modality on an as-needed basis to individual families for the parenting challenges that arise regarding their particular teen. We typically offer parenting sessions as a short-term modality; many parents feel they receive substantial help in 6–12 parent-focused sessions, whereas some opt to continue longer. The parent-training therapist then becomes the parent's telephone skills coach. While we offer the mode to one or both parents from a family, a team could consider offering walking the middle path–based parenting skills as a separate group modality for parents as well. Note that if a family does not opt for parent training sessions, one can still offer the parents telephone coaching with a skills trainer who is not the teen's primary therapist. Research is needed to investigate the incremental validity of parenting sessions in adolescent DBT.

A NOTE ABOUT MANAGING SUICIDAL BEHAVIORS

We believe it is imperative that clinicians working with emotionally dysregulated, multiproblem patients learn the components of assessing and treating suicidal behaviors. Even patients who at first present without suicidal ideation or behavior may become suicidal as circumstances change. Thus, if one is providing skills training without an individual therapy component, it remains critical for the skills trainer to assess for suicidal risk factors at intake, recognize signs and risk factors during treatment, refer for individual therapy when suicidal behavior emerges, and handle a suicidal crisis competently should one arise. A detailed discussion of intervention for suicide risk is beyond the scope of this skills manual. However, many books and chapters on this topic exist, and we recommend, at a minimum, reading Linehan's original text (1993a); becoming familiar with more recent, comprehensive assessments, including the LRAMP (Linehan et al., 2012); and considering intensive training in DBT, as starting points to learning to manage suicidal behaviors.

We urge readers providing DBT skills training to read further and partake in intensive DBT training. Practitioners need to familiarize themselves with key treatment planning steps with suicidal patients (Linehan, 1999), including (1) knowing and assessing for long-term and imminent suicide risk factors, (2) obtaining detailed descriptions of suicidal behaviors, (3) monitoring ongoing behavior, and (4) conducting detailed behavioral chain analyses and solution analyses of suicidal behaviors. Solution analyses could include finding ways to prevent precipitants, replacing crisis responses with more skillful responses, and tolerating distress. Furthermore, they must include the adolescent's commitment to follow through on strategies developed with the therapist. Linehan's general guidelines for treating suicidal behaviors include being more active when suicide risk is high (Linehan, 1993a, 1999), being more flexible in considering responses, being more conservative, openly and matter-of-factly talking about suicide, remaining aware of individualized risk factors, presenting suicidal behavior as an ineffective response/solution to a problem, involving significant others (especially parents, in the case of teens), maintaining frequent contact, and scheduling sessions (and family sessions) as frequently as needed. Linehan recommends maintaining a strong therapeutic alliance with one's suicidal client and consulting with colleagues whenever managing a suicidal crisis.

OUTCOME RESEARCH ON DBT PROGRAMS

Research on DBT with Adults

Multiple randomized controlled trials (RCTs) have demonstrated DBT's comprehensive superiority to treatment as usual for problems associated with BPD (Linehan, Armstrong, Suarez, Allmon, & Heard, 1991; Linehan, Heard, & Armstrong, 1993; Linehan et al., 2006; Koons et al., 2001; van den Bosch, Koeter, Stijnen, Verheul, & van den Brink, 2005; Verheul et al., 2003). DBT has been shown to improve treatment adherence rates, decrease inpatient psychiatric days, and reduce frequency and severity of suicide attempts, nonsuicidal self-injurious behaviors, and suicidal ideation (Bohus, Haaf, & Simms, 2004; Linehan et al., 1991, 2006; Lynch, Morse, Mendelson, & Robins, 2003; Koons et al., 2001; van den Bosch et al., 2005; Verheul et al., 2003). Reviews of this research can be found in Scheel (2000), Robins and Chapman (2004), and Lynch, Trost, Salsman, and Linehan (2007).

Research on DBT has been conducted with various adult populations, including outpatient (e.g., Linehan et al., 1991, 1993, 2006; van den Bosch et al., 2005; Verheul et al., 2003), inpatient (Barley et al., 1993; Bohus et al., 2000, 2004; Linehan et al., 1999; Koons et al., 2001; Simpson et al., 1998), and forensic populations (Berzins & Trestman 2004; Bradley & Follingstad, 2003; Evershed et al., 2003). DBT has been shown to have applications for adults with comorbid BPD and substance abuse problems (Linehan et al., 1999, 2002; van den Bosch et al., 2005), comorbid BPD and eating disorders (Palmer, 2003), as an independent treatment for eating disorders (Safer, Telch, & Agras, 2001; Safer, Telch, & Chen, 2009; Telch, Agras, & Linehan, 2000), as an enhancement treatment for habit reversal treatment for trichotillomania (Keuthen et al., 2010), and as a treatment for depressed geriatric outpatients with mixed personality features (Lynch, 2000; Lynch et al., 2003).

Research on DBT with Adolescents

In a recently published review article, Groves, Backer, van den Bosch, and Miller (2012) summarized 12 adolescent DBT outcome studies published between 1997 and 2008. Since 2008, two additional adolescent DBT studies have been published. None of these studies was an RCT. However, three RCTs are now completed and another large RCT is under way.

Cooney and colleagues (2012) conducted a small randomized controlled feasibility study in New Zealand. These investigators assigned adolescents ($N = 29$) who had at least one suicide attempt or history of self-injury in the previous 3 months to either DBT ($n = 14$) or treatment as usual ($n = 15$) for 6 months. In this study DBT consisted of weekly individual therapy, weekly multifamily skills training, family sessions as required, telephone coaching to both teens and parents, and a therapist consultation team. These investigators used Linehan's (1993b) skills training materials and blended in some of our adolescent DBT handouts (e.g., Walking the Middle Path Skills). DBT sessions in this study were coded for adherence by expert raters. Cooney determined that the treatment was feasible to administer and well tolerated by adolescents and families in New Zealand.

Lars Mehlum and colleagues (2012, 2014) conducted a large randomized controlled trial in Oslo, Norway, comparing 16 weeks of outpatient DBT to enhanced usual care (EUC) for suicidal and self-harming adolescents who also met at least three out of nine BPD criteria. EUC consisted of any non-DBT therapy coupled with suicide risk assessment protocol training. In addition, the blinded research assessors would notify the EUC therapists any time an adolescent endorsed suicidality during the assessment. The Norwegian research team translated our adolescent DBT skills manual into Norwegian. Similar to our original outcome study (Rathus & Miller, 2002), their DBT condition consisted of weekly individual therapy, weekly multifamily skills training group, telephone coaching for adolescents, as-needed family sessions, and weekly therapist consultation team meetings.

The sample consisted of 77 adolescents with recent and repetitive self-harm and borderline features, treated at community child and adolescent psychiatric outpatient clinics. Treatment retention was generally good in both treatment conditions, and the use of emergency services was low. DBT was, however, superior to EUC in reducing self-harm, suicidal ideation, depression, and BPD symptoms. Effect sizes were large for treatment outcomes in patients who received DBT, whereas effect sizes were small for outcomes in patients receiving EUC. DBT sessions were coded for adherence to DBT by expert raters. Mehlum and colleagues intend to conduct a 1-year, 2-year, and 10-year follow-up study of these youth and their families.

Goldstein and colleagues (2012) conducted a small RCT of DBT comparing DBT ($n = 14$) to treatment as usual ($n = 6$) for suicidal adolescents diagnosed with bipolar disorder. Goldstein and colleagues used our adolescent skills manual and added several additional handouts containing psychoeducation on bipolar disorder. In this study DBT was delivered 1 week with an individual therapy session alternating with 1 week with a family skills training session, so that each was received every other week for 12 months. Results indicated that participants receiving DBT had significantly greater reductions in depression and trends toward significantly greater reductions in suicidal ideation and emotion dysregulation. The DBT group was more severe at baseline and the study was not adequately powered to expect significance. Thus, even the trends toward significant reduction were noteworthy.

Linehan, McCauley, Asarnow, and Berk are currently conducting a large multisite RCT (Collaborative Adolescent Research on Emotions and Suicide [CARES]) comparing comprehensive DBT to supportive therapy for recent and repeated suicidal behavior in adolescents with at least three BPD features. The DBT intervention spans 6 months and employs a multifamily group format with telephone coaching for teens and parents. These investigators use Linehan's skills training materials coupled with some content from the Walking the Middle Path Skills module (Miller et al., 2007).

In addition to these RCTs, three quasi-experimental studies on DBT with adolescents have been conducted to date, all of which indicate that the treatment is promising in reducing numerous target behaviors found among suicidal multiproblem youth (Fleischhaker et al., 2011; Katz, Cox, Gunasekara, & Miller, 2004; Rathus & Miller, 2002). These studies demonstrated feasibility and promising outcomes, including the results from a 1-year follow-up conducted by Fleischhaker and colleagues (2011).

Numerous open trials have also been published of DBT with adolescents with various problems and disorders: (1) multiproblem, multidiagnosed adolescents with suicidal and nonsuicidal self-injurious behaviors (Fleishchhaker, Munz, Böhme, Sixt, & Schulz, 2006; James, Taylor, Winmill, & Alfoadari, 2008; Sunseri, 2004; Woodberry & Popenoe, 2008); (2) adolescents diagnosed with bipolar disorder (Goldstein, Axelson, Birmaher, & Brent, 2007); (3) adolescents diagnosed with externalizing disorders in both forensic (Trupin, Stewart, Beach, & Boesky, 2002) and outpatient settings (Nelson-Gray et al., 2006); and (4) adolescents diagnosed with eating disorders, including bulimia, binge eating, and anorexia nervosa (Safer, Lock, & Couturier, 2007; Salbach, Klinkowski, Pfeiffer, Lehmkuhl, & Korte, 2007; Salbach-Andrae, Bohnekamp, Pfeiffer, Lehmkuhl, & Miller, 2008).

Other open trials highlight the application of DBT to various treatment settings beyond traditional outpatient, short-term inpatient, and forensic settings. These include applying DBT to adolescent girls in a residential treatment facility (Sunseri, 2004); adolescents receiving long-term inpatient care (McDonell et al., 2010); children and adolescents in school settings (Mason, Catucci, Lusk, & Johnson, 2009; Perepletchikova et al., 2010; Sally, Jackson, Carney, Kevelson, & Miller, 2002); and youth in a children's hospital who are noncompliant with treatment for their chronic medical conditions, such as renal disease, diabetes, sickle cell disease, and obesity (Hashim, Vadnais, & Miller, 2013).

The common denominator in all of these studies appears to be the adolescents' deficits in emotion regulation and the subsequent engagement in impulsive or avoidant behavior. The problematic impulsive or avoidant behavior is often a consequence of emotion dysregulation or an effort to re-regulate. As we described previously (Miller et al., 2007), we believe that the profile of emotional and behavioral dysregulation in adolescents makes DBT a relevant treatment modality across diagnoses and behavioral problems.

Results reported from experimental and quasi-experimental studies to date indicate that DBT appears to reduce suicidal behavior, depression, and BPD features, as well as have strong treatment feasibility, acceptability (i.e., well tolerated), and reasonably strong treatment retention rates (Cooney et al., 2012; Goldstein et al., 2007, 2012; Groves et al., 2012; Mehlum et al., 2014; Rathus & Miller, 2002). We anticipate the results from the Linehan and colleagues CARES study will further advance the evidence base of DBT for suicidal and multiproblem adolescents.

In the next chapter, we describe how skills training is organized, including the overall treatment course, the session structure, and the setting-up of a skills training group.

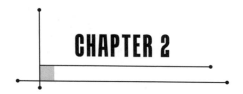

CHAPTER 2

Structure of DBT Skills Training

In this chapter we describe the structure of DBT skills training programs for adolescents, highlighting the multifamily skills training group format. We address topics such as treatment length, group composition, and session format. We conclude the chapter by discussing variations in adolescent DBT programs by setting.

SKILLS TRAINING TREATMENT COURSE: TREATMENT MODULE CYCLES

Interpersonal effectiveness skills, emotion regulation skills, distress tolerance skills, and walking the middle path skills are each typically taught over 4 weeks. An orientation to new group members and mindfulness skills is taught in a 2-week block that repeats before the start of each of the other four modules.

Thus, a group schedule might look like that shown in Table 2.1: Orientation and Mindfulness Skills (Week 1), Mindfulness Skills (Week 2), Distress Tolerance Skills (4 weeks), followed by a repeat of Orientation and Mindfulness Skills (2 weeks) and then Walking the Middle Path Skills (4 weeks) modules. The 2 weeks of orientation and mindfulness skills repeat again before the Emotion Regulation Skills module (4 weeks) and the Interpersonal Effectiveness Skills module (4 weeks).

An alternative schedule is to teach mindfulness and orientation skills in 1 week and devote 5 weeks each to the other modules. For either option, a complete course through all the modules lasts 24 weeks (6 months). Assuming a group with rolling admissions, the 24-week cycle would then repeat. Importantly, although we present the skills teaching notes in Chapters 5–10 in the prior format (2 weeks for Orientation and Mindfulness Skills modules and 4 weeks for each other skills module), a practitioner can easily change this to reflect the 1-plus-5-week format, allowing 5 weeks for each module other than Mindfulness Skills. The skills trainer would simply cover about one fewer handout or skill per group session to allow for a slower pace.

Note that families repeat the orientation material as well as the mindfulness skills before the start of each new module. Orientation includes an explanation of DBT, including DBT's

**TABLE 2.1. Sample Treatment Schedule
for Multifamily Skills Group**

2 weeks: Orientation and Mindfulness Skills modules
4 weeks: Distress Tolerance Skills module

2 weeks: Orientation and Mindfulness Skills modules
4 weeks: Walking the Middle Path Skills module

2 weeks: Orientation and Mindfulness Skills modules
4 weeks: Emotion Regulation Skills module

2 weeks: Orientation and Mindfulness Skills modules
4 weeks: Interpersonal Effectiveness Skills module

24 weeks completes one cycle through all modules

biosocial theory, the rationale for skills training, DBT treatment assumptions, and group guidelines. We believe it is important to give existing group members the chance to revisit problem areas and consider their progress while reviewing treatment assumptions and group rules. In addition, we often enlist senior group members to help orient newer members by explaining the importance of a rule or explaining an assumption. In the case of closed groups, leaders might not choose to repeat orientation content, or might review it less often. Note that even in rolling admission groups, it may be possible to conduct separate orientation sessions for new families and review orientation points more briefly during group time. In standard outpatient DBT with adults, clients repeat the 6-month cycle of skills for a total of 1 year of skills training. For adolescents, a number of possibilities exist. Some outpatient programs follow the standard model for 1 year of treatment. In others, therapists determine, on a case-by-case basis, who will go through the skills training a second time. This decision is based on the current severity of the adolescent's problems and the progress taking place; those who have successfully reached the Stage 1 targets of safety and behavioral control (see Miller et al., 2007) and who wish to graduate after one full cycle may do so. Those still engaging in self-harm or other impulsive, risky behaviors should be urged to remain and repeat some or all skills modules. Still another option is to allow patients to graduate after a single course of skills training but provide for a continuation phase with graduate-level skills groups (see "A Model for an Adolescent Graduate Group," below).

Breadth versus Depth in Teaching Skills

Determining how many skills to cover and in what time frame raises the issue of breadth versus depth. Teaching fewer skills in greater depth helps increase clients' expertise in those skills, whereas teaching many skills in a short time exposes clients to the skills but with little time for mastery or practice. On the other hand, it allows exposure to many skills, which a primary therapist can then reinforce during problem solving, phone coaching, and family sessions, if a client receives comprehensive DBT. Exposure to a wide range of skills is important because not all skills may work for all clients, yet all clients seem to find some skills that work for them. We also do not have an empirical basis for determining which, if any, to cut. Ultimately, skills trainers must attend to the learning styles of their clients, and move at a pace that does not overwhelm them and result in little learning.

We attend to depth of skills training by giving each skill adequate didactic explanation and practice. Practice occurs during group and with homework. Our skills groups run 2 full hours, allowing for 50–55 minutes of a mindfulness practice and thorough homework review in the first half, and 50–60 minutes for teaching new material. Therapists can also make tradeoffs to include more skills in a shorter time when needed. For example, the skill of Cope Ahead could take an entire group session or be only one of a few skills taught in a session. One can teach Cope Ahead quickly by providing an example and asking clients to bring the skill into individual therapy to practice as part of a solution analysis for examining problematic behaviors and upcoming challenging situations. It may also be possible to slightly alter the structure to create more time for certain skills content. For example, if there are no new families entering the group, and the group members are sufficiently familiar with the orientation content, then some of this content can be abbreviated, with 1 week on orientation and mindfulness and 5 weeks devoted to the following module.

A Word about Duration of Skills Training

Linehan, Armstrong, Suarez, Allmon, and Heard's (1991) original research with adults was based on a 1-year treatment. Some may wish to shorten the length of treatment with adolescents to enhance the willingness to commit and the likelihood of treatment completion, as many adolescents tend to complete only a limited number of therapy sessions (e.g., Trautman, Stewart, & Morishima, 1993). In addition, the behavior patterns of some adolescent clients may not always be as severely entrenched as emotionally dysregulated adult clients. Although we previously published data and program descriptions based on a shortened length of treatment (e.g., see Rathus & Miller, 2002, for an initial quasi-experimental study in which skills were covered in 12 weeks, and Miller et al., 2007, that describes covering skills in 16 weeks), we have since increased the length of our skills training program to 24 weeks. This increase is partly due to the addition of the Walking the Middle Path Skills module and partly due to our experience that the shortened formats did not allow enough time to adequately cover the material; too many skills were sacrificed. We now only slightly shorten standard DBT skills (Linehan, 1993b) to accommodate the Walking the Middle Path Skills module to fit into a 6-month curriculum. Although various lengths of treatment have been tried and appear promising (e.g., Goldstein et al., 2012; Mehlum et al., 2014; Rathus & Miller, 2002), the optimal length of treatment with adolescents remains an empirical question, and may depend on the setting, length of each scheduled skills training session, severity of the targeted problems, and learning abilities of group members.

SETTING UP A SKILLS GROUP

Group Size

We recommend having two skills trainers per group regardless of group size. A small group (two to three families, or four to nine members plus leaders) provides more individualized attention, more leader awareness of individual patient reactions and struggles, more time for practice and opportunity for engaging in role plays with leader feedback, more intimacy, and thus possibly a greater comfort level. Also, such a group may be practical for clinicians in settings with a slower referral flow. However, such a group size may feel "too close for comfort" to some group members, and one or two absences on a given day can derail the sense of "group." It also might be tempting, in such a small setting, to address individual issues that members raise, detracting from the focus on skills acquisition and practice.

A large group size (six to eight families, or 12–24 clients in the room) may be efficient in terms of cost and resources, may provide a degree of anonymity within the group for socially anxious members (although a large group could also raise social anxiety), may provide a social support network for families, and may provide a strong buffer against the effects of family absences. However, skills acquisition and strengthening can easily be sacrificed in a large group where there is less time for engaging each member in review of between-session assignments and *in vivo* practice of particular skills. Also, opportunities for therapy-interfering distractions abound with many group members, and there may be less ability for leaders to handle problems as they arise.

A useful rule of thumb is to plan for 3–5 minutes for homework review per group member, including parents. So, if 45 minutes are allotted for the homework review portion of the session, 9–15 members are optimal (three to five families, or up to six, if all are two-parent families). Alternatively, for slightly larger groups, we recommend breaking into two separate groups for homework review, with half (randomly divided) going with a leader into a separate room. In that way, leaders can provide ample time per person for feedback, and afterward everyone can come together for the rest of the session.

Rolling Admissions versus Closed Groups

Open and closed groups each offer advantages and disadvantages, but we recommend open groups, allowing new families to join at the start of each Orientation and Mindfulness Skills module, when feasible. When groups are ongoing, it does not matter at what point in the cycle a family enters treatment. At the end of 6 months, all members will have been exposed to the same sets of skills. When new members enter group, a culture of a well-functioning group (i.e., a supportive atmosphere where learning takes place) has already been established; in this sense, veteran members set the tone as much as skills trainers do.

A second reason to keep the group open is that these adolescents need practice adapting to changes in their environment. Adolescents with BPD features or problems with emotional dys-regulation, like their adult counterparts, have great difficulty handling change. Thus, the open group allows for exposure to controlled but continual change in a therapeutic context.

A third reason to keep the group open is that it creates a seniority system within the group. By allowing new members into the group at the start of each Orientation and Mindfulness Skills module, the group creates a culture in which senior members can help orient junior members do DBT. We have found that the seniors provide coping models and will often volunteer ways in which the skills have helped them, thus helping to build commitment in newer members. The senior group members also model skillful behavior as well as give constructive feedback to the more junior members. Finally, the junior members can see that there is an end in sight, and that many people who commit themselves to DBT do improve and ultimately graduate. This last point cannot be overemphasized; we find that seeing other families successfully complete group and report on their treatment gains to be a powerful motivator that provides hope for overwhelmed families just beginning this process.

In closed groups, members start and remain together until all the modules are completed, without the addition of new members. The primary advantage of a closed group is that the members get to know each other better, may come to trust each other more, and therefore may be more likely to participate more openly. A disadvantage is that once clients feel too comfortable with one another, it may become more difficult to keep the focus on behavioral skills training and more likely for the group to drift into process issues. It is incumbent upon skills trainers to maintain the focus.

Heterogeneity versus Homogeneity of Group Composition

Structuring a DBT skills training group for adolescents requires decisions about how the client population will be defined. Age, gender, diagnosis, and culture are important population parameters that will warrant consideration in determining a program's inclusion and exclusion criteria.

Age

Adolescence is generally defined as ages 12–19 (Berk, 2000) or even older. However, this range does not comprise a homogeneous group. Early adolescence, roughly ages 11/12–14, is characterized by recent entry into puberty; often first-time experimenting with behaviors such as dating and tobacco, drug, and alcohol use; and attending middle school or junior high school. Middle to late adolescents, roughly ages 14–18, are typically attending high school and are often facing increased demands, pressures, and responsibility. The oldest adolescents might be considered to range from roughly age 18–20, 21, or even as old as 25. For example, Arnett (1999) has defined the period from ages 18–25 as "emerging adulthood" or "transitional adulthood."

In our programs, clients typically range in age from 13 to 18 years of age. (Note that we make occasional exceptions for youth who are slightly younger or slightly older but still living at home. Some programs create a young-adult track for those above 18, with separate support groups or skills offered to parents.) We have found that older clients will often play a big sibling role to younger clients, coaching them and imparting advice and wisdom. This is inspirational for younger attendees and a source of pride and motivation for older attendees. One risk of this approach is that older group members might expose younger members to new risk behaviors, such as sexual promiscuity or drug use. For this reason we discourage teens from disclosing their treatment target behaviors in detail in the group or in outside friendships (see Chapter 5 on orientation and group rules). Another risk in mixed-age groups is having an outlier in age. For example, a 19-year-old in a group of mostly 14- and 15-year-olds can end up feeling alienated. To prevent this, the skills trainer can encourage the older teen to play a special role in the group to capitalize on the age discrepancy. Other alternatives are referring the adolescent to another group or conducting skills training individually.

Advantages to limiting treatment to particular age groups within adolescence include increased homogeneity of life issues, possibly leading to a greater connection to peers in group settings. However, a setting must have enough of a referral base that it can afford to either turn away adolescents outside a specific age range or staff multiple groups, each favoring specific ages. Some settings might have several groups running simultaneously and might thus choose to divide them into two or more age groupings (e.g., 12–15, 16–19). Some settings, such as hospitals, might have institution-wide criteria for ages, whereby those clients 17 and younger are treated in a child/adolescent program and those clients 18 and above automatically receive services in the adult outpatient, day treatment, or inpatient department. Many programs include young-adult groups for adults in their early to mid-20s, who are likely struggling with common developmental issues such as completing college, living independently, finding work, and connecting with romantic partners. Still other settings without a large enough teen referral base may include adolescents ages 16 and older in adult programs.

Gender

Gender is another factor to consider. Will your program include both girls and boys, and if so, will it place them together in groups? Some inpatient or residential treatment settings are limited to treating one gender, or else separate the genders into different residences. But most other settings admit boys and girls. Similar to issues concerning age, limiting skills group to a single gender may allow for greater homogeneity of issues brought into group and, for some, perhaps greater comfort with self-disclosure. Furthermore, it may minimize the degree of disruption or distraction for some due to sexual interest or increased social anxiety due to the presence of the other sex. The issue of sexual interest could obviously remain for lesbian, gay, bisexual, and transgender (LGBT) adolescents regardless of group type.

In our programs, we combine genders for several reasons. First, this practice allows us to treat boys in settings that get a low percentage of male referrals; there might not otherwise be enough male participants to fill a group. In our settings, only 15–20% of our DBT referrals are male, resulting in about one male adolescent per group of five or six clients and their families. This ratio is typical, given the much higher rates of BPD diagnosis, suicide attempts, and nonsuicidal self-injury behaviors in females. Second, the presence of both genders allows for developing skillful opposite-sex friendships, role-playing boyfriend or girlfriend conversations with an opposite-sex participant, and gaining insight on issues from another gender's perspective. This promotes generalization of skills. Third, combined groups allow for inclusiveness of LGBT clients without consideration of gender identity or sexual orientation. In mixed-gender groups, it is important to orient members to the possibility that both boys and girls will join the group even if there are no boys in the group at some points.

Diagnosis

Highly homogeneous groups may be hard to come by since individuals with emotion regulation difficulties tend to be characterized by multiple problems and multiple comorbidities. Mixed diagnostic groups may be beneficial; more evidence is emerging that DBT can be successfully adapted for a range of populations and target behaviors (see Miller & Rathus, 2000). The range of populations includes, but is not limited to, mood disorders, substance use disorders, disruptive behavior disorders, eating disorders, and anxiety disorders. Many of the youth we treat carry several of these diagnoses. Target behaviors may include drug or alcohol use, binge or purge behavior, school refusal, family conflicts, or suicidal or nonsuicidal self-injurious behaviors, to name a few. Although casting a wider net has the potential to benefit more people, certain cautions are warranted in combining diagnostic groups or having varied inclusion criteria. First, certain diagnoses, although appropriate for DBT, might be better served in a more specifically tailored DBT program. Examples include primary diagnoses of eating disorders or substance abuse. Second, certain diagnostic groups may not be best served in group settings. For example, recent evidence finds that antisocial and conduct-disordered youth fare *worse* when treated in group formats due to the modeling, training, and peer validation of antisocial behaviors that occur (Dishion, McCord, & Poulin, 1999). Third, if entry criteria become too loose, individuals' severity and treatment targets may be so different that the group skills training loses its focus; the biosocial theory underlying the treatment may no longer apply, and the group may disintegrate. Thus, we recommend having a clear, unifying theme to group membership.

Common exclusion criteria consist of active psychosis, severe learning disabilities, or severe cognitive impairment.

Ethnicity and Culture

In our experience, a program's ethnic and cultural composition tends to be shaped by setting and geography. For example, one of our programs serves an inner-city population consisting of mostly lower-socioeconomic-status (SES) adolescents who represent ethnic minority groups (predominantly Latino, African American, and Caribbean American). Another program in the suburbs consists of mostly white, middle- to upper-SES teens. Thus, the cultural makeup of the groups sorts itself out organically. However, cultural factors might be disparate enough within a setting that there would be reason to consider assigning members to different groups on this basis. One factor might be the primary language spoken by the family; for example, some settings have implemented skills groups taught in Spanish to allow family members' participation when little or no English is spoken. Another factor might concern group cohesion, for example, by placing together groups that have common characteristics, such as recent immigrant status or primary medical diagnoses. On the other hand, definition of culture varies widely (see discussion of culture in Rathus & Feindler, 2004), and culturally diverse groups have the potential to enhance members' experience. We thus do not generally consider culture a priori, when assigning members to groups.

Flexible Admissions to a Multifamily Skills Training Group

On occasion, one might have reason to accept an adolescent without family members, or to accept parents without their adolescent child, to the multifamily group. We've allowed adolescents to join our groups without parents on rare occasions when the teens are living geographically away from their parents, are estranged from their parents, or when the relationship is so conflicted that the parents' presence would significantly disrupt or destroy treatment. In such cases other families have at times "adopted" the lone teens during group time, and the teens have tolerated this arrangement reasonably well. However, problems can arise, often in the form of the lone teen's sensitivity to discussions about parents, envy of group members whose parents are present, and persistent feelings of being an outsider. Nonetheless, when faced with the choice of allowing a teen to join group alone or not receiving skills training, we recommend allowing the teen to join the group.

Similarly, on rare occasions we have allowed one or both parents to participate in the multifamily group without their teen. We have permitted this when teens have been away (perhaps in a residential program or receiving DBT at college), or when a teen has graduated from group and entered the graduate group but the parents feel they could benefit from another round of skills. This has generally worked well, and the rare parent in the group without a teen often becomes a supportive figure for other teens. One has to be careful that the parent–teen ratio does not get too out of balance, though. If a group already has two parents for every teen and then another set of parents is admitted, there might be only three or four teens and eight or 10 adults in the room; such an imbalance could inhibit teen group members. Ideally, skills trainers can refer parents seeking skills training (without their teens present) to a DBT parenting group nearby if one exists.

SKILLS TRAINING SESSIONS

Setting Up the Room

Trainers often conduct skills training in whatever room is large enough and available in the setting. However, when one has a choice in the arrangement, we believe several factors facilitate skills training. First, we prefer a large, conference-style table around which group members sit. This format encourages members to keep their notebooks of handouts and worksheets (see below) in plain sight of leaders, and it makes it easier for members to write notes in their books. Second, members at the table should all be able to see a large whiteboard or other large writing surface. If no table is available, place chairs in a large circle, oval, or U-shape facing a whiteboard. This shape facilitates group feedback and interaction. Third, skills trainers should sit opposite each other to facilitate eye contact and communication and allow for leader proximity to more group members. This positioning also allows for better observation and engagement of members while discouraging therapy-interfering behavior (discussed in more detail in Chapter 3). Fourth, it is helpful to use a room large enough for the leaders and group members to move around. We encourage group members to stand up and even move around the room while teaching to heighten engagement. At times group members will break into small groups for role-playing exercises, and space is needed for this.

Other Materials Needed

Leaders should bring a small bell (consider a Zen *singing bowl*) to each session that they ring to signal the beginning and ending of mindfulness practices. Leaders give group members handouts, worksheets, and loose-leaf binders in which to keep the handouts. A three-hole punch is also useful. The papers can be distributed in a variety of ways. Members can be given handouts and worksheets at each session that cover the session content and homework assignment, or members can be given packets of all module materials at the beginning of each module. Alternatively, members can be given complete notebooks with extra homework sheets at the beginning of treatment. Keep loaner notebooks, extra homework sheets, and pens in the group room so members can always participate even if they have forgotten to bring their materials.

Technology is appealing to teens and can enhance the teaching of skills. Including a smartboard or computer with projection screen, when available, can allow for access to music, movie clips, YouTube videos, and the like. One can use such media for teaching a variety of DBT skills, such as mindfulness exercises, for illustrating states of mind, for practice in distracting and soothing oneself, for identifying and labeling emotions in response to evocative stimuli, for illustrating acting in an opposite manner to emotion-based urges, for demonstrating challenging interpersonal situations and both skillful and nonskillful means to handle them, and for illustrating how walking the middle path can provide solutions to family dilemmas. For example, a skills trainer could select a Beatles song to self-soothe, a funny *Modern Family* video clip to help teach distraction with other emotions, or a clip from the TV show *Glee* to demonstrate keeping self-respect using FAST skills. Other possibilities include devising computer-based games or quizzes to test group members in skills knowledge. Advantages are the almost limitless possibilities and the opportunity to offer diverse formats for teaching that keep the material fresh and engaging.

Session Structure

Skills training group sessions with adolescents and their families usually run 2 hours with a 10-minute break in the middle. This is shorter than the 2½ hours of standard DBT (Linehan et al., 1993) skills training sessions. Adolescents have a somewhat shorter attention span than adults, and we find that 2 hours better fits parents' work schedules and kids' homework demands. Except for orientation sessions, the first half of the skills session is devoted to review of homework. The second half is devoted to teaching and practice of new skills.

When skills training is conducted one on one with a single family, it is often shorter (1–1½ hours). Homework review, discussion, and practice of new skills require less time with only one family, though the skills trainer would cover the same material as if in a group. In some programs, especially in settings with captive audiences or settings where the participants have limited scheduling blocks (i.e., inpatient, school, residential, and juvenile justice settings), skills training is divided into two shorter sessions over different days of the week: one session for teaching new skills and one session for homework review and practice.

Table 2.2 lists the two types of skills session formats. Sessions that begin with orientation content have their own format. Orienting information is presented in the first half of the session, and mindfulness skills are taught in the second half, following a break. All other sessions follow the second format, which begins with homework review and teaches new content in the second half. Chapter 5 describes how to conduct orientation module sessions in detail; Chapter 3 outlines the second format.

Final Skills Session: Goodbye Ritual and Graduation Ceremony

In an open group, at the end of the final week of each skills module, some group members will have completed the rotation. In a closed group, all members complete a rotation at the end of the contracted skills training period. In either case, we recommend providing some type of goodbye ritual or ceremony to mark the completion of skills training. The allocated time is worth the reinforcement it provides for those completing skills training as well as the vicarious reinforcement and motivation it provides the remaining members.

In our outpatient open group, participants and skills trainers engage in a goodbye ritual typically lasting 30–60 minutes, whenever people complete the skills rotation. On these nights, leaders stop teaching content approximately 30 minutes early in a 2-hour group format, in order to initiate the ceremony within the group time. Nights containing graduation ceremonies often extend at least 30 minutes beyond the standard group time period, so members should be forewarned the week before that they may end up staying later. The goodbye ritual often starts with group leaders, and sometimes other family members, bringing special treats to eat, including fruit, baked goods, etc. Then the group leaders and each remaining group member offer specific constructive and encouraging feedback to the graduates about the work they have accomplished as well as what potential pitfalls to anticipate upon graduation. Following this go-around, the graduate says goodbye to each remaining member as well as to each peer and family member who is also graduating. These goodbyes are opportunities for adolescents, family members, and therapists alike to share their feelings and provide constructive feedback. These exchanges are

TABLE 2.2. Multifamily Skills Group Session Format

Orientation session with start of mindfulness skills training (2 hours)
50–55 minutes
  Introduce all group members and skills trainers.
  Review limits of confidentiality.
  Present rationale for why these adolescents were chosen for this program.
  Present group treatment goals.
  Orient members to DBT biosocial theory and assumptions.
  Orient members to group guidelines and format.
  Ask adolescents and family members to sign contract.

Break: 10-minute snack

50–60 minutes
  Present didactic material on mindfulness skills.
  Assign homework exercise.
  Session wind-down exercise.

All other skills sessions (2 hours)
50–55 minutes
  Mindfulness exercise.
  Announcements and overview of session content.
  Homework practice review.

Break: 10-minute snack

50–60 minutes
  Presentation of didactic material on new skills.
  Assign homework exercise.
  Session wind-down exercise.

typically taken quite seriously; the comments are thoughtful and poignant. It is important that the parent receive the same goodbye and acknowledgment of accomplishment after completing the program. The ritual ends with a graduation ceremony. Graduating clients and their families are each awarded a diploma for successful completion of the DBT program. Teen graduates also receive a token gift, such as the *Wise Movement* CD that contains DBT skills put to rap music, a self-soothe kit, or some gift that relates to a skillful behavior or interest of the client (e.g., journals, sketch pads, music).

OPTIONS FOR ADOLESCENTS FOLLOWING GRADUATION FROM SKILLS TRAINING

Many comprehensive DBT programs offer skills training graduates opportunities to further enhance their gains and remain connected to the program by entering the next phase of treatment. For example, standard DBT is typically followed by exposure treatment addressing Stage 2 targets for trauma when needed. Standard DBT and other, adapted programs have also incorporated continuation phases such as "graduate groups." The appropriate next steps for each graduate should be discussed with the primary therapist. The importance of additional treatment is supported by research with depressed adolescents, which suggests that a continuation phase of therapy enhances the longer-term gains of a short-term treatment (Birmaher et al., 2000; Brent, Baugher, Bridge, Chen, & Chiappetta, 1999). Thus, for working with suicidal or multiproblem adolescents, we have recommended the use of a second group phase of treatment. It not only makes clinical sense to have a continuation phase in treating such adolescents, most of whom have an affective disorder, but the continuation can also help titrate them out of therapy.

Assuming exposure therapy for trauma is made available for clients who need it, it can be beneficial to also offer an optional graduate group. This group can follow numerous formats, but therapists who implement it generally have as goals skill maintenance, generalization, and strengthening along with opportunities for problem solving and peer support. This group can be conducted in a structured format with planned didactics for each meeting, or in a process-supportive format, where the group follows its own course but where application of DBT skills is worked in whenever applicable.

A Model for an Adolescent Graduate Group

Our model of a graduate group helps taper adolescents from Stage 1 group skills training by reducing the group leader's role through greater use of peer coaching and problem solving. In our optional graduate skills group, the primary goals are (1) to promote skills maintenance by reinforcing the progress made in the previous skills training group, (2) to help clients continue to practice and generalize the skills, and (3) to increase behaviors instrumental to quality of life while decreasing behaviors interfering with quality of life.

Group therapy is an especially powerful therapeutic tool with this age group because peer relationships promote the development of social skills and identity formation (Brown, 1990). Moreover, the transition from Stage 1 of treatment to the Stage 2 graduate group is characterized by increased responsibility for group members who now participate without parents, take active skills teaching and consulting roles in group, and practice problem solving with peers. These changes mirror the adolescent developmental trajectory toward separation, individuation, greater self-sufficiency, and the importance of peers. Note that participation in a graduate group can occur concomitantly with standard DBT Stage 2 individual therapy focused on emotionally processing the past. See Miller and colleagues (2007) for in-depth discussion of the graduate group model.

ALTERNATIVES TO THE MULTIFAMILY GROUP MODEL

Despite the benefits of conducting skills training with multiple family groups, other formats are at times more practical for given settings or situations. We next discuss skills training with teen-only groups, parent-only groups, and individual family skills training.

Teen-Only Groups

Some programs do not include family members in skills training, due to limitations of the setting or because of the team's preference. Family participation is impractical in inpatient, day treatment, residential, or forensic settings. Other options for parents might include family meetings or workshops to orient family members to skills. Whatever the format, we recommend as much parent orientation and information as possible so that they can support the goals of skills training and recognize and reinforce their teen's attempts at more skillful behavior.

Some teams prefer not to include parents in skills training groups because teens may reveal more and participate more without a parent present. Additionally, teens might be less likely to become angry, dysregulated, or triggered. However, this format risks the possibility for increased therapy-interfering behavior since there is an imbalance of teens and adults in the room (although at times, parents can engage in as much treatment-interfering behavior as the teens). There is also less opportunity for teens to practice skills with and receive feedback from their own and other parents. Similarly, there is less opportunity for parents to learn skills and benefit from the perspective of their own teens as well as the perspectives of the other families. Therefore, this format risks the possibility of less skills generalization.

Clinicians should also be aware that while teens may initially resist the notion of participating in a group with their parents, teens often get used to the format and become more comfortable with having their parents in the room with them. At the end of treatment they often provide positive feedback on the strong benefits of this format, noting their improved communication with participating family members, the shared time they've spent, and the increased skillfulness on the part of their family members.

Family-Member-Only Groups

Some settings with teen-only skills training conduct separate groups for parents. These might take the form of parallel skills groups in which parents are seen separately but taught the same curriculum (e.g., see Ritschel, Cheavens, & Nelson, 2012). Alternatively, some programs have separate parent groups with overlapping but not identical content; for example, emphasis on biosocial theory, parent training, psychoeducation, interpersonal effectiveness skills, walking the middle path skills, and supportive or other material might be included. In addition to such group programs we have run in our own practices, there are several examples of strong family-member-only programs. First, the National Education Alliance for Borderline Personality Disorder (NEA-BPD) sponsors the Family Connections Program (cf. Hoffman & Steiner-Grossman, 2008), a family-member-led group that teaches DBT skills to family members of those struggling with a diagnosis of BPD. Second, the Treatment and Research Advancements (TARA) for BPD organizes psychoeducational groups for caregivers and family members of those with BPD (Porr, 2010).

Primary reasons for separating parent skills training groups include a lack of access to teens who are receiving DBT in inpatient, residential, or other settings; belief in the importance of covering material specific to family members of the identified patients; belief that inclusion of parents might inhibit adolescents' self-disclosure (or parents' ability to speak freely); or, in the case of families with severely dysfunctional interactions or abuse, belief that family members' presence might have a treatment-destroying effect in the group.

Individual Family Skills Training

For clinicians working in settings where it is not feasible to start a group due to client flow or other factors, or if a family cannot make the scheduled group time, one might consider teaching skills to a single family (e.g., see Goldstein et al., 2007). Skills training with one family is feasible as long as it is delivered in a regular weekly session, *the sole agenda of which is skills training.* If the primary (individual) therapist serves as skills trainer in comprehensive DBT, we recommend scheduling a separate session each week to address skills. If commuting to the setting is an issue, we suggest scheduling double sessions in which the first focuses on skills and the second, preceded by a short break, focuses on individual behavioral analysis and problem solving. We recommend this clear boundary between modes to ensure a separate focus on each important treatment function, without confusion. The teen and family should be oriented ahead of time about the nature and format of each session, and the skills trainer must take care to avoid drifting into individual therapy targets during the skills session.

It is important to keep visits for skills training distinct from individual therapy and other family therapy work (see Miller et al., 2007, on family sessions in adolescent DBT), or else family crises may emerge that derail skills training. The functions for these modes are more easily kept separate when the family skills trainer is someone other than the adolescent's individual therapist or a family's therapist. Skills training with individual families allows for flexibility, such as placing greater emphasis on skills especially needed in a given family or adjusting the pace to a family's needs. However, it does not offer the camaraderie or modeling potential of a group format and may make it easier for the therapist and family to use skills training time for purposes other than skill acquisition.

VARIATIONS IN ADOLESCENT DBT SKILLS TRAINING BY SETTING

Outpatient settings lend themselves most easily to weekly skills training with family participation. However, DBT has been adapted to a variety of other adolescent treatment settings, including psychiatric inpatient, residential, partial hospitalization, forensic, foster care, and medical inpatient and outpatient clinic formats (Hashim et al., 2013; Mason et al., 2009; Miller et al., 2007). The methods, modes, and dosage of skills training vary depending on the setting. Each setting impacts the degree of family participation in the treatment as a whole and in the skills training component in particular, though our overarching belief remains that it is most effective to enlist families into the treatment to the greatest extent possible.

Inpatient

DBT studies conducted in both acute and long-term inpatient settings (Katz et al., 2004; McDonell et al., 2010) focus on teaching skills to their patients in different formats. The targets of inpatient treatment are different from those of outpatient treatment, in that the focus is primarily on Stage 1 targets addressing life-threatening and egregious behaviors that prompted the inpatient hospitalization. Typically, inpatient DBT providers do not target quality-of-life-interfering behaviors, leaving those for the patient to address with future outpatient providers. Hence, it seems necessary to teach only those skills needed for adolescents to get out of the hospital, back to their lives, and reduce the possibility of a "mental patient" identity.

In an acute 2-week inpatient setting (Katz et al., 2004), researchers chose to teach mindfulness skills and select distress tolerance and emotion regulation skills. New skills were taught every other day in a 45-minute skills training group. The assigned homework was reviewed on alternate days in a 45-minute homework review group. Katz and colleagues (2004), and other inpatient programs, have involved families in the treatment to enhance the family members' capabilities while also enhancing skills generalization. Inpatient providers may consider including the following components when involving families: (1) engaging them in pretreatment orientation and commitment, which includes learning the biosocial theory; (2) helping them understand treatment target behaviors and the corresponding skills modules; (3) teaching an introduction to dialectics and validation skills to improve communication and relationship behaviors; (4) identifying family-related dysfunctional behaviors that are key links in the adolescent's life-threatening or egregious behaviors; and (5) encouraging parents to participate in identifying and troubleshooting solutions to prevent relapse upon discharge. This is one model to consider when offering short-term inpatient hospitalization.

Residential and Forensic

Residential (and forensic) settings can be considered a hybrid of inpatient and outpatient settings; they are typically longer-term and often less restrictive (Sunseri, 2004; Trupin et al., 2002). These settings can be considered fertile ground with ample time and opportunity for adolescents to learn and generalize new DBT skills. Although frequency and length of skills training sessions will vary, it is essential that they do not encourage discussion of nonsuicidal self-injurious behavior (NSSI) that can inadvertently become iatrogenic in such settings (Springer, Lohr, Buchtel, & Silk, 1996). When possible, we recommend inviting family members to participate at whatever frequency possible—especially if the plan is for the youth to return to his or her home upon discharge. Given the long distances some family members need to travel to access the residential (or forensic) settings, it is not always logistically possible to have frequent face-to-face interactions. Some solutions to such problems are to (1) schedule a pretreatment orientation and commitment session with the family members when the youth arrives to the program; (2) schedule a half-day skills training workshop to teach family members the biosocial theory and validation skills; (3) provide some time for multiple families to get support and validation from each other and the staff; and (4) teach other DBT skills to families. Some such settings use conference calls with families, teens, and therapists, as well as Skype or another form of video conferencing, to maintain contact and to practice and generalize skills.

Schools

Given the earlier onset of psychiatric disorders among youth coupled with the fact that school districts are being given mandates to keep their emotionally disturbed youth within their districts to save money, many superintendents, principals, and directors of special education have sought solutions to this problem. Many districts around the country have identified adolescent DBT as a viable solution, given the flexible and comprehensive nature of targeting a range of emotional and behavioral problems, the use of a skills training curriculum (i.e., conducive to classroom-type learning), and its focus on the management of crises. Applying DBT in a school setting offers both unique advantages and disadvantages (Mason et al., 2009; Mazza, Dexter-Mazza, Murphy, Miller, & Rathus, in press; Perepletchikova et al., 2011). One advantage is having a "captive" audience; students can be pulled from classes or their lunch period, resulting in less frequent therapy-interfering behavior than one might find in a standard outpatient setting. Another advantage is the prospect of providing primary and secondary prevention interventions to youth by teaching DBT skills as part of the educational curriculum (e.g., health curriculum). Mazza and colleagues (in press) have developed a class-length DBT skills curriculum for teachers to deliver in middle and high schools.

The primary challenge to administering DBT in this setting is that most school programs can only afford a 42-minute class period to conduct skills training groups. As a result, skills trainers in schools typically need to reduce the standard outpatient 2-hour group format to less than half the length. This allows less time for homework review, behavioral rehearsal, and the teaching of new content, which inevitably results in lengthening the duration of the group to an entire school year. The key point for those starting a school program is to never drop homework review or give it short shrift in the service of teaching new content. Otherwise, one runs the risk that students will not practice or understand the effective application of the new skills.

Engaging families in school DBT programs is challenging. As is outlined in the inpatient section above, we have found some schools that invite family members for specific 1- to 2-hour skills workshops throughout the school year to review (1) orientation to DBT, (2) biosocial theory, (3) validation, (4) dialectics, (5) learning principles, and (6) distress tolerance. In addition, some school DBT therapists will conduct family sessions to help with *in vivo* skills practice for all parties, with special attention paid to interpersonal skills, validation, problem solving, and troubleshooting.

Medical Settings

In recent years, Hashim and colleagues (2013) have begun to adapt DBT for youth who are noncompliant with treatment regimens for their chronic medical condition. DBT was identified as a useful treatment approach, given its skills-based focus coupled with the emphasis on therapy-interfering behaviors and commitment strategies used to extract new prosocial behaviors. At the Children's Hospital at Montefiore (CHAM), in New York, we have applied a modified version of DBT skills training for obese youth who are at high risk of morbidity and mortality. In addition, a targeted individual six-session protocol has been developed for medically high-risk youth diagnosed with renal disease who were removed from the kidney transplant list due to their noncompliance with medical treatment. Results from a preliminary open trial of this intervention are promising (Hashim et al., 2013). Adaptations for noncompliant youth with diabetes and sickle cell disease are in the planning stages.

CONCLUSION

This chapter outlined the structure of skills training groups, including the overall training course, group composition, session structure, and alternatives to the multifamily group model. Once a group program is established, skills trainers must focus on running the group. The following chapters focus on effectively managing the multifamily skills group.

CHAPTER 3

Managing Skills Training Group Sessions

The previous chapter detailed the structure of skills training, and this chapter explains how skills trainers can effectively deliver skills training content within that structure. We begin the chapter by reviewing initial orientation and commitment to DBT skills training for teens and families. The rest of the chapter focuses on skills training targets in more detail and how to best use the session format to increase the learning of behavioral skills.

We begin with pretreatment and the evaluation and intake process wherein the therapist targets orienting teens and families and obtaining their commitment to treatment. We then discuss how to manage the typical group session in a way that addresses treatment targets.

THE INITIAL CONTACT AND EVALUATION

We often tell the family member who calls to arrange the "intake for DBT" that we are happy to arrange a consultation to evaluate whether the youth is appropriate for DBT; however, we let the person know that there is no guarantee DBT will ultimately be the treatment recommendation.

Never presuppose a new referral to your setting is "definitely a DBT case." In keeping with good standard health care practice, clinicians must conduct a comprehensive diagnostic evaluation at the outset to determine presenting problems, diagnoses, and specific behavioral problems. Only from this assessment can one appropriately determine treatment recommendations, including those for DBT. This process typically involves spending time with the adolescent alone as well as spending time with the parents alone collecting family history and data specific to the youth. Including family members in the initial consultation is essential for several reasons. First, they can corroborate the youth's self-report. Second, they can often fill in gaps in the youth's story and provide more precise time lines regarding onset of problematic behaviors. This part of the assessment may include sharing important information about the adolescent's school performance or legal difficulties that he or she may not otherwise self-disclose in a first visit. Third, their presence allows for rapport building with them as well as with teens.

During the first consultation, we typically invite the adolescent and parents in to the therapy office and allow a few minutes for each member of the family to describe the presenting problems. We often ask the teen to return to the waiting room and complete self-report measures in order to allow private time with the caregivers so that we can elicit developmental history and family history as well as current concerns. This time alone with caregivers provides the clinician with relevant information to better engage a teen who may reveal little about his or her problems (see Miller et al., 2007, for further elaboration of the intake process). It also allows the clinician to spend time validating the caregivers, who inevitably have been experiencing a range of emotional and practical stressors with regard to their teen.

When meeting with the teen, we recommend the administration of a semistructured diagnostic interview such as the Kiddie Schedule for Affective Disorders and Schizophrenia (K-SADS; Kaufman et al., 1997) and a personality measure (e.g., the Structured Interview for DSM Personality Disorders [SID-P]) to formally assess for a range of disorders, including BPD. When there is little time for formal structured interviews, one might use a brief self-report screening tool for BPD features, such as the Life Problems Inventory (Rathus, Wagner, & Miller, 2013) and conduct a thorough clinical interview to establish diagnostic impressions. These steps would ultimately assess the five major problem areas associated with BPD in adolescents: (1) confusion about self, (2) impulsivity, (3) emotional dysregulation, (4) interpersonal problems, and (5) adolescent–family dilemmas. These five problem areas are the source of key symptoms of pervasive emotional and behavioral dysregulation. Each of the five problem areas has a corresponding DBT skills module to address it.

Guidelines for Assigning Treatment

We have adopted some general guidelines to help make treatment assignment determinations. In a clinical setting if a youth endorses all five problem areas, then it is clear the treatment recommendation should be comprehensive DBT. In fact, based on our clinical experience, if the youth (and family members) endorses at least three of the five DBT problem areas or endorses suicide attempts or repetitive NSSI, then a recommendation for comprehensive DBT should also be made.

DBT skills can benefit those who endorse fewer than three problem areas. For example, if someone identifies "interpersonal problems" as the primary difficulty, we would likely recommend the DBT skills module on interpersonal effectiveness and mindfulness. If an individual endorses only confusion about self, including a lack of awareness of current experience and goals, with little to no impairment in other functioning, we would likely recommend DBT mindfulness training. If another youth endorses "emotional dysregulation" and is experiencing significant depression, anger, shame, or anxiety, we would employ one of the relevant evidence-based cognitive-behavioral therapy (CBT) protocols while also teaching the full range of DBT skills. Medication might also be recommended depending on the severity of the condition. Assuming the adolescent is not engaging in Target 1 (life-threatening behaviors) or Target 2 (treatment-interfering behaviors), the DBT therapist would address Target 3 (quality-of-life-interfering behaviors) by using relevant treatment protocols (e.g., Hope, Heimberg, Juster, and Turk's [2000] *Managing Social Anxiety Client Workbook* or Morin's [1993] sleep hygiene protocol).

ORIENTING AND OBTAINING COMMITMENT

The pretreatment stage of orientation and commitment to DBT begins once assessments are complete and the adolescent has been found appropriate for multifamily DBT skills training, whether as part of a comprehensive DBT program or a less comprehensive treatment. In comprehensive DBT with adolescents and families, the individual therapist provides the initial orientation to DBT treatment as a whole, including the different modes and functions of treatment.

Clinicians orient teens, one on one, by folding their presenting problems into DBT's five problem areas: confusion about self, impulsivity, emotional dysregulation, interpersonal problems, and adolescent–family dilemmas. Once the adolescent recognizes the problems characterized in this way, the DBT therapist links each of the problem areas to its corresponding skills module, intended to address these problems (e.g., emotion regulation skills to reduce emotional instability). Note also that all skills modules facilitate progress with all of the DBT problem areas; for example, regulating emotions and reducing impulsivity no doubt improve interpersonal relationships. The therapist then elicits the adolescent's long-term goals and links these to Stage 1 treatment targets (see Miller et al., 2007, for a fuller discussion of this process).

Obtaining commitment from adolescents and parents to attend skills training takes place before they begin group. "Selling" commitment can be especially challenging with adolescents, since they are often brought in by parents or referred by other practitioners, as opposed to discovering DBT for themselves and seeking the treatment. Linehan (1993a) developed a set of DBT commitment strategies used in initial pretreatment sessions to secure commitment, and reapplied in later sessions to renew and strengthen that commitment.

Commitment Strategies

DBT specifies a set of strategies that can be used to obtain commitment or recommitment to the treatment. The therapist needs to be flexible and creative while employing one or more of the following: (1) selling the commitment by evaluating pros and cons; (2) playing devil's advocate; (3) the foot-in-the-door and door-in-the-face techniques; (4) connecting present commitments to prior commitments; (5) highlighting freedom to choose and absence of alternatives; (6) cheerleading; and (7) shaping. (See also Linehan, 1993a, and Miller et al., 2007, for a fuller discussion.)

Evaluating the Pros and Cons

Using this strategy, the therapist elicits from the client the advantages and disadvantages of pursuing treatment versus continuing life without it. To assist with the latter point, the therapist elicits the client's counterarguments for treatment, based on the client's reservations. These are likely to arise later, when the client is alone and has no help in defusing doubts. The therapist helps to highlight the short-term benefits to not pursuing treatment versus the long-term benefits of pursuing treatment. When the client has articulated his or her own reservations as well as the need to embark on treatment, the resolve is strengthened.

Playing Devil's Advocate

The therapist poses arguments against making a commitment to treatment, with the intent that the client will make his or her argument *for* participating in treatment. This should only be used when there is at least minimal agreement to initiate treatment; the strategy then strengthens the adolescent's sometimes superficial commitment.

Foot-in-the-Door/Door-in-the-Face Techniques

With the foot-in-the-door technique, the therapist can increase compliance by making an easy first request, followed by a more difficult request. Using the door-in-the-face technique, the therapist first asks for something very difficult, and then something easier, with the expectation of taking something less.

Connecting Present Commitments to Prior Commitments

This technique is useful when the strength of a previous commitment seems to be waning. The therapist reminds the teen (or parent) of the previous commitment and discusses whether he or she still has that commitment.

Highlight Freedom to Choose and Absence of Alternatives

The idea behind this strategy is that commitment and compliance are enhanced when adolescents believe that they have chosen freely and when there are no other alternatives to reach their goal. Hence, the therapist should enhance the feeling of choice, while at the same time stressing the lack of effective alternatives.

Cheerleading

The point of cheerleading is to generate hope and encourage the teen that progress is possible. Cheerleading may also be required when the devil's advocate strategy falls flat.

Shaping

Shaping refers to reinforcing even the slightest movement toward commitment, when a client is initially reluctant or unwilling to consider participating in treatment. Skills trainers will sometimes settle for a partial commitment at the outset with the hope of shaping a stronger commitment over time.

The overall pretreatment goal is to obtain and strengthen as much commitment as possible before the teen enters the skills group. An adolescent's lack of commitment will easily become therapy-interfering or even therapy-destroying behavior. There is nothing to be gained by rushing this process and simply hoping for the best. Note that an adolescent might be in the pretreatment and commitment stage for weeks before beginning skills group.

Once adolescents are sufficiently oriented and committed to joining the weekly skills group to learn these new DBT skills, we then ask them to (1) explain the relevance of these new DBT skills to their personal lives and (2) invite their parents or other caregivers to join them in learning these new skills. If an adolescent is unable to explain the five problem areas and corresponding skills modules, even with "Goals of Skills Training" (Orientation Handout 2) in front of them as a guide, the therapist assists in explaining how the DBT skills modules are applicable. The therapist might use this opportunity to invite the caregiver to assess his or her own problem areas. For example, one parent might report that he or she could benefit from learning and practicing specific interpersonal effectiveness skills with the teen. Another might report problems with emotional dysregulation, and yet another might report problems in all of the areas. This acknowledgment not only helps normalize these problems for the teen but also can enhance parents' commitment to participating in skills group. The following section addresses caregivers' commitment to skills training in more detail.

Obtaining Commitment from Caregivers

We attempt to orient and get commitment from family members by the end of the initial evaluation. We enhance their motivation by linking treatment to their own goals and troubleshooting barriers to treatment by generating solutions. Thus, the specific DBT commitment strategies described above are often applied to caregivers as needed. Many caregivers are willing to participate in the skills training group and do not require significant orienting and commitment; other caregivers are reluctant or initially unwilling. Sometimes it is a matter of problem-solving child care for the adolescent's siblings during the group time, or temporarily adjusting parent work schedules. Some families have been involved with child protection agencies and are worried that information may be disclosed in group that might adversely affect them. Other families see this as a "teenager" problem and not a family problem and do not sufficiently understand the importance of their role in the treatment. Some caregivers are worried about crossing paths with other group members outside the sessions or that these other members will not maintain confidentiality. All of these concerns need to be taken seriously and considered before a family enters a group.

It is important for caregivers to understand that their positive attitude toward and participation in treatment will likely result in better treatment outcomes (Halaby, 2004). In order to enhance willing participation, it is critical to spend time validating parents' experiences with their teens and their concerns about treatment. Caregivers often arrive with many strong emotions themselves, such as anxiety, anger, frustration, hopelessness, shame, or guilt. Conveying that these emotions make sense given the challenges they have experienced helps the parents feel understood and not blamed for their adolescent's problems. As such, they can move into treatment with a more open and willing attitude. In general, taking the time to enhance parents' motivation and commitment has been shown to improve parenting adherence, commitment, and retention (Nock & Kazdin, 2005).

IDENTIFICATION OF APPROPRIATE FAMILY MEMBERS FOR SKILLS TRAINING

Part of the pretreatment and commitment stage involves determining which family members will attend group with the adolescent. We normally recommend at least one parent, and two if parents are together and both available. We have also included stepparents, parents, and others in caretaker roles such as grandparents and even older siblings or foster parents (although we normally limit caregiver involvement to two selected caregivers per teen). Identification of appropriate family members involves choosing someone who is living with the teen at least part-time—someone who is a stable and influential part of the adolescent's environment. Importantly, the caregiver must also be able to come to the skills training sessions on a weekly basis and abide by the same attendance policy as the teen (see "Skills Training Group Guidelines," Chapter 5). Many parents have asked us whether they could alternate who attends or attend group intermittently because of work schedules. We do not recommend this type of intermittent attendance for three reasons. First, it fails to model commitment to treatment. Second, it seriously compromises the skills acquisition process, since so much material is missed. Third, it tends to be disruptive to other group members, who come to rely on the presence of their fellow group attendees.

Marital Discord

When an adolescent client's parents are going through relationship distress or are divorced or separated, there are several potential challenges. Careful screening, orienting, and problem solving ahead of time are crucial to admitting such families to group, so that problematic interactions do not interfere with, or destroy, therapy for other members or themselves. Relevant factors to consider include the following: Is it feasible and/or clinically appropriate to invite both parents to skills training group? Is there too much animosity for both of them to be in the same room? If the answer is yes, then which caregiver should be invited to share the group experience with the teen? We recommend inviting the caregiver with whom the adolescent has the most discord. Although this choice may seem counterintuitive, it offers the opportunity to significantly enhance the relationship and thus reduce the teen's invalidating environment. This shift can improve family discord as well.

Other solutions might also work well, such as teaching one parent the skills separately from group, or admitting parents to consecutive complete sets of modules (i.e., one parent joins with the teen for 6 months, and then the other parent attends with the same teen for the next 6 months).

ORIENTATION TO THE MULTIFAMILY SKILLS GROUP

Once families have committed to participate in skills training, the skills trainer's first task is to conduct a specific orientation to this modality's goals, format, treatment assumptions, and guidelines, as well as to educate participants about the biosocial theory that underlies the treatment (see Chapter 1). Whether skills training is conducted for a single family or in a multifamily format, skills trainers elicit commitments from each participant at the end of the first skills training session. These commitments include (1) to complete the 24-week skills training curriculum, (2) to attend each session on time, (3) to complete the weekly homework assignments, and (4) to adhere to the group guidelines and rules, which include information regarding confidentiality and respecting other members, to name a few. These commitments are outlined in the skills training contract signed by each participant and skills trainer at the end of the first session (see Chapter 5). Skills trainers also provide role induction at the beginning of each skills lesson as an orienting strategy. When a specific skill is taught, the skills trainer explains the purpose of the skill; how it relates to adolescents' and caregivers' life problems, values, and goals; and what they can expect if they use and practice the skill. The skills trainer can reduce potential negative feelings toward treatment by targeting misinformation or unrealistic expectations about the application of skills. For example, when teaching the distress tolerance skill called "Distract with ACCEPTS," the skills trainer often makes clear at the outset that "these crisis survival skills are not intended to make you feel better; rather, they are intended to stop you from making a difficult situation worse than it already is. It's like a tourniquet; it keeps you alive, but you don't necessarily feel good during the process."

A second orienting strategy involves shaping expectations with the participant about practicing a new skill. For example, when introducing distress tolerance crisis survival skills, the skills trainer may tell an adolescent:

"Some of these skills help some of the teens, some of the time. So, if one skill doesn't work, try another. And if one skill works for only 5 minutes and you still need to reduce your distress, switch to another. It is useful to choose several of these 'distract' and 'self-soothe' skills to create a 'crisis survival kit' so you can access them immediately on an as-needed basis."

It is often necessary to review exactly what is expected using step-by-step instructions in order to help an emotionally dysregulated teen use a new skill both in and out of group.

At the end of each session, the skills trainer elicits a commitment from each member to complete the assigned homework. When applicable, the skills trainer asks each individual to report precisely which piece of the skill he or she will practice. For example, after the session on mindfulness "What" skills, the teen or parent may say, "I commit to practicing 'participate' and 'don't judge' skills this week." In another case, the member might say, "I commit to practicing my PLEASE skills and to focus on improving my sleep and eating behaviors each day of the week."

Eliciting adolescents' and caregivers' recommitment to completing and sharing their homework, coming on time, participating during group, and attempting to stay focused during group are often targets the skills trainer revisits throughout treatment. The skills trainer may use commitment strategies with the entire group during a session or with an individual before or after the session or during the break. If problems in these commitments persist, the skills group leader may enlist the help of the primary therapist to target these behaviors during individual therapy sessions (or sometimes during a family session) as therapy-interfering behaviors.

PRIMARY TREATMENT TARGETS IN SKILLS TRAINING

Skills training treatment targets differ from those in individual DBT. The skills training treatment hierarchy sets the following priorities: (1) reducing treatment-destroying behaviors, (2) increasing behavioral skills, and (3) reducing therapy-interfering behaviors.

Reducing Treatment-Destroying Behavior

DBT behavioral skills training functions primarily to increase clients' capacities. However, if a treatment-destroying behavior occurs, by definition, skills acquisition will not occur, and group members' treatment is jeopardized or stopped. Treatment-destroying behaviors literally threaten to destroy treatment for the client engaging in them or for other group members. Thus, these behaviors become the primary target when they arise, and group leaders must stop them immediately. Two leaders handle such behaviors more easily than just one. Treatment-destroying behaviors include arguing loudly with a family member; toppling chairs, throwing, or breaking something; hurting oneself or threatening to hurt oneself during group; hurting or threatening another group member; screaming, cursing, and using threatening body language toward other group members and group leaders; persistently disparaging the treatment program as a complete waste of time (particularly when done by a parent); not responding to skills trainer redirection or coaching when engaging in invalidation of other group members; presenting strong emotional or retraumatizing triggers to other group members (e.g., revealing a freshly cut arm); getting high with other group members during break; taking calls during group; repeatedly exiting and entering the room; and other behaviors that bring teaching to a halt or threaten the perceived safety of other group members.

Both skills trainers may need to pause the group to control or stop the behavior, or skills trainers may be able to address the behavior directly in the group with a directive. Depending on the nature of the treatment-destroying behavior, one skills trainer may need to escort a member outside the room and address the egregious behavior privately. When this is an adolescent, the skills trainer may then suggest the primary therapist be called so the teen can receive individualized skills coaching and get re-regulated enough to return to the group. With parents who are not in their own individual therapy, it is up to the skills group co-leader to provide coaching.

If the therapy-destroying behavior is directed at another group member, it might be necessary for the member to make a "repair" before being allowed to return to group. One example of a repair is a written letter of apology with a recommitment not to engage in the problem behavior and identification of the specific skills to use next time the emotions become activated. Group leaders may allow the person to make his or her repair at the start of a session, which should then proceed with the standard mindfulness practice and without allowing further processing of what happened other than "I was upset that you said [or did] . . . and I now accept your apology and repair." Group leaders may also need to follow up both in the session and individually with the other clients to do "damage control." In rare cases, when a client has not been able to respond to remediation for the behavior, he or she may not be admitted back into the group, and skills training may need to be continued separately.

Handling Group Member Relationships and Contacts Outside of Group

Outside relationships have the potential to be therapy destroying for individuals who engage in them in ineffective ways. We address these relationships in group guidelines (see the section "Skills Training Group Guidelines" in Chapter 5), limiting them to nondating and nonprivate relationships, where no discussion of, or engaging in, high-risk or target behaviors is permitted. When we orient families in the group at the start of each module, we emphasize the limits of outside relationships and the potential for harm. We have experienced group members becoming increasingly suicidal, refusing to return to group, attending group but with high levels of anxiety and distraction and increased target behaviors such as substance use because of outside contact with group members in person or online. For these reasons, we take a firm stance on these limitations. Even something as seemingly innocuous as "friending" one another on Facebook or connecting through other online social media can trigger group members as they read highly distressed posts or blogs about one another. Outside contacts that violate the group guidelines result in a behavioral analysis and problem solving in individual therapy. Leaders also warn teens that they could be dismissed from the program if contact continues.

Note that when members follow the group guidelines for periodic, noncrisis outside contact, it can be experienced as supportive. We especially find this the case for parents; we have observed much lower risk and high levels of social support from such contacts. Sticking within the guidelines as well as moderation seems to be the key for successful management of outside contact.

Increasing Behavioral Skills

When therapy-destroying behavior does not arise, increasing clients' capacities through behavioral skills training is the priority target, through teaching the skills of mindfulness, distress tolerance, interpersonal effectiveness, emotion regulation, and our new skills module, walking the middle path. Skills training proceeds according to Chapters 5–10, and group leaders do not allow minor annoyances or distractions to derail the process. Skills trainers teach skills to clients through utilizing didactics, handouts, questions, role plays with coaching and corrective feedback, and experiential exercises. Trainers keep to a schedule of modules and topics and teach the skills in order. To ensure that skills acquisition occurs, trainers need to keep this focus and maintain the pacing. Focus and pacing take priority over process issues or small disruptions.

In order to increase client capabilities, trainers must address three subtargets: skills acquisition, skills strengthening, and skills generalization and maintenance.

Skills Acquisition

Skills trainers ensure skills acquisition using didactics, role plays, and other experiential exercises that "drag out" new skills. The teen's individual therapist promotes the acquisition of new skills in individual sessions and in coaching calls. This might include offering a didactic on a skill not yet covered in group—which happens often with distress tolerance crisis survival skills (Chapter 7).

Skills Strengthening

Skills strengthening involves enhancing the robustness and thoroughness with which one knows the skills. This occurs through in-group behavioral rehearsal with corrective feedback and re-doing the skill to reach mastery, between-session homework and in-session homework review with feedback, phone coaching regarding skill use, and integrating skills into individual therapy, family, or parenting sessions.

Skills Generalization and Maintenance

Skills generalization refers to applying the skills to all relevant situations and contexts in clients' lives. *Maintenance* refers to ensuring a steady level of skill knowledge and application, and working to prevent the fading of skill knowledge and use with time. Clinicians enhance generalization and maintenance through assigning and reviewing skills training homework (which involves applying skills to real-life situations), including family members in skills training, and at times recommending a repetition of the skills modules a second time. When applying comprehensive DBT, skills generalization and maintenance also occur in the reinforcing of skills through behavior and solution analyses in individual sessions, phone coaching, and by offering family and/or parenting sessions to achieve a more validating and supportive family context.

Reducing Therapy-Interfering Behaviors

Reducing therapy-interfering behaviors is the third priority in skills training. With multiple teens and their families in one room, therapists can anticipate a steady stream of therapy-interfering behaviors, such as giggling, whispering or side conversations, eye rolling, interrupting, texting, "zoning out," getting out of one's seat, doodling on one's notebook, nonparticipation, not completing homework, coming late, and so on. If therapists addressed each of these behaviors as they arose, there would be little time to teach and practice skills. Group leaders can address these therapy-interfering behaviors in a variety of ways, most of which involve being mindful of behavioral principles operating in every interaction within the group and to reinforce, extinguish, or punish behaviors as needed.

First, leaders convey group rules during the orientation session (see Chapter 5). These rules include putting away cell phones during group, refraining from mean or disrespectful behaviors toward other members, etc. Thus, leaders aim to prevent problems by promoting a prosocial and respectful group culture and encouraging members to police themselves in this regard. Early on leaders need to reinforce courtesy toward others; tone of voice (avoid sarcasm, freshness, etc.); and self-management skills such as coming on time, clearing away snack plates/cups, etc. Such skills are not only helpful for managing group but are also undoubtedly helpful life skills. Teaching and modeling dialectical thinking also provides a way for group leaders to reduce or prevent therapy-interfering behavior. Leaders model "both–and" rather than "either/or" positions, helping to deflect conflict or negative feelings about having alternative points of view. When group members make judgmental comments about family members or, just as often, themselves, leaders immediately stop them and ask them to rephrase their comment in a nonjudgmental manner. Over time, this process reduces extremes in thinking.

Second, leaders can put many therapy-interfering behaviors on an extinction schedule. That is, leaders can ignore certain behaviors if they are relatively harmless and would be more disruptive to address in the group than the behaviors themselves. Leaders can ignore such behaviors as doodling, spacing out, occasional cross-talking, pacing, standing up and leaving the room for a short break, criticizing the therapist, or an eye roll at one's parent or another teen. Leaders can orient parents to "strategic ignoring" ahead of time by informing group members that the leaders will often ignore such behaviors so as not to detract from group time. Otherwise, parents may perceive the skills trainers to be naïve about what is going on or unable to control the group, rather than strategically electing to ignore certain behaviors. Many behaviors will diminish on their own if not reinforced.

Third, some therapy-interfering behaviors can be handled by gradually shaping more functional alternative behaviors through a reinforcement schedule. To do this, the skills trainer needs to mentally retain a shaping hierarchy of each group participant so that when a more adaptive behavior shows up, it can be reinforced immediately. A therapist might ignore one participant sitting quietly with his eyes downcast while another time choosing to reinforce a different quiet member with downcast eyes, since that behavior reflects significant progress from laying her head on the table or spinning in her chair. If a patient refuses to speak in group, the therapist might ask for a small gesture and reinforce that, such as sitting at the table instead of the back of the room. The next week, the group leader might ask the patient to read a line from the handout aloud, reinforce that level of participation, and so on.

Regarding how to reinforce group members, leaders might try praise, a small piece of candy, a chance to lead a mindfulness exercise, a cool sticker for their notebooks, or even a smile and approving nod of the head. Skills trainers must be aware of what each member finds reinforcing. Adolescents, especially those diagnosed with BPD, sometimes find praise aversive and thus not positively reinforcing, since praise may be associated with heightened expectations or with abandonment. Thus, skills trainers need to remain mindful of each participant's reaction to praise so as to (1) observe whether or not praise is aversive and (2) if it is reinforcing, use it judiciously. It is important not to satiate the individual; move soon to an intermittent reinforcement schedule.

As Pryor (2002) admonishes in her book *Don't Shoot the Dog!*, punishment does not teach new behavior. Hence, skills trainers should reserve the use of punishment for times when positive reinforcement and extinction are neither effective nor appropriate. For example, when a parent failed to bring in her homework 2 weeks in a row despite the positive problem solving and encouragement in the prior weeks, the skills trainer effectively applied two mild aversives: looking dismayed and conducting a brief behavioral chain analysis regarding what was getting in the way of her completing her homework. In another case in which an adolescent had not completed homework, the skills trainer asked the teen to generate a homework example on the spot. After eliciting that example, the skills trainer said, "Now that you appear to understand the homework so well, I'm going to reassign this sheet to you, and this time I'd love for you to fill it out and bring it for next week—in addition to the other assignment we're going to give you this evening." Having double homework was an aversive consequence, as communicated by the teen's disappointed face upon hearing the news. In a third example, an adolescent who had been in the group for several months was increasingly talking to peers during the sessions. The skills trainer approached the teen at the break and said, "Steven—you're killing me in there. I can't focus on my teaching while you're talking to your peers, and I'm feeling frustrated that I'm not doing a good job." This mild aversive got the adolescent's attention and stopped the behavior. It was especially effective since the skills trainer had a strong relationship with the teen.

Fourth, leaders can more covertly address therapy-interfering behavior in the following ways: by increasing the intensity or engagement level of the material; redirecting a distracted group member to read the next point on the handout or participate in a role play; or walking around the room (a normal part of leaders' styles) and lightly placing a hand on the shoulder of a disengaged member. Leaders may occasionally reorient to the group rules if members are drifting away from abiding by them. If the behavior persists, leaders can address a member privately during a group break or model the interpersonal DEAR MAN skill for effectively requesting something from another (see Chapter 10). Leaders should address cases of persistent problematic behavior directly with the patient during break or after group, or a co-leader can address it outside the room while group is running. Clients should be urged to address these behaviors with their individual therapists when receiving comprehensive DBT. In addition, persistent cases of problematic behavior would be brought to the therapist consultation team in order to develop a strategic approach for addressing them. This approach will typically include the individual therapist addressing the therapy-interfering behavior(s) with a behavioral analysis in individual therapy (see Miller et al., 2007, on conducting behavioral analyses in individual therapy).

A general maxim for leaders of skills training groups is that therapy begins 15 minutes before the session formally starts, includes the break, and continues 15 minutes after the session's formal conclusion. These times can be critical for checking in or repairing relationships with dysregulated or disengaged group members, enhancing parent commitment, and answering questions or clarifying material that clients won't raise in a group setting. Even chit-chat during break can facilitate emotion regulation in preparation for learning new material. We have found that making oneself available at these times enhances connection and prevents or addresses problems.

Absences

If a group member calls the day of the session and says he or she (or the family) will be absent, it is important to find out why. We have found that same-day cancellations are often impulsive or mood-dependent; some phone coaching and cheerleading can work to motivate them to change their minds and come. If a group member is a no-show without a call, it can be helpful for a co-leader to excuse him- or herself and call the family. Some coaching may be able to get the member to the session, even if late. Absences from group should be addressed primarily as therapy-interfering behavior in individual therapy, however.

Caregiver Therapy-Interfering Behavior

Some caregivers appear highly motivated at the outset but then their commitment wanes. Indicators for this problem include coming late, not attending group for consecutive weeks, not completing skills group homework, or appearing disengaged and nonparticipatory in group. We find several strategies effective in managing this problem. First, the skills trainer can employ contingency management strategies, such as positive reinforcement, or mild aversives such as a behavioral analysis regarding noncompliance with homework or highlighting, in a concerned way, how many times the parent has missed group. Second, the skills trainer can pull aside the identified parent before or after group, and do a concerned "check-in" to see how things are going and share the observation that the parent seems less engaged as compared to a few weeks ago. Third, it is sometimes useful to enlist the adolescent and encourage him or her to use the DEAR MAN interpersonal effectiveness skill to spur the parent to come on time. If these brief interventions fail, one may schedule a family or collateral visit (i.e., parent alone) to assess the problem and find solutions.

Once parents are engaged in the group, it is useful to intermittently reinforce their prosocial behaviors such as sharing observations in group, completing and sharing their homework, volunteering to lead a mindfulness practice exercise, and giving helpful feedback to the other parents and teenagers. It behooves skills trainers to give as much attention to caregivers as they do adolescents—before, during, and after group. Showing interest in the caregivers' lives, careers, hobbies, and life challenges is an important attachment strategy. Parents should not be considered merely extensions of their adolescents. View everyone at the table as a skills group participant, regardless of age. Everyone is expected to come to group on time, be prepared with materials and homework, and to participate fully. Skills trainers use positive reinforcement and shaping to increase these desired behaviors; they are also ready to employ extinction and punishment, as necessary, for problematic behaviors that arise.

MANAGING THE GROUP SESSION TO MEET PRIMARY TARGETS

Most skills training sessions begin with a mindfulness exercise followed by brief announcements. The session then moves to a review of homework and skills practice until a midsession break. The second half of the session is devoted to teaching new skills. This basic format is followed regardless of setting or whether the teaching of new skills follows directly or on a different day.

Mindfulness Exercise and Announcements

We begin each group with a 3- to 5-minute mindfulness exercise, plus a few additional minutes for taking observations, questions, and discussion. With teens, we recommend starting out with very brief mindfulness exercises (1–2 minutes) and gradually working up to longer ones. Then we move to brief announcements, during which we account for any absent or late members if we have information (e.g., "Keira and parents called to say they are running late, but they are on their way," or "James and his father couldn't make it tonight but they will be back next week"). There is no need to offer reasons for family's absences, unless they have shared them themselves (e.g., "We won't be able to be here next week because we are celebrating my uncle's birthday"). In these cases leaders can remind group members of the members' announcements from the week before. Leaders also orient group members each week by mentioning the skill that will be addressed that night, the skill coming up the following week, when a new module will start, or that a new family will be joining group. In addition, leaders make any special announcements, such as a change in the group schedule due to an upcoming holiday.

Reviewing the Homework Assignment from the Prior Week

Following mindfulness practice and announcements, group leaders devote the first half of the session to homework review. Homework makes up an important part of skills strengthening and generalization, and is thus just as important as the teaching of new skills for acquisition. Homework review offers a chance to ascertain whether clients have correctly learned the skills, provide behaviorally specific feedback, have clients redo a skill to attain mastery (e.g., restate the "negotiate" part of the DEAR MAN skill after receiving feedback), review concepts in which clients need extra help, and reinforce clients for making efforts to practice. It is important to review homework with each member in order to reinforce the importance of outside practice and to help with difficulties implementing the skill. A large group can break into two smaller groups for homework review, with a skills trainer meeting with each smaller group. Group members can then reconvene in a larger group for the teaching of new skills in the second half.

If there is time and need, homework review can begin with a very brief (i.e., 5 minutes) review of the skill taught the week before. Otherwise, leaders ask for a volunteer to start and typically proceed around the circle. We prefer going decisively in a circle for homework review rather than waiting for volunteers, as this approach reduces long pauses and avoidance.

Engaging the Whole Group during the Homework Review

We allot about 3–5 minutes per person for homework review. The review should be thorough enough that leaders can assess skill understanding and provide corrective feedback but short enough for the group to move at an engaging pace with no one omitted from going over homework. Group members should be shaped to write their homework on the worksheets. This helps ensure thinking about it prior to group and focuses their reporting while reviewing it. As a person reviews homework, therapists provide corrective feedback to further strengthen the behaviors being discussed. Group leaders or the person with homework under review can ask other group members to provide brief constructive feedback to engage other members, increase learning from others' examples, and decrease daydreaming while awaiting their turn. For example, Carlos reports, "I didn't really use any of my DEAR MAN skills this week." Then he reports a discussion with his teacher in which he indeed did use some good DEAR MAN skills, but the teacher did not grant him his request. The group leader might ask: "Hold on—you said that you didn't use *any* DEAR MAN skills, but I thought I picked up some in there. Group members, which skills did you hear Carlos using with his teacher?" This approach allows group members to engage in the discussion while reinforcing Carlos (who, incidentally, was making a common error of discounting his skill use because it did not lead to the desired outcome).

Leaders can also comment on a member's practice and its applicability to others as a way of engaging people during the homework go-around. For example, a leader might say, "Great job catching yourself and using a distress tolerance skill before saying something impulsive to your teacher, Kevin. It reminds me of what we were all talking about last week." Leaders can engage other members by asking them to write down one thing they learned or thought applied to them during others' reports of homework. Finally, leaders must remember to move homework along at a swift pace, avoiding long pauses between members' reports, blocking overreporting of homework, and helping to focus long-winded reports of homework.

Problems That Emerge during the Homework Review

A number of problems may impede homework review. These problems include not completing the homework or not reporting it because the person finds it aversive and avoids it. Problems can also involve the style of reporting on homework.

If the client has not done the homework, leaders briefly assess what happened to understand what interfered. In fact, we have often found that clients who say "I didn't do the homework" actually did it in some form or to some extent. Shame about the homework's lack of perfection or failure to produce desired results (as in the example of Carlos above) may lead parents or teens to say they did not do it. A client might also wish to "pass" during homework review because he or she has not completed the assignment or is reluctant to report on it out of shame or anxiety. It is critical to assess reasons rather than make assumptions about them. If some or most of the homework has actually been completed, it is important that the client reports on that portion, and leaders can reinforce the effort or the effective parts of it (or elicit this reinforcement from group members). If not, the leader should quickly generate a solution with the client for completing it next time. Solutions might involve providing a clearer explanation of the homework if it was not understood, having someone else read the homework sheet aloud if a client is too anxious, problem-solving about when during the week to do the homework if there was no time, or figuring out a place to leave the notebook with the homework so the teen remembers to bring it in if it was left home. After quickly assessing what happened, leaders can also spend time asking the member about his or her use of the skill during the previous week anyway, that is, whether he or she tried it, thought about it, or had a situation where he or she could have used it. The important point is not to skip the client who reports not doing the homework entirely and to demonstrate the importance of the homework through the seriousness and time leaders allocate to it. If not completing homework becomes a pattern for an individual, it can be brought up in the therapist's consultation team and also discussed with the primary therapist as a therapy-interfering behavior.

The style in which teens report on homework can become a problem. Some clients are tangential and long-winded. To manage this style, we orient clients at the start of each homework review, explaining that each person will have 3–5 minutes, so that each gets time to report. We also ask people not to supply a "back story" to the homework, but to please dive in directly to use of the skill. We also ask people to read from their homework sheets because that helps focus them. If we see that they are speaking extemporaneously, we will redirect them to what they wrote on their sheets. We also gently interrupt people and try to refocus them. If we know that certain group members typically lose track of time during the review, we will pick a focused, concise group member as a model to go first, and then give feedback that his or her report was focused and to the point. Finally, we use a shaping model, reinforcing small steps toward brevity for our wordy clients and reinforcing more sharing in the more reserved clients.

Session Break

Following the first 50–55 minutes of the session, groups generally take a 5- to 10-minute break. We have found that this break is important for several reasons. First, it is a practical necessity to allow participants to use the restrooms or return a quick phone call. Second, informal conversation takes place during this time that inevitably strengthens the alliance between participants and co-leaders. On some occasions, parents compare notes as to how they are coping with their adolescents' behaviors. Adolescents often discuss activities occurring at school, peer group issues, and weekend plans. The break also serves as a periodic opportunity for the skills trainers to check in on members who came in late or who appear emotionally dysregulated, or to give specific feedback to someone about his or her behavior. Finally, the break serves as reinforcement for attending group. For adolescents especially, the break provides necessary "downtime" and a chance to enjoy snacks and beverages.

Other settings structure the break in different ways. For example, some programs separate parents and teens, and each co-leader sits with them during break, while providing snacks. In some settings practitioners may be concerned about teens leaving the building or the area and being unsupervised; high-risk behaviors could then occur alone or in groups of teens. Some programs therefore may wish to implement rules about leaving the area or other break policies.

Teaching New Skills

Following the break, new skills are introduced. Skills trainers introduce skills with a story, question, or rationale that will engage group members and get them to consider how the skill could be useful for them. Leaders should explicitly relate the skill to members' problem behaviors and offer how it will get them closer to their goals. Leaders then provide didactic material in which they define and explain the skill and then quickly move to modeling, role playing, and other exercises for practicing the skill. Next leaders focus on "dragging out" new behaviors from clients. In Chapters 6–10, each skill is introduced in this manner. It is also important to weave self-management strategies in with discussion of skill use, such as the need to review the skill, practice the skill, and try it in new situations.

Leaders need to prepare before each group, know the handouts they will cover, homework sheets they will assign, and approximate time to allocate to the teaching of each skill. Without this plan, session material can easily wander off topic, planned material will not be covered, and clients will not learn the requisite skills. Sometimes the teaching will not go according to plan because group members elicit more discussion on a topic. If leaders believe that such discussion will enhance rather than sidetrack learning of the skill, it might be worth the extra time, which will have to be made up at some later point.

Leaders may want to prepare supplemental exercises, along with multiple examples and alternative teaching methods, for the following reasons:

- There may be extra time in which to illustrate or practice.
- Group members may not understand a concept and need additional explanations, demonstrations, or practice.
- The second time through a skills module with the same group, leaders may want to teach the same concepts in varied ways to maintain engagement.
- Using new examples or practice exercises helps prevent leaders from getting "stale" or burning out.

In the chapters detailing the skills training modules, we provide multiple examples and teaching exercises for the skills. Leaders will not have time to cover all of these in one group session or one pass through the modules; rather, they are meant to provide additional teaching options, and they are used to vary or support teaching as needed and at leaders' discretion.

As skills trainers teach a skill, it is helpful to be aware of clients' maladaptive patterns and address them, albeit indirectly. For example, if a skills trainer knows that three families in the room are experiencing significant struggles with explosive anger, she might use anger explosions as an example of applying Pros and Cons or Opposite Action (ER 20) without referring to anyone's specific situations. Similarly, if a skills trainer knows that some group members are struggling with saying no and making it stick, he or she might be sure to role-play the interpersonal DEAR MAN skill using a scenario where the goal is to say no effectively.

Dragging Out New Behaviors

After a new skill is introduced, role plays and practice can occur with the whole group or in smaller groups. The leaders walk around, listen in, and provide coaching and feedback. If smaller groups are preferred for this part, the group can be divided in half with a leader working with each half for more individualized practice. Still smaller groups can consist of dyads or triads such as two people and a "coach," or people playing two parents and a teen, or three friends, etc. We recommend strategically planning such smaller group memberships ahead of time and assigning people to their groups. People who clash should not be placed together because they are likely to dysregulate themselves and other members and to deflect learning. Putting together small groups that are likely to "click" can work wonders for increasing cohesion, disinhibiting shy group members, discouraging cliques, building new alliances, and making newer group members feel more connected.

A common mistake we have observed in new therapists or those without strong behavior therapy backgrounds is to spend time talking *about* the skill or simply reading from the handout rather than having clients *use* and *rehearse* the skill. It is not uncommon for clients to be able to describe a skill perfectly but not be able to apply it. Until skills trainers observe a client implementing a skill (e.g., in a role play, mindfulness practice, or other demonstration), they have not assessed and cannot determine the client's ability to apply the skill. Skills trainers teach skills to clients through coaching and specific labeled feedback on role plays and other frequent experiential exercises. After leaders provide feedback, they can ask the member to reattempt a skill, until mastery is reached. This opportunity for redoing an exercise in an improved way is critical for correct understanding and application of the skills. The importance of such practice, rehearsal with feedback, and repetition to mastery cannot be overstated.

Coaching and Feedback

Skills trainers need to coach clients' attempts to use the skills. Coaching can occur during the rehearsal of new skills or during homework review; it involves explaining to clients how their behavior is discrepant from a more accurate or effective performance of a skill, as well as specifically how to improve.

It is critical for coaching to be behaviorally specific. If a client role-plays the interpersonal DEAR MAN skill (Describe, Express, Assert, Reinforce, be Mindful, Appear confident,

Negotiate), the leader should *not* say, "That went pretty well, don't you think?" Instead, leaders should say something along these lines:

> "I liked how you described and expressed your feelings of being demoralized, asserted by asking directly for what you wanted, and reinforced by telling him that giving what you wanted would make you more motivated to work hard. And you definitely appeared confident with your voice tone and eye contact, and you stayed mindful. What was missing was the negotiation. Can you think of a way to negotiate what you are asking for? Let's try that now. You are off to a great start; you have most of it down!"

Because clients might feel criticized or experience shame for not using a skill perfectly, it can be helpful to surround negative feedback with positive feedback, as in the above example, which ends with an example of cheerleading.

Even if a client is highly subject to fear or shame, it is important that skills trainers continue to give corrective feedback. Otherwise, avoidance will be reinforced and no new learning will take place. It is best to provide repeated exposure to the cues of corrective feedback (including modeling corrective feedback to others!) so that urges to escape will decrease. Skills trainers can apply a shaping paradigm using reinforcement to encourage successive approximations toward participating, rehearsing skills, or sharing homework.

Behavioral specificity means giving feedback on the client's actual performance rather than on any assumed motives. If a client did not appear confident while practicing DEAR MAN, a skills trainer can say, "Can you try it again? Remember to work on your body language and voice tone so that you appear confident." The trainer should not say, "You were embarrassed, weren't you?"

After knowing a group member for some time, trainers can identify his or her patterns of skill use and so help identify what he or she might practice. For example, some clients might have an easy time applying skills at work but struggle using them with family members. When using the GIVE skill (be Gentle, act Interested, Validate, use an Easy manner), some might be gentle but struggle with validation. Leaders can point out these patterns to encourage practice toward further mastery of skills.

Leaders should reinforce clients' positive behaviors toward other group members. If a client spontaneously praises, encourages, or validates another group member, whether within the same family or not, leaders can attend to and reinforce that gesture; this creates and maintains a supportive group culture.

Finally, if group members get discouraged or find a skill challenging, emphasize practice. Practice should occur both inside and outside of group, at times with the help of the members' individual therapists. Homework continues the learning process through helping with rehearsal and generalization.

Managing the Assignment of Homework

After completing the teaching of a skill, leaders assign homework that will strengthen and help generalize the new skill. Homework assignments are provided for each skill in Chapters 6–10. Skills trainers should clearly explain the assignments and can even write them out on the whiteboard. Assign one or two homework sheets per session. Review the specific worksheets with group members and ask for questions about the assignment. We find it helpful to ask someone to summarize the assignment to ensure that it was conveyed clearly. The more time spent on carefully defining and explicating the homework, the more likely it will get done properly.

Managing the End of Group: The Wind-Down

Each group session ends with a process-observing wind-down lasting about 3–5 minutes. It functions as an additional practice of a mindfulness, or distress tolerance skill, or to enhance commitment. It also helps ensure that clients are sufficiently regulated emotionally before they leave group.

A skills trainer rings the mindfulness bell and asks all group participants (including parents), in no particular order, to nonjudgmentally describe any observation they had about anything relevant to that day's group experience. Participants are instructed not to respond to anyone else's descriptions, and the skills trainers also participate, often adding an observation of concern about any member who did not attend that day's group. Group members typically enjoy this opportunity to share one nonjudgmental observation about themselves, the group, or other members, even though it is initially challenging for them to apply their skills in this format. This exercise brings a quiet, thoughtful closure to the group and strengthens mindfulness practice.

Skills trainers give feedback to shape closing observations in a way that is consistent with nonjudgmental observation and description, and not inference. For example, a leader might say, "That observation sounded a little judgmental to me. Can you try it again, observing and describing without the judgment?" Or a leader might say, "You said that Sophia seemed happy tonight, but remember that we cannot observe another person's mood. Can you say specifically what you observed? [e.g., a lot of smiling, laughing, and energy]." The trainer would then reinforce a more descriptive and less judgmental comment, modeling a nonjudgmental observation if needed, to enhance the central mindfulness skill of observing. Observations might range from "Even though I wasn't initially in the mood to come, I noticed an improvement in my mood and I observed having the thought 'I'm glad I came'" to "I observed the thought that Katie worked hard today when talking about her relationship problems" to "I'm noticing a feeling of happiness and sadness after hearing that AJ's family will be graduating soon" to "I observed having the thought that I'm probably not using enough validation when I speak with my daughter."

Some programs may choose to end group with other closing exercises, such as leading clients through a relaxation, guided imagery, meditation, or breathing exercise. Alternatively, they might invite closing statements on commitments to accomplishing something for building mastery, engaging in a pleasant event, following through on a commitment made during skills group, or practicing a new skill. Examples of closing commitments might include: "I'm going to work on radically accepting that my classmates are unable to handle the news that I am gay"; "I'm going to submit one college application by next group"; and "I'm going to commit to using my DEAR MAN skills with my friend, who keeps wanting to discuss her self-injuring with me, since it really upsets me." A variety of closing practices can serve to end an often emotionally intense group on a calm, focused, effective, and more regulated note.

CHAPTER 4

The Art of Conducting DBT Skills Training
Balancing DBT Strategies and Managing Dialectical Tensions

BALANCING DBT STRATEGIES TO ENGAGE THE GROUP

To effectively teach DBT skills to emotionally dysregulated adolescents (with or without their family members), one must engage the participants. Without an effective and at least somewhat entertaining teaching style, content becomes irrelevant because no one listens to, let alone learns, the material. This consideration is all the more important when working with adolescents in the 21st century who are accustomed to constant stimulation. Additionally, skills groups with adolescents (and families) typically occur around the dinner hour or later to allow time for teens and families to get home from school and work and then travel to group. Since many multifamily skills groups tend to be held after participants have already completed long days at school and work, skills trainers have to work even harder to maintain participants' interest.

Teaching skills effectively involves flexibly applying (by overlearning) all of the DBT treatment strategies and applying them in a balanced way. Funny skills trainers must balance humor with serious moments just as the flamboyant skills trainer needs some quiet moments. It is this dialectical stance that makes for good theatre and thus better potential for learning. Ultimately, we believe that an effective skills trainer has to "fully participate" (a mindfulness skill), which means throwing oneself fully into the moment: passionate, focused, and non-self-conscious. This takes practice.

At a minimum we want the group members to be engaged at a cognitive level, but we hope to engage them at an emotional level as well. Teaching is more effective when learners are engaged emotionally. The more the skills trainer can tap into his or her own emotional experience with the skills, the more he or she can breathe life into the material and the less didactic and dry it will feel. Skills trainers who regularly use the DBT skills in their own lives are most able to share emotionally engaging personal examples and discuss how the skills work from a first-person vantage point.

DBT skills trainers employ all DBT treatment strategies when conducting skills training. The core treatment involves balancing acceptance and change strategies with an emphasis on validation (acceptance) and problem solving (change). DBT stylistic and case management

53

strategies each contain some reflecting acceptance and some reflecting change. Dialectical strategies permeate treatment, and they can be especially helpful when the skills trainer and the client or family member become polarized.

Balancing Validation and Problem-Solving Strategies

Validation

As Linehan has written: "The essence of validation is this: The therapist communicates to the client that her responses make sense and are understandable within her current life context or situation. The therapist actively accepts the client and communicates this acceptance to the client" (1993a, pp. 222–223). There are six levels of DBT validation. The skills trainer employs all six levels while conducting skills training:

- Level 1: Unbiased listening and observing; listening and attending with interest.
- Level 2: Reflection, showing that you understand through paraphrasing the other's communication.
- Level 3: Mind reading by reading facial expression, body language, and articulating the other's thoughts or feelings that have not directly been expressed in words.
- Level 4: Acknowledging that the other's experience makes sense given his or her past learning history.
- Level 5: Communicating that the other's behavior makes sense given the current context.
- Level 6: Radical genuineness, by speaking in a way that conveys your view of the other as an equal and capable of handling direct and honest feedback.

For example, when a teen becomes tearful and momentarily speechless, the skills trainer employs Level 3 validation (i.e., mind reading) by saying, "I see you're feeling sad right now and it is difficult to speak." An example of Level 5 validation from a skills trainer might be: "Susan, I can see why you are having trouble staying focused when there are so many distractions at your end of the table." It is especially critical for the skills trainer to employ Level 6 validation, "radical genuineness." When therapists convey their honest feelings and reactions without couching them in watered down or patronizing "therapist-speak," clients feel validated. For example, when a group of teens and parents show up without anyone having completed homework, a radically genuine therapist might say, "I'm so demoralized that you guys didn't do your homework after committing to do it, especially since I know that these skills are the key to helping you get your lives back on track." When they show up the next week with homework completed, it is radically genuine to say, "You guys really made my day—seriously!" Another example is a skills trainer who allows himself to shed tears during a graduation ceremony in which a 15-year-old daughter genuinely expresses gratitude and relief to her previously absent father for his participation in the skills training group and for how much their relationship has improved the quality of her life. Intermittent and appropriate self-disclosure regarding the skills trainer's personal use of DBT skills in response to life's challenges is another example of radical genuineness. It might be sharing a decision-making dilemma via pros and cons, the application of mindfulness skills when feeling overwhelmed, the use of radical acceptance to cope with the loss of a loved one, or the application of DEAR MAN with a friend or relative—in all these ways, a skills trainer can demonstrate radical genuineness to the group. Each is validating and a good use of modeling and coping.

It is important to strike a balanced emotional tone when being radically genuine and using self-disclosure to illustrate skills use. Leaders want to avoid being either too emotionally distant or too emotionally vulnerable—the group should not feel the need to take care of the skills trainer. Self-disclosures will ideally have enough emotional content and detail while concluding with a demonstration of coping. Leaders thus serve as coping models, using skills to address life problems, and not as either mastery models, who always make the right choice or behave perfectly, or persons in need of care, who may not seem competent to handle group members' struggles.

Problem Solving

Skills trainers need to help teens and parents acquire and strengthen new behavioral skills. To accomplish this goal, they also need to briefly problem-solve whatever gets in the way of participants' learning and practicing of new skills. This problem solving can take the form of "dragging out" new behavior from clients, teens and parents alike. For example, in one group a 14-year-old girl with attention-deficit/hyperactivity disorder (ADHD) began shredding paper and spinning in her chair. The skills trainer said to her:

> "I know it's really hard to sit still for so long—especially late at night . . . and, I'm hoping you can hang in there for another 30 minutes so I can teach you and the rest of the group some really important emotion regulation skills. So, can you please try to use your mindfulness skills to stay focused on what I am saying? And when your mind and body start to wander, try to notice and gently refocus your attention . . . OK?"

It is often useful to provide clients with soothing or validation before attempting to elicit a new behavior, as shown in this example.

The primary role of the skills trainer is to help teens and families acquire and strengthen new behavioral skills through didactics, modeling, role plays and other experiential exercises, and homework review. When participants are not engaged in group or not doing homework, skills trainers use a number of strategies to increase their engagement and compliance. Chapter 3 contains a discussion of how to manage therapy-interfering behaviors.

Balancing Reciprocal and Irreverent Communication Strategies

Reciprocal communication is directly responsive and takes the client's agenda and wishes seriously. It is friendly, reflecting warmth and engagement. It is usually validating and acceptance-oriented. *Irreverent communication* is used to push the client off balance, get his or her attention, present an alternative viewpoint, or shift an affective response. It is change-oriented and is particularly useful when the client is immovable or when therapist and client are stuck. Although it is also responsive to the client, it is almost never the response the client expects (Linehan, 1993a).

Skills trainers employ several reciprocal communication strategies. For example, "Wow, Bill, it sounds like you had a very challenging week, so I am especially glad you were able to attend group tonight and are participating to the best of your ability." At times, it is also useful to employ the reciprocal communication strategy of "self-involving self-disclosure," in which the skills trainer communicates to the patient, "I feel X, when you do Y." For example, an intelligent and funny adolescent male in one group had a history of blurting out in class and offending teachers and peers; the skills trainer told him, "Although I am a big fan of yours, Bill, I feel invalidated when you try to make jokes and make faces toward other group members when I'm trying to convey a serious teaching point. I want you to use your marvelous sense of humor—just more mindfully and selectively. When you do that, I enjoy your contributions all the more."

In a group context, skills trainers use irreverent communication in different forms—always with the goal of getting the patient's attention, shifting his or her affective response, or helping him or her see another perspective. For example, one teen was asked to role-play asking for what she wants clearly and directly. Shaking her head, the teen replied, "I *never* do that—I am never assertive; maybe someone else can do this one." The therapist responded, "You could have fooled me! You're demonstrating your assertiveness skills by telling us you don't want to do this!" At times, irreverent communication may take the form of an offbeat response to a teen's sarcastic question. At other times, it involves oscillating intensity, such as varying one's voice tone or volume. For example, the skills trainer may choose to become very quiet or even silent for a few moments to catch the attention of a few disruptive cross-talking teens who have lost awareness of the group. As soon as they stop talking, the leader picks up where he or she left off without any comment.

Using another form of irreverence, the skills trainer acknowledges his or her own fallibility in life. One of us tells of a medical condition that was profoundly difficult to accept before ultimately, after some degree of suffering, being able to move toward radical acceptance. Every participant hangs on each word as this story is told since most of them are unaccustomed to therapists revealing personal stories. We call another form of irreverent communication used in the group "plunging in where angels fear to tread." Here, the skills trainer speaks directly and bluntly about serious and sometimes emotionally laden subject matter, such as sex, drugs, and self-harm. For example, the skills trainer may describe sexual and drug experimentation as "typical adolescent behaviors" while teaching Walking the Middle Path Skills to adolescents and caregivers. Talking about the subject matter in this manner elicits emotional reactions that infuse what could otherwise be a very didactic, less engaging discussion.

Case Management Strategies: Balancing Patient Consultation with Environmental Intervention

The spirit of the consultation-to-the-patient strategy is epitomized in the adage "If you give a man a fish, he eats for a night; if you teach a man to fish, he eats for a lifetime." Particularly when working with minors, mental health practitioners can overrely on environmental interventions to the detriment of adolescents' skill-building progress. Consultation-to-the-patient strategies teach the client how to interact with his or her environment. The bias of DBT therapists is toward this change-oriented approach. However, there are times when it is necessary to move to the acceptance side of the dialectic and provide environmental intervention, with the clinician consulting, on the teen's behalf, with family, school, other professionals, etc. Environmental intervention strategies are generally used when substantial harm may befall a client, the client lacks abilities, the environment is too powerful, or time is of the essence.

DBT skills trainers often use consultation-to-the-patient strategies in group when an adolescent or caregiver requires in-group feedback or coaching. For example, one teen reported having a problem with a teacher at school and expressed frustration and hopelessness. The teen's parents volunteered to take care of the problem. The skills trainer invoked the consultation-to-the-patient strategy by saying the following:

"I think even more helpful would be for Olivia to talk to her teacher by using the DEAR MAN skills taught last week. She can meet with her teacher to convey her frustration and to ask the teacher to be less critical of her in front of her class when she asks questions. Olivia, I know this may be difficult, but I think if we role-play and practice a few times, you may be able to get what you want without others having to do this for you!"

In another example, a teenage boy expressed frustration about a verbally abusive teacher. The boy had already attempted to resolve the conflict, only to be harshly criticized by the teacher. Given the fact that (1) the adolescent had already tried to use skills, (2) the environment was too powerful, and (3) it was becoming dangerous emotionally for the teen to continue, it was evident that environmental strategies were indicated. Thus, the skills trainer coached the parent to use her DEAR MAN skills first with the teacher and then with the assistant principal if the situation was not remedied immediately.

Using Dialectical Strategies

DBT skills trainers teach and model dialectical thinking, acting, and feeling throughout the course of the skills group. Behavioral extremes and rigidity may be signals that emotions are running high, the teen or caregiver may be polarized, and a synthesis must be achieved. The therapist helps the client move from an "either/or" to a "both–and" position. The key is not to invalidate the first idea or polarity when asserting the second. For example, a 17-year-old girl asked how to reconcile her parents' strong opinion with her own. "I told my mother I wanted to join the National Guard since I'm struggling in high school and I don't think I'm ready for college. She said I shouldn't even think about joining the National Guard since I'm too small and I'll get hurt or killed . . . so I guess I should listen to her and forget about my idea." The therapist replied by asking, "Could you consider this situation more dialectically by using 'both–and' so you don't invalidate yourself? In other words, could you try to say to yourself, 'I have my own idea of joining the National Guard for a variety of reasons, and, at the same time, my parents have expressed concerns about my safety if I pursue this plan. Both points have validity, and I can consider them both."

DBT includes a number of dialectical strategies, and we describe a few here (for complete discussion, see Linehan, 1993a). In "playing devil's advocate," the therapist presents a position opposite from the desired goal with the expectation that the teen will counter it and thereby argue for the desired goal. "Making lemonade out of lemons" finds a positive in, or makes meaning out of, a negative. For example, a socially anxious teen reported in group that it is too difficult to share homework because of her anxiety. The skills trainer might say, "How fortunate for you to be in a DBT skills group where you can receive coaching while working to overcome your anxiety. This is the place for you!"

Another dialectical strategy is called "movement, speed, and flow." DBT skills trainers, just like individual therapists, often get polarized and stuck on one issue with one client. It is important for the trainer to remember to keep things moving quickly in a group so as not to get stuck with one person. When one parent said, "None of the five DBT problem areas applies to me presently or in the past," the skills trainer quickly asked both playfully and skeptically, "Are you sure there's nothing that applies?" The parent said, "Nope." The skills trainer said "OK," while withholding some warmth (mild aversive) and swiftly moved on to the next group member and asked, "How do any of these five problem areas relate to you?" It is not effective for a skills group leader to get bogged down with a teen or parent who is not willing or able to answer a question. Thus, if one or two strategies do not work, move on and engage the next person. Remember, though, to positively reinforce an individual who reengages and adopts a more willing stance as soon as it occurs.

Many parents who learn about DBT enter the skills group hopeful and enthusiastic that this therapy will be the one that will finally restore quality of life for both the teens and families. Although skills trainers need to instill hope and confidence, it is important to adopt a balanced, moderate level of enthusiasm in words and tone. Many of the teens with whom we have worked enter the group thinking that if an adult (parent or therapist) likes something this much, it can't be good for them.

To retain participants' attention, it is helpful for the skills trainer to get comfortable standing at the head of the table (or front of the room) as well as moving around. Being seated and completely stationary for 2 hours can reduce the liveliness of teaching. Standing also allows the skills trainer to view the entire room more clearly and more easily make eye contact with each member at a large table.

In sum, new skills trainers not only need to overlearn the DBT skills content but also the DBT treatment strategies so that their teaching style embodies DBT, engages participants in the learning process, and models the skills *in vivo*. Effective skills trainers not only teach in a clear and organized manner, using frequent examples that breathe life into the skills, they are also theatrical teachers who vary their teaching styles by using irreverent and reciprocal communication strategies, dialectical strategies, and validation and problem-solving strategies. Observe seasoned skills trainers in action whenever possible. We encourage new staff to serve as co-leaders in these groups so that they can learn through observation as well as supervisory feedback until they gain proficiency with both content and style.

MANAGING DIALECTICAL DILEMMAS

A number of behavior patterns can emerge in skills training that interfere with running the group smoothly. Three of these patterns consist of the original dialectical dilemmas identified by Linehan (1993a) and described in Chapter 1:

- Emotional vulnerability versus self-invalidation
- Active passivity versus apparent competence
- Unrelenting crises versus inhibited experiencing

An overarching dilemma when observing these patterns in teens is to decipher when the behavior pattern represents normal adolescent behavior and when it should become a clinical target. For example, aspects of these patterns, described below, can reflect teens' typical struggles with mood fluctuations, dependency versus autonomy, and sense of urgency and intensity regarding interpersonal and other problems. One guideline to consider is this: When the pattern significantly impacts functioning, continually relates to other target behaviors, or repeatedly interferes with participation in the group, the pattern likely requires targeting by an individual therapist and/or by the skills trainers, as described below. We discuss these issues in relation to their application to skills training in Miller and colleagues (2007) as well as below.

Other patterns represent dialectical dilemmas specific to adolescents and their families targeted by the walking the middle path skills. These are normalizing pathological behaviors versus pathologizing normal adolescent behaviors, excessive leniency versus authoritarian control, and fostering dependence versus forcing autonomy. Each of these behavior patterns is associated with a set of secondary treatment targets. Unlike the primary treatment targets in DBT skills training, these secondary targets are addressed by therapists when they are related to other important therapy targets (e.g., learning new skills, behaviors that interfere with therapy, a client's personal targets for change).

These behavior patterns represent extreme imbalances in group interactions. Clients can fluctuate between opposite poles or primarily display one extreme. Family members can also polarize each other. (See Rathus & Miller, 2000, or Miller et al., 2007, for detailed discussions of the original dialectical dilemmas and their corresponding treatment targets as they apply to teens.) Managing these behaviors requires paying close attention to members' individual patterns and keeping them in mind while teaching. These patterns can guide who is selected to role-play certain skills, who is chosen to volunteer an example for demonstrating a particular skill, and what specific feedback is provided during homework review. Leaders can also spontaneously coach a member to apply a skill in the moment. Thus, some of these behavior patterns can be addressed by practicing skills, *in vivo*. This is an area where having a co-leader can be invaluable; while one trainer is actively teaching, the other can focus on group members' behaviors.

The following material describes how to manage the specific dialectical dilemmas as well as other dialectical tensions that can arise during skills training sessions.

Addressing Emotional Vulnerability and Self-Invalidation

Emotional vulnerability refers to the tendency to become highly distressed or emotionally aroused, a central experience for people entering DBT. Such clients can be highly sensitive and reactive, and they often experience intense emotions during group. Their inability to regulate emotional arousal during skills training leads to dysregulated behaviors (e.g., crying, yelling, leaving the room) and impaired cognitive processing that interferes with attention and learning. Advance preparation and coordination with the adolescent's individual therapist through the therapist consultation team can effectively address this problem. With the client in individual sessions, the individual therapist can plan and help the client practice skills for coping with episodes of dysregulation, such as by acting opposite to the current emotion, by applying mindfulness skills, or using distress tolerance skills such as distraction. Skills trainers can then remind members of these coping plans before group or during break. Skill use can also be briefly encouraged while in the session, with skills leaders briefly coaching the client to employ a skill to help tolerate the distress, refocus attention, or attempt to change the emotion by throwing him- or herself into skills training. The distress could also be ignored in the group but then addressed by a group co-leader outside the room or during break so as not to detract from the more primary target of increasing behavioral skills.

Self-invalidation refers to the dismissal of one's own emotions, perceptions, and problem-solving approaches. For example, when reporting on homework, a teen might say, "I shouldn't have felt that way," or in the midst of answering a question, the teen might retract the answer, saying, "Never mind—this is stupid." When this behavior appears, leaders can redirect the client to nonjudgmentally observe and describe his or her emotions, or to act opposite the self-invalidation by replacing such statements with self-validating ones.

Addressing Active Passivity and Apparent Competence

Active passivity refers to being passive in addressing one's own problems while actively eliciting the help of others to solve those problems. An additional problem is that these individuals are often not skillful in soliciting the help of others, and may do so in an off-putting or otherwise ineffective way. In skills training, a teen may identify numerous life problems coupled with an unwillingness to actively engage in problem solving or doing homework. Often, the skills trainer asks an actively passive client, "So, what skill might you use here?" and a common response is, "I dunno—what am I supposed to say?" The teen may be overly reliant on a parent, for example, repeatedly asking, "What page are we on?" or having a parent ask the skills trainer the question for the teen. Skills trainers can address this style by cheerleading and cajoling practice and by shaping an increase in active problem-solving efforts. In response to the "What should I say?" comment, a leader could reply, "Come on—I know you can do this! Where would you start? Can you give me one idea of a skill you could use?" After the client generates a brief response, the leader reinforces, perhaps saying, "Nice job! I knew you'd come up with something!" Skills trainers can also gently block parents or other group members from continuing to do the work for the patient. In the therapist consultation team, the skills trainer can also suggest to the individual therapist that conducting a behavior and solution analysis to increase problem-solving skills could be helpful.

Apparent competence refers to the tendency of clients with chronic emotional dysregulation to seem, at times, to be more competent, in control, and effective, and less in need of help, than they actually are. This presentation typically results from either of two conditions. First, the client's behavior may be mood-dependent; that is, the client is truly competent to perform a skill in the group when emotionally regulated but unable to successfully use the skill when dysregulated. For mood-dependent behavior, skills trainers can encourage clients to "cope ahead" by using, for example, imaginal rehearsal and to develop backup plans for when one coping plan does not work. They can also remind clients to call their primary therapists for coaching when in challenging situations. Apparent competence can also result when the client's facial expression and body language do not accurately reflect the level of experienced distress. In these cases, the client has likely learned to suppress emotion expression, as explicated in the biosocial theory (see Chapter 1). Skills leaders can help these clients become more adept at communicating emotional states. For example, trainers can coach and shape clients to mindfully observe and describe their emotions, thoughts, and action urges in group, using the Emotion Regulation Skills module's "model of emotions" (see Chapter 9).

Addressing Unrelenting Crises and Inhibited Experiencing

Unrelenting crises refers to repeatedly engaging in risky or impulsive behaviors to avert pain. This "crisis-of-the-week" syndrome sets up the conditions for additional painful emotions and aversive consequences and possibly for impulsive reporting of these behaviors in group. Sometimes, the crises are generated by excessively chaotic and invalidating life experiences and are not self-generated. Regardless of the origin, this pattern can result in a myriad of disruptive behaviors: for example, group members bubbling over with information about personal crises, appearing highly self-conscious or self-focused in group, engaging in risk taking with other group members, arriving to group in the midst of heated conflict with family members, or impulsive absences from the group. In response to this pattern, group leaders can emphasize (1) mindfulness skills (the practice of observing emotions and urges rather than acting on them in the moment), (2) emotion regulation skills to alter extreme emotional reaction, and (3) distress tolerance skills to avoid impulsive responding to emotional distress. Additional strategies, such as addressing faulty judgments, increasing the thinking through of consequences, and increasing insight and problem solving regarding maladaptive patterns, are best handled in individual therapy.

Inhibited experiencing refers to the pervasive avoidance of emotional pain. In response to subtle cues that evoke past losses or trauma, individuals in this pattern shut down the normal progression of emotions and never become habituated to their intense sadness, shame, grief, or anger. This pattern may present as numbness, a shut-down demeanor, or nonacknowledgment of emotions or distress during group. Substance abuse or other high-risk behaviors might be occurring regularly to help blunt emotions.

Inhibition of Others' Emotional Experiences

We have also observed a tendency for clients with inhibited experiencing (especially caregivers) to invalidate other group members. Such a group member might say things like "I don't understand why my [daughter, son, partner] gets so upset in these situations. It's just a math test. You bear down and do what you have to do. I don't get why there's all this drama." Note that sometimes such invalidating statements come from parents who live much of their lives in what we term *Reasonable Mind*, perhaps because of their own less emotional temperament along with possible modeling of their own invalidating environment.

For clients displaying the behaviors of inhibited experiencing, it can be helpful to emphasize the mindfulness of current emotions skill, which focuses on awareness of emotion without attempting to change it. Distress tolerance skills such as "radical acceptance" of the emotion, "self-soothe with six senses," and "distract with 'Wise Mind ACCEPTS'" temper the distress of an emotion so that it can be tolerated. Escape through some type of shutting down is then not the only option. Skills trainers can also suggest exposure work to the primary therapist on the consultation team. When clients invalidate other clients, skills trainers can briefly remind them about the different states of mind, the biosocial theory, and encourage them to notice what happens to others when their emotions are questioned or judged. Reliably, the other person's emotional intensity increases and so the strategy backfires if the goal is to reduce the emotion.

The adolescent–family-specific dialectical dilemmas discussed next are explicitly targeted within the Walking the Middle Path Skills module (see Chapter 10). Nevertheless, these behavior patterns may arise during the teaching of other skills, and skills trainers may need to address them. Note that these patterns tend to emerge during homework review when content from the week comes up, when role playing, or when soliciting examples in order to demonstrate skills. We present the dilemmas and their targets below.

Normalizing Pathological Behaviors versus Pathologizing Normal Adolescent Behaviors

In skills training, this dilemma comes up typically in the form of questions asked, often by parents, regarding what is developmentally normative for adolescents and what is a sign of a clinical problem. Such questions might arise when role-playing interpersonal effectiveness skills regarding a topic (e.g., whether a teen's boyfriend or girlfriend can sleep over) or when conducting a group example of the pros and cons (a distress tolerance skill) of trying marijuana at a party. This dilemma might also arise when skills trainers notice a parent discussing something, perhaps in the homework, that minimizes an adolescent's risk behavior (e.g., promiscuity, drug use, stealing). Group members can be referred to "What's Typical for Adolescents and What's Cause for Concern?" (Walking the Middle Path Handout 6) as a general guideline. However, the issue can be too complex to explore in skills training for several reasons. First, there may not be information available about what is typical for every behavior at every age. For example, what is normative for 17-year-olds may not be normative for 14-year-olds, such as attending a concert until 2:00 A.M. It may be increasingly common for teens to get tattoos and body piercings, or spend time on particular websites, but does this make it normative or effective?

Second, one must consider the family's culture, religion, and family subculture. For example, for more conservative families, experimenting with smoking or initiating sexual behavior may be out of the question, even though these behaviors may be occurring with some same-age peers. In a family with a "helicopter parent" or "tiger-mom" subculture, increased independence in decision making, desired privacy, receiving average grades, or spending time with peers might be discouraged, despite adolescent norms. In other family cultures, including in some European countries, parents are more hands-off and accepting of their adolescents' behaviors. For example, drinking alcohol with their family at dinner, spending time with a girlfriend or boyfriend, and allowing younger kids to walk unsupervised around town may be more normative.

Finally, one must consider an individual teen's history, vulnerabilities, and risk factors. For one teen, attending a party might be a sign of improved mood and social functioning; for another, the party might signal reconnection with a problematic peer group and may be best avoided. Skills trainers may briefly explain these points in group when related questions arise, and refer to the primary therapist for family sessions for more in-depth handling of such issues. We sometimes offer separate parenting sessions (ideally with a therapist other than the teen's primary therapist) to help parents navigate such issues.

Excessive Leniency versus Authoritarian Control

This behavior pattern often displays itself in a skills group when parents provide examples of parenting behaviors that are overly permissive (e.g., letting the teen smoke pot or come home obviously intoxicated with no consequence) or authoritarian (e.g., cutting off Internet use and phone use for 1 month for a poor test grade). Skills trainers can handle such behavioral extremes in a number of ways. First, these patterns are directly addressed in the Walking the Middle Path Skills module, and trainers might offer brief interventions in the group, such as referring the parent to "Dialectical Dilemmas" (Walking the Middle Path Handout 4). Trainers might ask if the parents can think of a less extreme, middle path response.

Second, a skills trainer can offer a quick didactic about the potential risks of one or the other extreme. For overpermissiveness, the trainer might say, "That response is likely to suggest to your son that this kind of behavior is fine to continue, which might make it harder for him to reach his goals and can lead to other problems." For authoritarian control, the trainer might say, "That response is likely to be demoralizing to Bryan, so that he stops trying so hard."

Third, the skills trainer could briefly ask about the impact of using that approach so far to highlight that it is not likely to work for achieving the parent's goals. For example, during homework review, a skills trainer might ask, "How does that usually work out? What do others think?" or "Has that very strong response been effective in stopping this behavior in the past?" Since a multifamily group is not the setting to belabor these points, we encourage caregivers and teens to bring the issue to an individual, family, or parenting session. Note that sometimes the teen can be the one applying overly loose or overly strict standards to him- or herself (e.g., not setting an alarm clock for the morning and repeatedly missing the bus for school; regularly restricting social activities to ensure that all schoolwork is perfect). This would be addressed in the group the same way and can also be brought to the attention of the primary therapist.

Fostering Dependence versus Forcing Autonomy

This behavior pattern is displayed in the group in two ways. The first is when family members are discussing homework, role-playing skills, asking questions, or making comments. For example, a parent says: "I had been driving her into the city for her class each week because of her fears [fostering dependence], and then finally I said, 'I'm done,' and just dropped her at the train station [forcing autonomy]." Second, group leaders may witness the pattern directly. For example, one parent regularly helped her 14-year-old find the appropriate page in the notebook, got up and got her tissues, and served her snack (fostering dependence). The skills trainer coaches the parent to give the adolescent a chance to be more autonomous inside and outside of group, by gradually withdrawing assistance while coaching the teen about how to become more self-sufficient. For example, the skills trainer can suggest to the caregiver to review the train schedule with her daughter and then accompany her to the city by train for the first time.

MANAGING OTHER DIALECTICAL TENSIONS IN SKILLS TRAINING

In addition to the adult and adolescent–family dialectical dilemmas described above, a number of other dialectical tensions often emerge when conducting skills training groups.

Undertalkers versus Overtalkers

Some group members say little and hardly participate, whereas others may dominate the discussion with high energy and wordiness. For taciturn members, shaping is often the best strategy. Requesting and then reinforcing small steps toward participation tends to work well for increasing participation; for example: "Would you join us at the table today, Marissa?" Or "Can you just read the first line? Nice, thanks!" For those who may be taking up too much group time with their questions, examples, and review of homework, group leaders can manage their verbosity by being sure to call on other volunteers in a balanced manner, or saying something like this: "Angelica, I know you've got this one, but I'd like to give somebody else a chance to answer. Who else would like to share an example?" See also Chapter 3 for more on limiting overtalkers' speaking time in homework review.

Too Boisterous versus Too Calm

It may be hard to create the perfect balance of energetic and engaged yet attentive and focused group members. Often leaders may find themselves trying to regain control of either a rowdy or dysregulated group (i.e., angry, open-family conflict; impulsive calling out or cross-talking). Conversely, group leaders may find themselves trying to invigorate and animate a group reticent because of depression, social anxiety, tiredness, or boredom. As a moderate level of energy is optimal for learning, we suggest that leaders use strategies to downregulate or upregulate group members' emotions and behaviors.

Activities that can be calming in an overly energized group include certain mindfulness activities (e.g., observing the breath, observing body sensations), paced breathing, muscle relaxation exercises, or *in vivo* self-soothing practice. These latter strategies can be applied within the group that teaches the pertinent skills content, such as IMPROVE the Moment, TIPP, or Self-Soothe exercises described in the handouts by those names). Group members can also be asked to quietly write individually during a skills-based activity, such as writing out steps for long-term goals in emotion regulation.

For a more withdrawn, internalizing group atmosphere, leaders can apply a number of energizing group activities. These include stories (e.g., introducing a skill by telling lively, emotional, or funny stories), small-group or dyadic exercises (e.g., interviewing the other group members about favorite short-term pleasant activities, best ways to build mastery, or breaking a goal into small steps), role plays (particularly with interpersonal effectiveness skills), co-leader role plays (a dramatic role play between co-leaders illustrating the need for an interpersonal effectiveness skill can get the group energized, laughing, and even applauding), mindfulness exercises that emphasize participation (e.g., singing, cheering for a favorite team, doing the hokey-pokey, playing soundball, snap-crackle-pop), or games (e.g., using Jeopardy as a model to review module content). Leaders should also make sure the content moves along swiftly and that homework review engages other group members and does not drag.

In the skills module chapters that follow, we note some activities as calming and soothing and some as high-energy ones; leaders can select as needed. It is helpful to monitor the energy level in the room and pull out, in the moment, teaching and engagement approaches that can calm or enliven group members. When the energy and engagement level is optimal, leaders can vary their use of quieting and animating teaching strategies and exercises, and vary their voice tone and volume, consistent with the DBT stylistic strategy of speed, movement, and flow.

Avoidance of Family Problems versus Overfocus on Them

Some clients steadfastly avoid any allusion to family conflict or "personal" examples in either role plays or homework examples. They refer only to school or workplace examples or other more "Reasonable Mind" matters. Others focus on family conflict so much that there is a risk of the group turning into a family therapy session. The family's emotions intensify; everyone squirms with discomfort; other group members can become triggered and storm out of the room or sit quietly but visibly seething. Teaching breaks down.

To address these extremes, skills trainers can give the family members some gentle feedback in the moment, during break, or after the session, depending on the need. Skills trainers can also prompt the family either to try to use their family situation as an example this time, or to firmly interrupt and redirect members who are getting too personal, provocative, or heated. When either extreme becomes an ongoing tendency, it can be discussed by the consultation team, tackled in a family session, or, if appropriate, addressed in individual therapy.

ADDRESSING IMBALANCES IN GROUP MEMBER AND LEADER ALLIANCES

A group can become imbalanced by alliances that form and create tensions among members. Examples include one member versus the rest of the group, the group leaders versus teens in the group, teens versus parents, pairs or triads of teens (even to the degree of forming cliques) versus other group members, and a leader's alliance with a particular parent or teen.

One Member versus the Group

This pattern emerges when a single group member, parent or teen, seems angry, skeptical, or withdrawn and has not connected with the group. This can occur when one parent, who is in favor of therapy, "drags" in a more reluctant parent. The reluctant parent can then come across as cynical and perhaps even hostile session after session. Marital tensions can become activated and one partner can withdraw out of anger or discomfort. For teens, this pattern can also occur out of reluctance to be in the group, despite prior commitment, which may wane. Family tensions may make it hard to be in the room with parents. Social anxiety, anger, or shame can make it hard to connect with and trust group members.

Leaders can address this problem by speaking compassionately to the teen or parent outside of group and briefly trying to understand and solve the problem. This might involve coaching and cheerleading the client to improve the group experience; pairing that member with a particularly warm, validating, or approachable group member in a role play; or activating behavior by asking the person to read or volunteer in a fun role play or exercise. The leader can try joking with the teen or parent or otherwise work hard to build rapport. Skills trainers can bring this problem to the consultation team and the attention of the primary therapist who can conduct detailed behavioral analyses of the problematic behavior, especially if it is by a teen. For parents, the skills trainer might have to spend more time reaching out. If the member is really stuck and nonparticipation or oppositional behavior in group becomes therapy-destroying for the group member or others, the member or family might need some more pretreatment work or individual skills training before continuing in group skills training (assessment and commitment strategies, as well as a selection of skills to promote effective participation and learning in group such as mindfulness skills, distress tolerance skills, emotion regulation skills such as Coping Ahead and Problem Solving, and interpersonal effectiveness skills such as GIVE).

Group Leaders versus Teens

At times, teens may band together and adopt a somewhat rebellious attitude toward group structures and group leaders. In one group, a cadre of teens did not return after break. They were found outside in the parking lot, hanging out together, some smoking, in no apparent hurry to return. At times, a group of teens develops some disruptive behavior such as giggling, note passing, inside joking, or nonattending during mindfulness. Several strategies can help, such as a light but firm DEAR MAN request to the group about the problem, one-on-one directives to the members before or after the session, or modifying group rules or structure to prevent recurrences. To address the group hanging in the parking lot, we stopped allowing members to leave the office suite during breaks. This quickly stopped the problem of returning late as well as preventing potential problems with risk behaviors and safety. Contingency management can work well too, such as offering, "If everyone returns from break on time, we'll have time to show our funny movie clip illustrating the Act Opposite skill." It is nearly always useful to ask clients to use a skill in the moment to resist engaging in whatever the problematic behavior is. For example, teens colluding in distraction or nonparticipation during mindfulness practice or homework review can be asked to each pick a skill to practice that will help them focus. Good choices here include the mindfulness "What and How Skills" skills of participating and doing what works, and distress tolerance skills such as one thing in the moment and willingness. If problems persist, the consultation team provides a great place to problem-solve. Individual therapists can also conduct behavioral analyses of this therapy-interfering behavior with their clients to understand individual triggers and functions.

Teens versus Parents

At times, teen group members will think the skills trainers are acceptable human beings, or even cool ones, and proceed to form alliances in opposition to parents. Parents are dismissed as annoying, the cause of their problems, or worthy of dismissal or disrespect. We see these various messages in the body language, facial expressions, or overt statements. Group assumptions and guidelines taught during the orientation session are intended to prevent these problems. For example, even parents are "doing the best they can," and "group members are not to engage in mean or disrespectful behavior." We return to these assumptions and guidelines before the start of every mindfulness module and as needed reminders, asking group members to comment on why we have that assumption or guideline; how it would be effective to follow it. We might also break kids into groups for practice exercises with their own or others' parents, to break their focus on their peers.

Pairs or Triads of Teens versus Other Group Members

This problem occurs fairly often in a benign way, simply because of the developmental stage and the normal occurrence of teens forming bonds with other like-minded kids. However, teens on the outside of such alliances are often exquisitely sensitive to feeling left out or concerned that they may be judged or talked about by those inside. Such sensitivity sometimes derives from realistic past experiences of being bullied or considered "outcasts" by their peers. In addition, sometimes these alliances reach the level of a clique, ripe with note passing, inside jokes, whispering during groups, and getting up together and leaving the room for break. This can make other group members feel unwelcome or unsafe, and needs to be tempered by leaders. In the orientation session, we teach that group members cannot form private relationships outside of skills group; we remind clients that this means we do not want relationships that are exclusionary; everyone needs to be included. Leaders can also strategically break up alliance members for small-group practice or engineer the seating to disrupt interaction among the alliance members. We might also talk to members privately and nonjudgmentally describe the behaviors we are observing and point out how they can make others uncomfortable and even detract from their own learning. We then request that they make more of an effort to include others.

Leader Alliance with a Particular Parent or Teen

At times a therapist might develop more empathy for a particular teen or parent (or set of parents) and ally with them more than the other family members. This alliance can be observed through repeated validating comments or other support offered to one person in the family with less tolerance and time spent on others in the same family. The leader may also empathically represent one party during the therapist consultation meeting, while not displaying empathy, or even expressing judgments, regarding the other party. When this unbalanced alliance occurs, the other skills trainers or therapists on the consultation team can point it out by asking the dialectical question: "What is being left out?" The team may be able to help the therapist increase compassion for the judged parent or teen. This is often facilitated by remembering the biosocial theory and viewing problematic behaviors as part of a transaction between the person and an environmental context.

MANAGING CHALLENGES SPECIFIC TO CAREGIVERS

Invalidation by Caregiver

Most parents genuinely love their children. However, even the most loving parents can fall prey to invalidating these very same children in the face of feeling anxious, impotent, hopeless, angry, depressed, confused, or attacked. The biosocial theory helps DBT therapists, caregivers, and teens better understand how this invalidation cycle happens. By the time some caregivers arrive in a DBT skills group, they are feeling "burned out" with the adolescent as well as with therapy and the mental health care system in general. They have often felt ineffective and disappointed by their child's mental health care providers. Some caregivers grew up in their own invalidating environments and know no other methods of communication. Some might feel that invalidation is somehow effective because it does not "spoil" or "enable" the children.

In a skills group, it is not uncommon for caregivers to engage in verbal and nonverbal behavior that invalidates their teens. These behaviors include using critical language to describe the teen, minimizing the teen's reported emotional reaction to an event, or oversimplifying the ease of solving a problem. Invalidating nonverbal behaviors displayed by caregivers include eye rolling, actively looking away or turning the back toward the teen, and loud sighing in response to what a teen is saying or doing.

Skills trainers are in a position to stop the cycle of invalidation in *both* directions. That is, skills trainers need to be mindful of invalidation directed at adolescents as well as coming from adolescents directed toward others, including skills trainers, peers, and other caregivers. If it goes unaddressed, it may appear that the skills trainer is condoning and thus tacitly reinforcing invalidating behaviors. How then does a skills trainer effectively target this behavior in a group context without people feeling judged or shamed?

Skills trainers can target caregiver invalidation in several ways. First, they can observe and describe the behavior nonjudgmentally as sounding like invalidation and ask the caregiver to try to communicate what he or she meant again without using the same language or behavior. If the caregiver gets defensive and states, "No, it wasn't," the trainer can respond by saying, "I took it that way; others may not have." If the group is familiar enough with one another and has had enough training together, it can sometimes be useful to involve the group, and add, "Was it just me or did other people hear it the way I did?"

Leaders can use humor to point out invalidation. A trainer might say: "As someone who spent many years of my life invalidating others before learning DBT, I tell you I can smell invalidation from a mile out. This smells invalidating [said with a knowing smile] and let me explain why. . . ."

Leaders can ask the recipient of the apparent invalidation, "Out of curiosity, was that experienced as invalidating by you?" If the individual says no, the skills trainer might say, "You have thicker skin than I, since I experienced it for you as invalidating."

The skills trainer can ring the mindfulness bell. The group members can learn that the bell rings for mindfulness practice as well as for "judgments" (both intentional and inadvertent) or invalidations (self and other) that are expressed in the group.

In each of these interventions, it's important to employ DBT communication and dialectical strategies simultaneously. That is, sometimes being serious, at other times gently humorous (depending on the extent of the invalidation), and sometimes being both. Movement, speed, and flow demand that the skills trainer draw attention to the invalidation by stopping whatever was being taught, before rapidly moving back to the content.

If the invalidation persists after these interventions have been made, it may be useful for the skills trainer to speak to the caregiver privately (before or after group, or even during the break). Sometimes reminding the caregiver of the consequences of pervasive invalidation is enough to help him or her attend more mindfully to the problem. Although it might appear that a family session is indicated, that suggestion can backfire unless the parent can display a reasonable capacity to validate and refrain from invalidation. Instead we might recommend a caregiver session (without the teen present) to review and practice validation skills.

If family sessions are called for other reasons and invalidation is persistent, the individual therapist is encouraged to spend the initial one or two family sessions teaching validation skills (whether they have been taught in group or not) to ensure that the adolescent and caregiver are able to use validation skills on benign topics (e.g., the weather, food likes and dislikes) *before* addressing any emotionally loaded family topics. The caregiver is often eager to dive into the problematic issues at hand; however, it is imperative that the therapist assure the caregiver and adolescent that they will get to those problematic issues as soon as the therapist is certain that everyone has been taught and is willing to apply validation skills during the session. This serves as a contingency management strategy as well.

Managing Caregiver Anxiety

Caregivers who have difficulty managing anxiety in skills group can express it by oversharing (spilling too much information) or undersharing. All can be influenced by, or be a consequence of, poor anxiety management. Skills trainers can behaviorally shape "oversharers" by gently cutting them off, saying, "That's a good point, and I need to give other people a chance to respond as well." Undersharers often require gentle coaxing and shaping of sharing anything, including work examples, to help them become more comfortable in the group.

Many parents are anxious about their ineffectiveness at changing their teens' behavior and some become dysregulated themselves by this anxiety. Other caregivers get appropriately worried about their teen's behaviors but are afraid to address it for fear that the teen may become dysregulated, not be able to focus, or may leave the group. In the latter cases, it is helpful to model interpersonal effectiveness skills with contingency management strategies added when necessary. For example, with one dysregulated teen becoming verbally threatening in group, and the parent trying ineffectively to soothe him, the skills trainer gently and firmly said to the teen:

> "Robert, I see you're having a tough time right now managing your emotions. I'm glad you're here so that you can learn some skills; however, I know that most people, when they are this upset, find it hard to learn. So, I want to give you a choice. If you can use your mindfulness and distress tolerance skills to help you regain control over the next minute or two, I'd like you to stay. If you feel that you are unable to regroup right now and need some breathing room, then I'd like you to step into the waiting room for 5 minutes to do just that and then come back in. What will it be?"

Managing Caregiver Anger

Caregiver anger is often a secondary emotion. It behooves skills trainers to use an easy manner and ask caregivers if the anger they are expressing, or referring to in their homework example, is primary or secondary. Skills trainers can explain that many caregivers in fact are feeling quite anxious or sad about their teens' well-being yet are less able to express that and instead express anger. The skills trainer can use the moment to encourage caregivers to more effectively communicate the primary emotion preceding the anger, when it appears that anger is not the primary one. For example:

> "In our society, it is often easier to express anger than it is to express worry or hurt to our teens. Therefore, what our teens experience is more anger—however, it might be more effective (remember the "How" skill *effectively*) to express your sadness, your hurt, your fear, guilt, or embarrassment, *instead* of the anger that is coming out verbally and nonverbally in an attacking manner. The challenge is that this makes you more vulnerable. By expressing hurt, you might become more hurt if the hurt isn't validated. Thus, we tend to avoid that and go with the anger—we're less likely to get hurt, right? I'd like you to try to observe and describe your primary emotions. When you feel ready, see if you can express it to others and notice what happens. I bet that you will be more gentle, and the responses you get will be less angry than those you have received in the past."

Regardless of whether the anger is primary or secondary, it is often expressed ineffectively. Group members can be encouraged to handle anger in skills training by remembering to apply skills such as "The Wave Skill: Mindfulness of Current Emotions" (Emotion Regulation Handout 18), "Opposite Action to Change Emotions" (Emotion Regulation Handout 20), and "Building and Maintaining Positive Relationships: GIVE Skills" (Interpersonal Effectiveness Handout 3).

Caregiver Emotional Dysregulation and Mental Health Concerns

Caregiver invalidation can be a skills deficit targeted by validation skills training, but it sometimes indicates emotional struggles and other skills deficits. Caregivers who display great degrees of emotional dysregulation and mental health–related problems in the group adversely impact not only their own learning but also their teen's and that of the group at large. Any therapy-destroying behaviors should be handled immediately, as described in Chapter 3. Skills trainers may choose to target less severe, more relatively benign caregiver emotional dysregulation in group when:

1. The behavior interferes in the teaching of the content (e.g., interrupting the skills trainer).
2. The behavior is consistently affecting other group members' ability to focus on the content (e.g., glaring at other group members, including their own family members).
3. The behavior is relevant to skills content and provides a direct illustration of the teaching point (e.g., teaching "don't judge" and the parent just made a judgmental statement; or teaching "Opposite Action to Change Emotion" [Emotion Regulation Handout 20] to emotion and the identified caregiver is in a very sad, withdrawn, nonparticipatory state).
4. The caregiver's behavior is a known dysfunctional link on the adolescent's behavioral

chain (e.g., the caregiver's assuming the worst tends to create fear in the adolescent, which is a link in her chain toward self-harming behavior). It requires a delicate balance to effectively target this behavior in the group and not make it a family session. If not easily done, it should be reserved for the family session.

Managing Caregivers with Problems of Severe Emotion Dysregulation

Caregivers sometimes acknowledge their own clinical diagnoses and multiple problems at the outset of treatment. In those cases, it may be useful to recommend that the caregiver seek his or her own therapist, possibly even a DBT program, in addition to participating with the adolescent in skills training. It is important to acknowledge the time and expense to participate in two programs simultaneously; it may be necessary and feasible to do them only in sequence.

At other times, the caregiver may appear to have features of BPD or severe emotional dysregulation but does not endorse having any mental health problems. In fact the person may have never been diagnosed. Although it is not necessary for the DBT skills trainer to make a diagnosis of a caregiver, it is helpful to have a good working knowledge of the caregiver's five problem areas so that they can be addressed effectively during the course of the group. It often takes some clinical finesse to help a caregiver consider the possibility, let alone recognize, that he or she may benefit from his or her own therapy. As the relationship develops and history is obtained by the DBT treatment providers, it should be left to a private discussion with the primary therapist (if there is one) to facilitate this discussion while taking a nonjudgmental, behaviorally descriptive, compassionate, hope-instilling stance.

Regardless of the caregiver's willingness to acknowledge the major problem areas and/or a BPD diagnosis, the DBT skills trainer will need to employ all of the same strategies used with an adolescent with BPD. Caregivers with BPD may be more emotionally sensitive, reactive, and have a slower return to emotional baseline than other caregivers. They may be more prone to experience invalidation, more prone to invalidate others in the group, and less able to help regulate themselves in group or model effective skill use. As a result, they may require more coaching in and out of skills group.

Managing Caregiver Depression

Caregiver depression is sometimes less overtly disruptive than other forms of caregiver emotional difficulties. There still may be effects both inside and outside of the group. Garber and colleagues (2009) have pointed out that caregivers' untreated depression can interfere with adolescent-only CBT treatment for depression. Not surprisingly, they found that depression remitted less among youth treated in an adolescent CBT group whose caregivers were actively depressed. In our experience, it seems harder for multiproblem adolescents in DBT to engage and make progress when their caregivers are depressed, whether outside or inside group. Caregiver depression can have adverse affects in group as well and may manifest by the parent (1) not coming to skills group, (2) not participating verbally in group, (3) not appearing interested or engaged, and (4) not completing homework assignments.

Skills trainers can sometimes coax depressed caregivers, as they would adolescents, to become more engaged using a variety of DBT treatment strategies, including validation, problem-solving, stylistic, and dialectical techniques. Brief problem solving with a caregiver who fails to arrive with homework is sometimes all it takes to get a parent activated. At other times, it is useful to validate the parents' apparent low energy while coaching them to use a skill such as "Opposite Action to Change Emotions" (Emotion Regulation Handout 20) to help them get the most out of this group. If some of these in-session interventions are ineffective, it may be necessary to meet with a parent outside of group to discuss effects on him or her and the adolescent if the caregiver's depression goes untreated. It is at this point that we may offer the caregiver a referral for his or her own treatment.

When the Parent Is Responsible for an Adolescent's Breaking DBT Rules

At times, teens will miss sessions because of their participating family member. This can happen when the adolescent is dependent on the parent for transportation or the parent arranges a scheduling conflict, such as scheduling a doctor's appointment during session time. Although it is unfortunate for an adolescent to be penalized for a parent's lack of commitment to the treatment, it is important to be consistent in applying policies such as those for missed sessions. If it is clear that a parent is interfering with or hindering the adolescent's attendance, the trainer can coach the adolescent on (1) interpersonal effectiveness skills to request that the parent make it to treatment or (2) problem solving to find other solutions (e.g., alternate means of transportation). For example, one adolescent whose mother had erratic work hours arranged, on several occasions, to get rides to group with another family who lived nearby.

CONCLUSION

There is no single effective teaching method. However, one of the keys to being an effective skills trainer is to vary one's delivery so as not to be predictable. The successful skills trainer makes ample use of movement, speed, and flow; irreverence; validation; and dialectics to keep group moving while attending to the skills content and the relationships with and among members. Ultimately, full participation in the moment by skills trainers, with attention to engagement, pacing, and content, helps balance dialectical tensions and yields the most successful outcomes. Arriving for group well prepared and organized, with knowledge of the skills being taught, teaching points to be made, exercises to use, and homework to assign helps a great deal.

The chapters that follow in Part II describe how to teach the specific DBT skills and provide stories, examples, exercises, and homework assignments.

PART II

Skills Training Modules

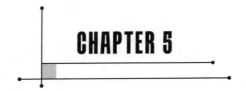

CHAPTER 5

Orientation to Multifamily Skills Training Group

SESSION OUTLINE

First Half of Session

▶ Introduction of Group Members and Skills Trainers

▶ What Is DBT for Adolescents?

▶ The Five DBT Problem Areas

▶ DBT's Five Sets of Skills

▶ DBT Skills Training Group Format

▶ Biosocial Theory of DBT

▶ DBT Treatment Assumptions

▶ Skills Training Group Guidelines

▶ DBT Contract

Handouts and Other Materials

▶ Orientation Handout 1, "What Is Dialectical Behavior Therapy (DBT)?"

▶ Orientation Handout 2, "Goals of Skills Training"

▶ Orientation Handout 3, "DBT Skills Training Group Format"

▶ Orientation Handout 4, "Biosocial Theory"

▶ Orientation Handout 5, "DBT Assumptions"

▶ Orientation Handout 6, "Guidelines for the Adolescent Skills Training Group"

▶ Orientation Handout 7, "DBT Contract"

▶ Whiteboard or other large writing surface and marker

TEACHING NOTES

> There are two mistakes one can make along the road to truth—
> not going all the way, and not starting.
> —PRINCE SIDDHARTHA GUATAMA (a founder of Buddhism),
>   563–483 B.C.E.

ABOUT THIS MODULE

Leaders typically conduct an orientation to the DBT skills training during the first half (45–75 minutes) of the session, and the second half introduces the mindfulness skills (see Chapter 6). Together, the Orientation and Mindfulness Skills modules are repeated before each of the other three modules. New families begin the group with this orientation, but the orientation is repeated whether or not new families join. The time needed for orientation may vary depending on the setting, overall length of the sessions, and the number of new participants in the group.

The teaching notes in Chapters 5–10 are generally written as suggested scripts for skills trainers addressing group members. Content addressed to the skills trainer is italicized or labeled "Note to Leaders."

This chapter ends with a discussion of challenges skills trainers may encounter when teaching this module, with advice on how to address those challenges.

INTRODUCTION OF GROUP MEMBERS AND SKILLS TRAINERS

Skills trainers first introduce themselves, modeling introductions, and then ask each member (including caregivers) to introduce him- or herself. Some skills trainers ask only for names and with whom the adolescent is attending (e.g., "My name is Mike and I'm here with my mom, Sarah"); others ask for more information, such as a brief statement of an interest, hobby, or favorite sports team.

EXERCISES (OPTIONAL)

Sometimes leaders use ice-breaking exercises in the initial group skills training session. These might include having the first person state his or her name, the second person repeats that name and then states his or her own name; the third person repeats the first two names and then adds his or her own, and so on.

In another exercise, members break into dyads (separating family members), exchange information for 2 minutes (name, grade, interests, etc.), and then each introduces the other partner to the group. Note that some adolescents enter group with extreme social anxiety and might find introductions difficult. With such teens, skills trainers accept whatever is possible for them in the first session and then shape participation with positive feedback. Trainers might also choose an introduction method that minimizes performance anxiety, such as just asking for names on the first day or asking each to introduce a partner rather than him- or herself. Teens tend to feel less self-conscious reporting on someone else than speaking about themselves. Ice breakers are used at the discretion of group leaders, since there may not be the time or need for them.

WHAT IS DBT FOR ADOLESCENTS?

Refer participants to Orientation Handout 1, "What Is Dialectical Behavior Therapy (DBT)?" Orient teens and families to this specialized program called DBT. It is important for them to understand why they were chosen for DBT and what exactly DBT is. Explain:

- DBT was the first effective treatment for adults with significant difficulty regulating their emotions and behaviors. Psychologist Marsha M. Linehan developed DBT in the 1980s (Linehan, 1993a, 1993b; Linehan et al., 1991). In the 1990s, DBT began to be used with adolescents and families who struggled to manage their emotions and behaviors (Miller, Rathus, Linehan, Wetzler, & Leigh, 1997; Miller et al., 2007).
- DBT skills teach adolescents and families to:
  - Regulate their emotions and behaviors.
  - Reduce problem behaviors and increase skillful behaviors.
  - Experience a range of emotions without necessarily acting on those emotions.
  - Improve relationships with family, school, and peers.
- The overarching goal of DBT is to help people create a life worth living.

What Does *Dialectical* Mean?

- Dialectical means that two opposing ideas can be true at the same time, and when considered together, can create a new truth, and a new way of viewing the situation.
- There is always more than one way to think about a situation.

From "Either/Or" to "Both–And"

To improve relationships and reduce conflict, we suggest that you move away from either/or, black-and-white, nondialectical ways of thinking and instead consider using "both–and" ways of thinking that honor other points of view. For example, instead of saying, "You're not trying, you have to make an effort," you could say, "You're doing the best you can in this moment, *and* I hope you can do better moving forward."

Instead of saying, "I'm right and you're wrong," you could say, "I feel strongly about my point of view, *and* I can see you feel strongly about your point of view too. Let's see how we can find a middle path."

It is also useful to apply dialectical thinking to yourself: "At times I am a leader, *and* at other times I am a follower"; "I struggle in some areas, *and* I do well in others."

> **DISCUSSION POINT:** *Ask participants to think about and share one example of dialectical thinking. Ask if anyone notices how thinking dialectically can help reduce the intensity of emotions.*

THE FIVE DBT PROBLEM AREAS

Refer participants to Orientation Handout 2, "Goals of Skills Training."

> **Note to Leaders:** If one or more families have been through orientation before, consider enlisting them to explain the five problem areas on Orientation Handout 2. If this is a

completely new group or the senior members are not skillful enough to explain succinctly, briefly orient members to the problem areas and then invite discussion on how each may relate to them.

Why was each of you chosen for this group? We selected you because we believe you experience at least some of the problems we are about to describe (i.e., problems to decrease). DBT is a treatment for this specific set of problems:

Reduced Awareness and Focus; Confusion about Self

• *Difficulty being aware of your own emotions*, *thoughts, and urges* in the moment; that is, not always knowing what is making you upset before shutting down or lashing out. A wave of emotion comes over you, and you're not sure how it got there so fast or intensely. Do you find yourself acting impulsively on that emotion and you don't recognize the urge before it's too late—and you've already acted?

• *Difficulty staying focused and participating fully in the present*. Do you ever find yourself worrying about what is going to happen tomorrow? Or being stuck in your sadness or regret about what happened in the past? A consequence of this past and future focus is that you miss out on living in the present moment, including opportunities to experience joy, happiness, and other positive emotions and experiences.

• *Not knowing what your goals are*. Do you feel unsure about who you want to be, what you want, or what your values are? Do you want to improve your family relationships? Do you want to graduate from high school and college? Do you behave according to your values, for example, with honesty, respect, and loyalty?

If you are having difficulty with these problems, there is a name for it: We call this *reduced awareness and focus and confusion about yourself*. When intense emotions get revved up, especially if they go from 0 to 60 in 5 seconds, the harder it is to see and catch them. The goal is to help you become aware of yourself at 5 mph then 10 mph, well before you get to 60 mph. This will allow you to choose to do something about it in time.

Emotional Dysregulation

• *Fast intense mood changes with little control*: for example, one moment feeling fine, then feeling a wave of anxiety for 15 minutes, then ashamed for 5 minutes, then moving to anger for 1 hour, and so on.

And/or

• *Steady negative emotional state*: for example, steadily depressed, steadily anxious, steadily angry.

Emotional dysregulation is the central problem for people in our program. We find that the remaining problem areas are often a consequence of people's difficulty with controlling emotions or their mood-dependent responses—when your behavior is based on the mood you are in rather than on your goals or what might be most effective.

Impulsivity

• *Acting without thinking it all through; escaping or avoiding emotional experiences*. Do you find yourself acting on an urge without thinking about the consequences?

Impulsive actions run the gamut: blurting out in class or at the dinner table; angry verbal and physical outbursts; impulsive eating, shopping, sex, sexting, drinking, or drugging; driving recklessly, self-harm, and even suicidal behavior. If you are engaging in any behavior without thinking beforehand about the consequences, you are likely engaging in impulsive behavior. As you can imagine, you are more likely to behave impulsively when intense emotions are activated.

Interpersonal Problems

• *Difficulty keeping relationships steady*. You feel intense shifts in connection; for example, today you love this person and tomorrow you feel angry, betrayed, and want to end the relationship. Or you have lots of conflict in your relationships.

• *Difficulty getting what you want from others*, including effectively saying no. You don't know how to effectively and skillfully convince people to give you what you want, whether it is asking for a later curfew from your parents or declining an invitation to a party without hurting the other person's feelings.

• *Difficulty keeping your self-respect*. Self-respect requires you to be aware of your values and to stick with them. It means not doing things due to peer pressure—for example, effectively saying no when you are asked to do drugs, engage in sexual activity, cheat on a test, or lie to your parents or friends.

• *Loneliness*. Difficulty controlling emotions or behaviors often affects the quality of relationships, which can lead to loneliness.

Teenager and Family Challenges

• *Extreme thinking*—that is, either/or, black-or-white, all-or-nothing thinking. At times you see only your own perspective as the "right one" and are unable to consider that another person's viewpoint can have validity (i.e., nondialectical thinking).

• *Extreme feelings and actions*—that is, making decisions in an emotional state that result in more extreme action. For example, telling your child "You're grounded for the next 6 months" or calling yourself "a complete idiot" (i.e., nondialectical actions).

• *Difficulty understanding another's reaction*—that is, difficulty validating others.

• *Difficulty conveying to yourself* that your feelings, thoughts, or actions make sense in the current context (i.e., difficulty validating yourself).

• *Difficulty rewarding others*—for example, difficulty praising a loved one when he or she does something you want (i.e., difficulty providing positive reinforcement).

• *Difficulty applying effective consequences*—for example, providing a time-limited and appropriate consequence when unwanted behaviors occur, and not overusing punishment to change behavior.

DISCUSSION POINT: *Invite all participants to take 3 mindful minutes to review the five problem areas on Orientation Handout 2, "Goals of Skills Training," and write down which apply to themselves (not their family members). Then ask them to describe briefly how they apply. Ask the most senior adolescent member to share how these problem areas apply to him or her presently or in the past; if no one is more senior than anyone else, ask the person who is most willing to share. Then invite the most experienced adult group member to share which of these five problem areas applies to him or her presently, in the recent past, or during his or her adolescence.*

Note to Leaders: The above discussion is intended not only as an informal self-assessment but also as a means to orient new members to the common areas that have brought them together in treatment. The reviewing of problem areas and goals is repeated when orientation repeats (i.e., every 5–6 weeks). For any members repeating the orientation, ask the client and the family to gauge how they are progressing on each of these problem areas. Skills trainers should also assess progress. Encourage participants making progress to acknowledge this improvement while indicating areas still in need of change. Be sure to praise progress and offer feedback about areas that still require attention.

DBT'S FIVE SETS OF SKILLS

Here's the good news—for each of the five problem areas, we have specific sets of skills that will help you remedy the problems and replace them with more skillful behaviors. Thus for reduced awareness and focus/confusion about self, we're going to teach you mindfulness skills. For emotional dysregulation, we're going to teach you emotion regulation skills. For impulsivity we're going to teach you distress tolerance skills. For interpersonal problems, we're going to teach you interpersonal effectiveness skills, and for teenager and family challenges, we're going to teach you what we call *walking the middle path* skills. Each of these skills modules also contributes to improving all of the other problem areas, not just the one with which it is identified. For example, without skills to regulate your emotions, it would also be very hard to use your interpersonal effectiveness skills and keep your relationships going smoothly.

Note to Leaders: This is an opportunity to instill hope by clarifying that we have the tools to reduce these problem behaviors and add new adaptive behaviors that will ultimately help them reach their goals.

DBT SKILLS TRAINING GROUP FORMAT

Refer participants to Orientation Handout 3, "DBT Skills Training Group Format."

Overall Course and Sequence of Skills Modules

This 24-week [*or use number of weeks in your program*] program covers five different skills modules. As you can see on the handout, the entry point for new group members is always orientation (half a session) and mindfulness skills (one to one and a half sessions), followed by 4–5 weeks of a skills module (for a total of 6 weeks). We then return to orientation and mindfulness before teaching another skills module—distress tolerance, walking the middle path, emotion regulation, or interpersonal effectiveness.

Why Repeat Mindfulness Skills?

You may ask, why do we keep repeating mindfulness skills again and again? The answer is simple: Mindfulness skills are the core of the treatment. Without mindfulness skills, you are not aware that you are feeling angry or sad and then cannot make an informed decision about what to do with your emotional state—whether to experience it as it is or do something to change it. Without mindfulness skills, you are not aware that you need to use a specific distress tolerance skill to cope with an impulsive urge you are having. Without mindfulness skills, you are not aware of what your goal is in a particular interpersonal interaction and consequently may be less likely to get what you want in that interaction.

Session Format

Each session is 2 hours long. The first hour involves reviewing homework (or what you practiced during the week) and then we'll take a 10-minute break. During the second hour we will teach you new material.

Bringing Materials to the Session

Please bring your handouts and worksheets each week. Complete your assigned DBT practice exercises directly on the worksheets.

Starting on Time

We start the group on time so that we can end on time. To help us start on time, we would appreciate it if you could come into the group room a few minutes early so that you can get settled in and ready to go. You don't want to come late because you will miss our interesting mindfulness practice exercises that begin each session, except for tonight's orientation. The mindfulness exercise could involve eating a piece of candy mindfully, listening to a piece of music mindfully, and so on. We will eventually invite volunteers to lead a mindfulness exercise so each of you will have a chance to practice leading one. We will explain more as we go along.

Biosocial Theory of DBT

Refer participants to Orientation Handout 4, "Biosocial Theory." Begin by referring to the five DBT problem areas.

How is it that this group of adolescents has such a similar constellation of problems? The answer can be found in the biosocial theory. If you understand the theory I am about to teach you, you will understand how adolescents develop these problems and how the problems are maintained, or how they get "stuck." As you hear the description of this theory, consider how it may apply to you.

Overview: Defining *Bio* and *Social*

Who can explain what *bio* refers to? [*Give participants a chance to share their thoughts.*] *Bio* refers to your biological makeup—in particular, the wiring in your brain that contributes to how you experience and control emotions, act on urges, etc.

Social refers to what? [*Give participants a chance to share their thoughts.*] *Social* refers to your social environments—to the people in your life. These social environments include family members, friends, teachers, coaches, therapists, people in the neighborhood, etc.

Sometimes other people are unable to understand where you are coming from. When this happens, you may experience these social environments as "invalidating." DBT's biosocial theory suggests that your difficulties are based on the transaction (or influences) between your biological makeup and an invalidating environment over time.

A Biological Vulnerability to Emotions

Increasing amounts of research suggest that powerfully emotional people like yourselves may be wired differently than some of your siblings and peers. Certain emotion centers of the brain appear different on brain scans for folks who are more often emotionally and behaviorally dysregulated. Let me say that there are some definite positives to being wired differently, as I will discuss in a few minutes. First, however, let me ask you if the following is true of you.

- *High emotional sensitivity.* Do you have high emotional sensitivity? Do things get under your skin more easily than other people you know? Do you feel your emotions quickly? For example, some people are *physically* sensitive—like being sensitive to tree pollen and starting to sneeze and having watery eyes as soon as spring has sprung, whereas other lucky individuals walk around completely unaffected. Another example: Imagine someone who has experienced third-degree burns on his arms, and he's lying in a hospital bed with the window open beside him. When the door opens, the air current blows from the window to the opened door. That air current blows on the burned arms and makes the patient cringe in pain. The person sitting in the chair beside the bed doesn't even notice the air current. This is what we mean by *sensitivity*, and some of you may be like this with your emotions.

> DISCUSSION POINT: *Briefly invite people to endorse this item or not.*

- *High emotional reactivity.* Do you have high emotional reactivity? Not only are some of you emotionally sensitive, but you may also be emotionally reactive. Do you find that your experience of emotions is intense, powerful? You don't just feel a little blue sometimes; instead you feel profoundly sad or depressed? You don't just feel mildly irritated about things; you are likely to get furious and then say or do hurtful things? You don't just feel a few butterflies in your stomach when you get anxious; instead you feel panic-stricken and want to avoid the situation completely? I am describing emotions that get to the high end of the emotional continuum.

> *Note to Leaders:* Draw a vertical line on the board with 0 on bottom and 100 on top. Refer to any emotion, such as anger, pointing out that mild irritability falls near the bottom of the line, anger in the middle, and rage at the top. (This will become the *y*-axis of a graph, as shown in Figure 5.1.)

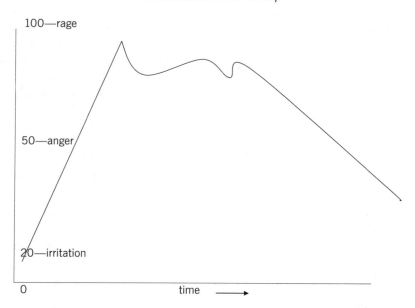

FIGURE 5.1. High emotional reactivity; slow return to baseline.

▓ **DISCUSSION POINT**: *Briefly invite people to endorse this item or not.*

• *Slow return to baseline.* Are your emotions slow to return to an emotional baseline? Not only are some of you emotionally sensitive and emotionally reactive, but you may also have a slow return to your emotional baseline once you get emotionally dysregulated. What does this mean? If you feel an intense emotion such as rage, shame, sadness, or fear [*point to top of the scale just drawn*], it may not come down in 5–10 minutes like it might for other people with different emotional wiring. When you get really emotional, it may take hours, or even a good portion of a day, before you come back down closer to 0 again.

> *Note to Leaders:* Draw an *x*-axis (time), as in Figure 5.1, along with the line indicating a rapid increase of intense emotion with very slow reduction in intensity over time.

• *Why does it take a long time for your emotions to return to baseline?* Think about a fire in a fireplace. If you already have a good fire under way, adding fresh logs will make the fire burn intensely for a long time. If you are already a powerfully emotional person at baseline, with high sensitivity and reactivity, it can be hard for your emotions to come back down quickly because you are sensitive to little things that reactivate your emotion again and again, like throwing another log on a hot fire.

▓ **DISCUSSION POINT**: *Briefly invite people to endorse this item or not.*

• *Being powerfully emotional can be a strength.* Feeling things intensely helps you be passionate about your interests, creative, engaged in your relationships, and motivated to do things that are important to you. Many emotionally powerful and passionate people become influential leaders. They can mobilize others as well as themselves to perform in sports; they motivate colleagues to work together toward a unified goal. We want you to experience and communicate these emotions—but in such a way that you control them rather than the emotions controlling you. Strong, powerful emotions become a problem when you don't know how to effectively regulate them.

An Inability to Effectively Regulate Emotions

Without emotion regulation skills, you are likely to end up engaging in problem behaviors. In the short term, using alcohol, drugs, avoiding school, self-harm, etc., often work to bring down anger, shame, fear, or whatever intense emotion you are experiencing. But in the long term these strong emotions tend not to be helpful and cause more problems than they solve. The good news is that we are going to teach you important DBT skills to effectively regulate your own emotions.

An Invalidating Environment

So we are saying that a set of common problems arises when an individual who (1) has a biological vulnerability to emotions, and (2) can't effectively regulate them, is (3) placed in an invalidating social environment. Let's discuss this next.

Invite participants to look again at Orientation Handout 4, "Biosocial Theory."

• **Define validation and invalidation**. What does *validation* mean? [*Invite comments.*] To validate is to confirm, to corroborate, to verify, to authenticate, to communicate an understanding of. *Invalidation*, therefore, is to disconfirm, to discount, to delegitimize, to communicate that what the other person is thinking, feeling, or doing does *not* make sense.

Invalidating social environments may include, but are not limited to, family members—parents, siblings, grandparents, aunts, uncles, cousins—as well as teachers, peers, coaches, therapists, and sometimes even yourself.

Invalidation means communicating that what you are feeling, thinking, or doing doesn't make sense, is considered inaccurate or an overreaction. The invalidating environment punishes or sometimes reinforces emotional displays and contributes to the person's suppression or escalation of emotions, and sometimes leaves the person feeling confused and unable to trust one's own emotion experiences (self-invalidation).

• **Everyone invalidates sometimes**. We all make invalidating statements from time to time, skills trainers included. [*Trainers might offer a personal example here. For example: "I'm fairly sure that I may have inadvertently invalidated my spouse, my kids, my colleagues, and even my co-leader on the other side of this table, at least once during the past week."*]

We're not saying, don't ever invalidate again. It would be nice, but that's not realistic. What we're saying is, don't be pervasively and persistently invalidating. Pay attention to what you say and how you say it. Also, what are you *not* saying or *not* doing that may be needed to communicate that you *do* understand or at least *want to* understand the other person's experience? The more you learn and practice validation skills, and the more you notice when you inadvertently invalidate others, the more validating you will become over time.

> *Note to Leaders:* At this point, offer an invalidating statement to the group to demonstrate. For example, you might say the following:
>
> > "There is a lot of stuff that I am teaching tonight. Since you're here for a reason, you should be learning this material quickly and easily. We expect you to be 100% focused. Your day isn't that long; you don't have anything else to do, and there's no place you'd rather be!"

DISCUSSION POINT: *Ask,* "How did each of you experience that comment? Do you think I accurately understand your experience tonight?"

If any of you had the experience—"He has no idea what he's talking about . . . he's making no sense . . . this biosocial theory is hard and it's been a long day; I have a lot of work to do and I'd rather be home or with friends"—then you know what invalidation feels like.

> *Note to Leaders:* Most people feel their emotions intensify when they experience invalidation and feel greater sense of ease when experiencing validation.

Now what if instead I said something like this: "I imagine it is hard to stay focused and to digest so much new material on your first night of group. What makes this experience even more challenging is that it's late, it's warm in here, and many of you haven't even had a chance to have dinner and probably have a lot of work to do"?

DISCUSSION POINT: *Ask,* "Did you think to yourself, 'She's got it and I appreciate that she's got it'? If so, that's what validation feels like. What was the difference in your emotions when you felt invalidated? How did that compare to how you felt when you experienced validation?"

Three Types of Invalidation

There are three common types of invalidation.

Type 1 Invalidation: Your Thoughts, Feelings, and Behaviors Are Indiscriminately Rejected

EXAMPLE

A teenage girl is very sad and disheartened about failing a test for which she believed she had studied sufficiently. The parent responds by saying, "It's your fault—if you had studied more, you would have passed." *Or* the parent responds by saying, "Stop worrying, it's not a big deal, Honey, it's only one test."

DISCUSSION POINT: *Ask,* "Why are these responses considered invalidating?"

THE NATURE OF THE PROBLEM

The problem with both responses is that they ignore how the girl is actually feeling about failing the test. The message of the first response seems to be that if you are somehow judged at fault, then you have no right to express feeling bad. In the second response, the message is for the girl to stop feeling the way she actually does feel about the test.

THE CONSEQUENCES OF INVALIDATION

The consequences of being frequently invalidated in either way are that the adolescent stops trusting what he or she feels and then (1) begins to self-invalidate by telling him- or herself that "what I am feeling/thinking/doing is inappropriate or inaccurate," and (2) scans the environment for clues about the "right way" to feel. In other words, the adolescent internalizes the invalidating environment and becomes his or her own worst enemy.

It is very depression-inducing to say to oneself over and over again, "I shouldn't feel this way. I shouldn't think this way." Who's to say what one should think or feel? We believe that "shoulding" on oneself is self-invalidating and can increase depression.

BARRIERS TO VALIDATION

Many people are reluctant to validate another person's emotions because:

1. They are afraid they will validate problem behaviors.
2. They're afraid that validating the emotion may make the person more upset.

> **DISCUSSION POINT:** *Ask,* "In the case above, what else could the parents have said to their daughter who was upset about failing a test?" *Discuss possible validating statements—for example, "I understand that you feel sad and worried about the poor test grade." Then ask the kids in the group,* "Would this make you more upset? Why or why not?" *Most will say that feeling understood does not make them more upset.*

Type 2 Invalidation: Lower-Level Expressions of Emotion Are Ignored or Punished and Emotional Escalation Is Sometimes Given Greater Attention (Intermittently Reinforced)

Let's take the same example of the teen who is sad and disheartened at failing a test. In this case, the parent responds by yelling "You're overreacting! What's the big friggin' deal?!" The adolescent begins to cry and then threatens not to go back to school. The parent then softens, and says, "OK, let's go out for a nice dinner tonight so you feel better; I'll help you study next time."

> **DISCUSSION POINT:** *Ask,* "Why is this example considered invalidating?"

THE NATURE OF THE PROBLEM

There are two problems with the above response. The parent's yelling, angry response dismisses how the teen feels, plus it is punishing. In response, the teen's emotion escalates. The consequence of this type of invalidation is that the teen tries to suppress emotion so as not to get punished *and* then becomes extremely emotional when suppression doesn't work. What's more, when the parent finally responds to the extreme emotion with an offer of help and dinner out, the parent is reinforcing the extreme emotion. That makes extreme emotion more likely to occur in the future. Occasional rewards (i.e., intermittent reinforcement) make a behavior more likely to be repeated and harder to stop.

Type 3 Invalidation: The Ease of Problem Solving and of Meeting Goals Is Overstated and Oversimplified

In this type of invalidation, the parent responds to the teen by saying nonchalantly, "Just study more next time and you'll do great." Nancy Reagan provides another example. When she was the First Lady of the United States, she chose as her special agenda to reduce substance abuse—a worthy goal. Her approach to the problem was announced with a great deal of fanfare. It was— "Just say no" to drugs.

DISCUSSION POINT: *Ask*, "Why might these two examples be considered invalidating?"

THE NATURE OF THE PROBLEM

Imagine having a 20-year addiction to heroin and someone tells you that the solution is "Just say no." That is the epitome of invalidation.

When you, as a parent, as a friend, as a therapist, as a coach, say to someone who is struggling, "Just do *x*, *y*, or *z*," and the person either gets angry or shuts down in response, you may be guilty of invalidation. Why?

EXAMPLE

[*Leaders might tell a personal story such as the following:*] In all fairness, we have been known on occasion to do something similar. I've said to a teen anxious about returning to his high school after being away at a therapeutic program, "Just tell yourself that other kids have done this, and then go to your guidance counselor. Tell her you're nervous about returning, and then . . . and then. . . ." My intentions were absolutely good; I intended to be helpful. Unfortunately, I underestimated how difficult it was going to be for this young person. I overestimated what he was ready to do, given the skills he had at that point. Just because I could do it didn't mean he could. Just because I can play a song on the piano, and I tell you to do it, doesn't mean you can do it.

A CONSEQUENCE OF TYPE 3 INVALIDATION

One consequence of oversimplifying problem solving and meeting goals is that the person forms unrealistic goals and expectations. "If I just say no to drugs, I should be able to resist and get off drugs." That's not realistic.

• *Poor fit as a cause of invalidation.* Sometimes there is a poor fit between a child's temperament and his or her family environment. For example, imagine a 5-year-old, Johnny, who has ADHD and whose temperament and biology cause him to want to run around continuously, bouncing and throwing a ball, singing loudly, and exuding boundless energy. Imagine that Johnny was born to a mother whose temperament was the opposite—low in energy, prefers things quiet or else she becomes anxious, and not interested in playing ball. When Johnny runs around bouncing the ball, acting appropriately for someone with his temperament, Mom says, "Johnny, can you please stop bouncing that ball and running around!" Johnny thinks to himself, "Hey, Mom, that's who I am. I love to run around and bounce a ball. If anything, you could liven things up around here." As you can see, Mom doesn't appreciate, understand, or validate Johnny's experience, and Johnny doesn't have the faintest idea of what Mom is reacting to. As Johnny gets bouncier, Mom tries to stop his activity. The more she tries to thwart him, the more upset he gets. The more upset he gets, the more upset she gets, and so on.

> *Note to Leaders:* Draw a diagram like that shown in Figure 5.2, depicting how a small amount of invalidation by Mom influences Johnny's biological predisposition by intensifying his emotional reactions. This in turn escalates Mom's invalidating behavior, and so on. Explain that over time, this adverse transaction between biology and environment can lead to increasing emotional dysregulation, behavioral dysregulation, self-dysregulation, and interpersonal dysregulation. Neither Johnny nor Mom intended to intensify the other's reactions; however, inadvertent invalidation inevitably has this effect.

• *Adolescents can invalidate others in their environments*. Moreover, it is important to recognize that adolescents can invalidate their social environments just as the environments can invalidate the adolescents. Neither Johnny nor Mom originally intended to invalidate the other but they lacked the ability to validate the other's experience (i.e., a skills deficit) and became increasingly invalidating over time. Even Johnny, in a sense, invalidated his mother, by not being able to heed her request and respond to her sensitivities.

DISCUSSION POINT: *Ask*, "Has anyone noticed this experience in his or her own life?"

• *Invalidation can be understandable in the context of high emotional dysregulation*. When someone is frequently emotionally intense, it takes much more work for those in the environment to stay validating—assuming they even have the skills. In the face of intense negative emotions, most people assume a defensive posture that may include attacking, escaping, or doing other things to attempt to deescalate the other person's reactivity. These efforts are usually experienced by the emotionally dysregulated individual as invalidating.

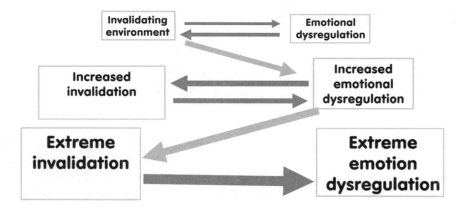

FIGURE 5.2. Ongoing emotion dysregulation results from transaction of biological vulnerability with invalidation over time.

• *Many adults have been invalidated growing up*. Many of the families that we work with report that they experienced extensive invalidation in their own families of origin. It makes perfect sense that if you, the caregivers, were invalidated growing up, it would be highly unlikely for you to be effective validators for your own children without being taught the skills elsewhere. You had no models of validation from which to learn. Many parents report being told by their own parents to "just suck it up," "brush it off," or "man up, and stop complaining." So, this is all you've known how to do when raising your own children. We are going to try to break that cycle starting tonight.

DISCUSSION POINT: *Invite caregivers to share their own experiences of validation versus invalidation in their own families of origin.*

> *Note to Leaders:* Some parents might not have experienced invalidation, but they still might find it difficult to validate an emotionally intense kid. Other parents might defensively reply, "Well, I'm no worse for the wear," suggesting that that style worked for them. It is important to highlight that what might work with one child doesn't necessarily work for another child. The question to ask such parents is, "How is what you are doing now with your child working for you?" If the answer is "Not so well," then maybe it's time for them to consider another approach.

• *Learning emotion regulation and validation skills will improve problem behaviors*. Here's the really *good news*. For those of you in this room who have trouble regulating emotions, we are going to teach you a whole host of skills to help you better regulate your emotions. And, for those in this room who tend to invalidate others or yourself, we are going to teach you a set of validation skills to better validate your loved ones as well as yourself. If we can accomplish those goals, you will quickly start to notice improvements in your relationships, your sense of self, and your emotion regulation capabilities.

DBT TREATMENT ASSUMPTIONS

Refer participants to Orientation Handout 5, "DBT Assumptions."

What are assumptions? Assumptions are unproven beliefs. We believe that it is helpful for each group member to consider these eight assumptions as true for the adolescents, caregivers, and the skills trainers in this room. If you "buy into" these assumptions, it is likely to improve the treatment process. Why? Because you will be more accepting and less judgmental of one another and of yourselves as you think and act dialectically.

> *Note to Leaders:* The first three assumptions can be used to highlight the core dialectic of acceptance and change in the treatment. This core dialectic simultaneously helps move everyone toward a synthesis by validating both the adolescents' and parents' perspectives.

1. *Everyone in the group is doing the best he or she can. Leaders should invite the parent that appears most distressed by his or her teenager's behavior to comment on whether the teen is doing the best he or she can. Assuming the parent says something like, "No way," the skills trainer should ask the following:*

"Do you think that when your teen, [e.g., Bill], was a child he thought, 'I can't wait to be in this treatment program when I get older'? In other words, if Bill could figure out how to manage his emotions and behaviors so that he wouldn't need this treatment, he would. Would you agree? [*If yes:*] By definition, then, Bill is doing the best he can in this moment as it is. I would assert that you [the parent] are also doing the best you can in this moment while you try to parent Bill during this difficult time. And, I believe that I am doing the best I can in this very moment trying to teach all of you a lot of material tonight."

DISCUSSION POINT: *Invite brief discussion about this assumption.*

2. ***Everyone in this group wants to improve.*** We are assuming that all the adolescents and parents in attendance are here because they want things to improve in their families.

DISCUSSION POINT: *Invite brief discussion about this assumption.*

> ***Note to Leaders:*** At this point, a parent whose teen was reluctant to join might say, "I don't think Abigail wants to improve." The leader can then refer to the first assumption and ask if this is Abigail's ideal way to spend an evening—to rush through dinner, drive 45 minutes, sit in group for 2 hours, get home, and stay up late finishing homework? And yet, she is here. At some level, everyone sitting in this room has demonstrated that he or she wants to improve.

3. ***Everyone needs to do better, try harder, and be more motivated to change.*** The third assumption appears to contradict the first two. However, even if you are doing the best you can and want to improve, this does not mean that your efforts and motivation to improve are up to the task. For numerous reasons, including past learning and lack of certain skills, you are doing the best you can at this point in time. However, you can learn new skills, do better, try harder, and become more motivated to change. Can you see how the first three assumptions can all be true at the same time? [*Allow responses and questions.*] These form the core dialectic in DBT: balancing (1) acceptance—each of us is doing the best we can in the moment and want to improve—with (2) change—we all need to do better, try harder, and be more motivated in order to reach our goals and function better.

> ***Note to Leaders:*** An adolescent whose parent refused to attend the group might state that his or her parent is not doing his or her best or wanting to improve based on not even making the effort to participate. What stance should be taken on family members who are not supporting the adolescent in treatment? We believe it is still useful to hold to the position that even those members who chose not to attend are doing the best they can at the present time, given their own situation and capabilities. Skills group leaders can also validate that it can be hard to see it that way sometimes, and it can still be painful when a loved one's "best" does not satisfy us. This may be the first time the adolescent has gotten the validation inherent in the transactional model of emotional dysregulation. That is, it is not just the teen who is "lazy, emotional," etc., but the parent who must also do better, try harder, and be more motivated to change.

4. ***People may not have caused all of their own problems, and they have to solve them anyway.***

DISCUSSION POINT: *Invite an adolescent to read this assumption and then express what he or she thinks of it. Adolescents sometimes balk at this assumption, saying, "That's not fair." Leaders might respond as follows:*

> "I agree that life isn't fair sometimes. Imagine the following scenario: I am walking along by the river carrying my laptop computer, wearing my work clothes, and a bicycle courier rides by quickly, knocks into me by accident, and I'm thrown into the water. Did I want to be swimming in the less than purified river water fully dressed with my laptop? No. Is it my fault that I am presently in the water? No. So, just because I did not put myself in the water does not mean that I still do not have to swim to get out."

Note to Leaders: It's helpful to also acknowledge that adolescents, by virtue of the fact that they are under 18, sometimes cannot solve their problems on their own to the degree that adults can. For example, unpaid medical bills, a family move to an undesirable residence, and a lack of transportation are all examples of problems that may be beyond the adolescent's capacity to solve. Parents or other authority figures (e.g., teachers, guidance counselors, other care providers) may be the only ones who can alter certain situations. In such cases, the group leaders should acknowledge that this may be the case at times. However, by presenting the idea that individuals need to solve their own problems, therapists are encouraging an active problem-solving approach and an openness to learning new skills.

    5. *The lives of group members are painful as they are currently being lived.* How could it be otherwise, given what everyone in this room has been through thus far and is going through? There are many challenges in life for the average person; however, when you add intense emotional, behavioral, interpersonal, self-dysregulation, and adolescent–family challenges, we all know it's extra hard.

DISCUSSION POINT: *Invite participants, both teens and parents, to discuss their reactions to this assumption. Allow them to briefly validate one another and themselves.*

Note to Leaders: This assumption is intended to validate the experience of adolescent clients and their family members. When considering this assumption, parents become more likely to see problematic behaviors as related to painful emotions rather than stubbornness, manipulativeness, vindictiveness, or laziness. Similarly, adolescents can come to see their parents' problematic behaviors as stemming, in part, from painful emotions rather than only negative qualities.

    6. *Group members must learn and practice new behaviors in all important situations in their lives.* It's all well and good to come to group each week and to talk about skills, have some laughs, and get support from one another. However, if each one of you in this room is willing to commit to learn *and* practice new behavioral skills *outside* of this room—in all of the places you need to practice them (e.g., at home with parents, brothers, and sisters; at work with colleagues; at school when you are distressed by a teacher or a peer)—this group will be especially helpful.

    Many of you engage in what we call "mood-dependent" behaviors. That is, you act in the way you feel. If you feel angry, you act angry. If you feel sad, you act sad. Practicing skills when and where you need them is critical in order to learn to manage emotions and behaviors differently.

We don't expect that you'll snap your fingers and "presto," you are able to do this on your own all of a sudden. [*If relevant:*] Teenagers, use your primary therapist as coaches, and parents, use the skills trainers as coaches so we can help you apply the appropriate skills at the appropriate times.

> **DISCUSSION POINT**: *Ask participants to share one thing they feel they do well—whether it is cooking, basketball, math, foreign language, driving a car. Say, "Each of these 'skills' takes practice. No one is born and then able to effectively drive a car or cook linguine with white clam sauce without learning and practicing."*

> **DISCUSSION POINT**: *Ask whether group members see the value of practice. Ask each member to commit to practicing these skills each week in all important situations in his or her life.*

7. *There is no absolute truth.* How many of you feel, especially when gripped by intense emotions, that you are "right," the sole proprietor of the truth, and that other people are flat-out "wrong"? Do you ever notice how when you think that way—I'm right and he's wrong—it gets you polarized, like standing on opposite sides of the Grand Canyon, and it becomes more difficult to reconcile the conflict?

We believe that both parents and teens have valid points to make and at any given time, a grain of truth can be found in either position. Yes, parents often need to make a final decision about things, but that does not mean they cannot search for the validity in the teen's perspective, validate it, and then try to move to a middle path when possible. We will teach you more about this when we teach you dialectical thinking and acting. We want you to search for a synthesis between opposite points of view.

> *Note to Leaders:* After reviewing the assumptions for the third time in group, one rather authoritarian father reported that since beginning the group, he had been carefully monitoring his tendency to assume an "absolute truth" stance with his daughter. He reported that trying to abide by this assumption helped to reduce some of their conflicts.

8. *Teens and their family members cannot fail in DBT.* Sadly, in some parts of the mental health world there is a tendency to blame the client and family if they are not getting better— "They're not motivated, they're not trying." That does not happen in other medical specialties. Pretend you have a friend who has a brain tumor and is receiving chemotherapy, but the tumor is not shrinking. Can you imagine the oncologist (i.e., the cancer doctor) coming to the patient and saying, "Clearly you're not trying hard enough since if you were, the tumor would be shrinking." No, the doctor would likely say that the treatment isn't working and we need to try something else. Likewise, in DBT, if you and your family are not making any gains after a round of this treatment, we're going to say that the therapy or therapist hasn't worked for you, and *not* blame you for it not working. Blame is not effective here. There are other treatments that may need to be considered.

Similarly, although this format may resemble a class, there are no tests and no grades. Thus, we simply want you to come and practice to your best ability.

SKILLS TRAINING GROUP GUIDELINES

Refer participants to Orientation Handout 6, "Guidelines for the Adolescent Skills Training Group." Ask each participant to read one guideline aloud and then ask the group for feedback on whether members disagree or believe that they cannot adhere to the guideline.

    1. *Information obtained during sessions (including the names of other clients) must remain confidential.* It is imperative that everyone in the room understands the importance of this guideline. Group members may run into each other at a party or at the mall, and if they do, they must not say, "This is my friend from my DBT group!" Similarly, teens must not reveal one another's identities to their friends outside of group, by saying something like this: "I met this really cool guy, Joe Smith, from Springfield, in my DBT program!" Invite a show of hands to verify that you are committing to not discussing anything that happens in the group outside of group, with the exception of discussing relevant skills content in individual therapy. The point is that the group needs to be experienced by everyone as a safe place, and if people breach each other's trust, it becomes a real problem.

> **Note to Leaders:** Handling confidentiality may at times present a challenge. Because of discussions in the weekly therapist consultation meetings, group leaders know more about clients than they may have revealed in group, and possibly more than their parents know. This can become even more complicated when a group leader is also the primary therapist. It is imperative that the group leader not divulge information obtained elsewhere because it can not only make the adolescent feel uncomfortable (i.e., not ready to have it shared in group), but it may also give the adolescent pause about "confiding" in his or her primary therapist in the future.

    2. *Clients are not to come to sessions under the influence of drugs or alcohol.*

    3. *Clients who miss more than five group sessions (absences) in a 24-week program (or more than four misses in a 20-week program) will be considered to have dropped out of treatment. They can apply to reenter after sitting out for one complete skills module. [Leaders may vary absence policy according to their own setting and group length. This rule is based on our policy for comprehensive DBT.]* The basis for this guideline is that if you miss 25% of the "dosage" of skills content, we do not believe you have received an adequate dose to claim you received the treatment. Imagine that you have an infection and you are prescribed antibiotics. What happens if you take the antibiotic every other day for 1 week rather than daily? It doesn't work. Thus, we recognize there are times you may be away for vacation or attending your sister's graduation, etc. That is why we figure in some absence—to allow for such occasions. However, on the sixth miss of group, you have "dropped out." *[For comprehensive DBT it is the sixth miss of either group or individual therapy in a 24-week program.]* This is why it is important to look at your schedule carefully, plan ahead, and not skip sessions lightly. If the teenager or the parent drops out, you can apply to reenter after sitting out for one complete skills module. Note that this rule applies to parents too!

    4. *Group members who come more than 15 minutes late will be allowed in the group but will be considered absent.* We recognize buses run late, construction delays occur on the roads, and you may in fact be running late from an important meeting. Thus, we grant you a 15-minute grace period, and we don't want you to turn around and go home if you are running late.

However, significant lateness counts as an absence because you will be missing mindfulness practice, homework review, and new content. It is important for you to receive the adequate "dosage" of treatment.

5. Clients are not allowed to discuss any risk behaviors with other clients outside of sessions. Sharing information about your risk behaviors with your peers can be triggering to them, and if they don't have the necessary skills, it may result in their engaging in that behavior. Thus, we want you to share this information only with your therapists.

6. Group members may not contact one another when in crisis and instead should contact their skills coach/therapist. It is not acceptable for a client to call someone from group and say, "I'm going to hurt myself or run away." This guideline helps to not trigger other group members or leave them feeling anxious and helpless. We ask that you try some skill that your therapist recommends and, in crisis, call your therapist rather than a peer from group.

7. People may not form private relationships (cliques or dating) with one another while they are in skills training together. We have this rule for two simple reasons: (a) If the relationship were to become unstable or dissolve, one or both members may feel uncomfortable attending group. For similar reasons, we do not allow clients to have their boyfriends or girlfriends serve as the accompanying "family member." (b) When people form private relationships in a group, others may feel excluded and uncomfortable as well. Thus, we ask that if the group members want to have a bite to eat after group, all members need to be invited. You are free to decline the invitation, of course.

8. Clients may not act in a mean or disrespectful manner toward other group members or group leaders. As has been said, we want this group to feel safe and comfortable for people to share, learn, and be supported. If people are mean or disrespectful, the remaining group members have greater difficulty accessing the help they are seeking.

> **DISCUSSION POINT**: *Name some disrespectful behaviors you think could affect this group (e.g., eye rolling, giggling, sarcastic jokes, teasing, texting). How might those behaviors lead others to feel and act? For example, they might shut down or not want to come back. We hope by this discussion you can see the value of this guideline.*

9. [*For teens in a comprehensive DBT program*] **Each adolescent must be in ongoing individual therapy.** Comprehensive DBT requires both individual therapy and skills training, so you cannot be in one without the other—at least, during the first phase of treatment. You need to complete the skills training group before you can be eligible for individual therapy only.

DBT CONTRACT

Refer participants to Orientation Handout 7, "DBT Contract."

Now that you have been oriented to the DBT rules, assumptions, biosocial theory, and treatment goals, we ask each of you to consider signing this agreement stating your willingness to commit to the DBT program. We, the skills trainers, will co-sign this contract as well.

Note to Leaders: Skills trainers also sign the contract to strengthen all members' commitment to the skills training group, the guidelines, attendance policy, and the homework. Orienting members to the fact that they will be subjected to a brief behavioral analysis if they do not complete their homework is useful to (1) clarify the contingencies and (2) improve motivation. When this approach is put into practice, it can be succinctly assessed with the questions, "What got in the way of your doing your homework? What can you do differently next time so that you are more likely to get your homework done?"

CHALLENGES WITH TEACHING ORIENTATION

Repetition

Sometimes families ask, "I've already been through orientation—do I have to come next week?" We clearly answer, "Yes," for several reasons, all having to do with the fact that the orientation itself is therapeutic:

- *It is an opportunity for members to review the problem areas that brought them in and to consider progress on these areas and present goals.*
- *It is therapeutic to review the DBT assumptions and consider whether they are questioning them or "buying in" to them.*
- *Reminding everyone of the guidelines prevents or reduces therapy-interfering behaviors.*
- *Families can always benefit from hearing the biosocial theory again, as it contains new ideas that can increase compassion, understanding, and hope.*
- *Mindfulness is taught in depth and practiced in the second half of orientation sessions!*

Too Much Material

Skills trainers may find that the above teaching notes contain too much material to cover. Some clients feel overwhelmed by the end of the session, given the mindfulness material presented in the second half. Our solution is to vary what we present for orientation, in terms of either the handouts we cover or the depth with which we cover them. When there are new families present, it is important to teach the problem areas, the biosocial theory, group guidelines, and the assumptions. If many group members have been in skills training for some time, we may briefly review problem areas, rules, or assumptions, without having a discussion about each point on the handouts. Additionally, we may omit some handouts such as "What Is Dialectical Behavior Therapy (DBT)?," the "DBT Contract," or "Biosocial Theory." These could possibly be taught every second, third, or fourth orientation, so that every family hears them at least once.

Another solution is to orient each family individually prior to entering group. The orientation materials can then be gone over briefly as a review, as the family will have already seen them. As such, they are less likely to feel overwhelmed by the many ideas presented.

CHAPTER 6

Mindfulness Skills

SESSION OUTLINES

Session 1

▶ Orientation to DBT Skills Training (see Chapter 5)

▶ Brief Mindfulness Exercise

▶ Homework Review

▶ Break

▶ Orientation of Clients to the Mindfulness Skills and Their Rationale

▶ Three States of Mind

▶ Assignment of Homework

▶ Session Wind-Down

Handouts and Other Materials

▶ Mindfulness Handout 1, "Mindfulness: Taking Hold of Your Mind"

▶ Mindfulness Handout 2, "Mindfulness: Why Bother?"

▶ Mindfulness Handout 3, "Three States of Mind"

▶ Mindfulness Handout 4, "Practice Exercise: Observing Yourself in Each State of Mind"

▶ Whiteboard or other large writing surface

▶ Mindfulness bell

Session 2

▶ Brief Mindfulness Exercise

▶ Homework Review

▶ Break

▶ Steps to Wise Mind

▶ Mindfulness "What" Skills

▶ Mindfulness "How" Skills

▶ How to Practice Mindfulness

▶ Assignment of Homework

▶ Session Wind-Down

▶ Mindfulness Exercises for Adolescents

Handouts and Other Materials

▶ Mindfulness Handout 5, "Mindfulness 'What' Skills"

▶ Mindfulness Handout 6, "Mindfulness 'How' Skills"

▶ Mindfulness Handout 7, "Mindfulness Cheat Sheet"

▶ Mindfulness Handout 8, "Practice Exercise: Mindfulness 'What' and 'How' Skills"

▶ Whiteboard or other large writing surface and marker

▶ Mindfulness bell

TEACHING NOTES

> Every moment is a fresh beginning.
> —T. S. ELIOT

> Everything has its wonders, even darkness and silence,
> and I learn, whatever state I may be in, therein to be
> content.
> —HELEN KELLER

ABOUT THIS MODULE

Mindfulness skills teach participants to increase nonjudgmental awareness of present experience and to improve attentional control. By learning how to participate fully in the present moment, clients are better able to reduce their own suffering and increase their capacity for pleasure. These skills form the core of the entire skills set, as individuals need these skills to be able to make use of the other DBT skills. As such, the module is repeated prior to the start of the other skills modules. By becoming aware of emotional states and urges, one develops the capacity to mindfully select a skillful response, rather than reacting impulsively.

This module is designed to be covered in two sessions. The material in Session 1 is taught in the second half of the Orientation session (Chapter 6). Mindfulness homework assigned at the end of Session 1 is reviewed in the first half of Session 2. Session 2's new material is taught in its second half following the break. Note that if less time is spent on Orientation (e.g., when a new module is starting and no new members join), the material can be covered within one

2-hour group session, leaving more time to cover material in the following skills module. With the exception of the Orientation session, every session starts with a brief mindfulness exercise. We offer one suggested mindfulness exercise at the start of Session 2 in this chapter's teaching notes, but trainers can also choose from the list of mindfulness exercises for adolescents at the end of this chapter. In addition to the relevant handouts and a whiteboard or other writing surface, bring a small bell (or "singing bowl") to the session and ring it three times to signal the start and one time to signal the end of mindfulness exercises.

SESSION 1

BRIEF MINDFULNESS EXERCISE
· · · ·
HOMEWORK REVIEW
· · · ·
BREAK
· · · ·

ORIENTATION OF CLIENTS TO THE MINDFULNESS SKILLS AND THEIR RATIONALE

Refer participants to Mindfulness Handout 1, "Mindfulness: Taking Hold of Your Mind."
Do you ever feel like your mind is controlling you rather than you are controlling your mind? Do you feel as though you have no control over your attention, your mental camera lens? [*Look through your hands as if looking through a camera. Move your hands around chaotically rather than steadily focusing on an image.*]

Do you ever notice that while you are trying to focus on doing one thing, other things seem to intrude into your mind? Do you find yourself texting someone while you're talking to someone else? When you try to do homework, do you get distracted by thoughts of events that happened at school that day? As you're listening to someone tell a story, does your mind drift to other things? As I am teaching right now, do you notice your mind drifting to what you're going to eat after group, or what homework you have to do tonight, or do you feel distracted by the heat in the room? Do you sometimes blurt things out in class or yell at someone and not realize that you were going to do that beforehand—like it just happened automatically without your realizing it? Do you find yourself saying and doing other things and not aware of what you're doing?

When these things happen, we call it living life with your eyes closed.

Being mindful is living with eyes wide open. It is being aware of things that you are experiencing (with all five senses, including urges) in the present moment, instead of getting pulled into the future or the past. It is taking hold of your mind and controlling it rather than it being in control of you.

What Is Mindfulness?

Invite a participant to read item 1 from Mindfulness Handout 1, "Mindfulness: Taking Hold of Your Mind."

Full Awareness

Mindfulness is being aware of your present moment (i.e., thoughts, feelings, and physical sensations) without judgment and without trying to change it. It is full awareness, having an opened mind.

EXERCISE: PRACTICE OPENED MIND

Orient group to the fact that you will now conduct a 2-minute practice. Lower the lights in the room if there are no windows or ask participants to close their eyes. Ring the mindfulness bell three times and ask the group to pay attention to their remaining senses—to the smells, sounds, tastes, physical sensations, both internal and external. Ask participants to describe their observations.

Attentional Control

Mindfulness means staying focused on one thing at a time. It means training our minds to focus on only one thing in the moment and not to "multitask." It is having control of your attention. When your mind is jumping all over the place and you are unfocused, what happens? Can you think of an example?

EXERCISE: PRACTICE FOCUSED MIND

Orient group to the fact that you will now conduct a 2-minute practice. You can choose from a menu of options here. You could ask them to focus on the experience of their feet touching the floor, or the experience of their buttocks touching the chair, or to hold up the palm of one hand and study it. They could also observe an object in the room (e.g., a picture or lamp), or observe the experience of eating a raisin or a caramel. Ring the mindfulness bell three times. Ask them to focus on only the selected activity, nonjudgmentally, and when their mind wanders to other things, ask them to notice it and gently bring their minds back to the one selected focus.

> DISCUSSION POINT: *Ask the group members about their experiences during the above exercise. It is very common for participants to say, "This doesn't work" or "I can't focus for more than 2 seconds before I get distracted." Validate and then explain:* The untrained mind is like a puppy that wanders all over the house or yard, attending to every new sound and smell, without sitting still too often. Mindfulness practice is like obedience training for the untrained puppy. We're asking the puppy—our mind—to "sit still" and "pay attention." We need to be patient with ourselves and practice a lot before our minds really *learn* how to sit still and focus for longer periods of time. If someone is training to run a marathon, play a new challenging piece of music, or learn a new sport, it takes a lot of practice to feel capable. The same is true for mindfulness skills. Try not to judge yourself when your mind wanders—the key is to notice when it happens and gently bring it back over and over again.

Mindfulness: Why Bother?

Refer participants to Mindfulness Handout 2, "Mindfulness: Why Bother?"

DISCUSSION POINT: *Elicit examples from participants about how not paying attention or not being aware of themselves or their surroundings impacts their lives over time. Next, elicit examples of times when they were more aware and more focused—how did that help them function better (emotionally, behaviorally, cognitively, interpersonally)? Why are full awareness and attention control useful skills to learn?*

1. ***Being mindful can give you more choices and more control over your behavior.*** Being fully aware is critically important if you are emotional and/or impulsive because it gives you time to catch yourself before you do something you might regret later. You can function better if you can make choices about how to *act* rather than impulsively *reacting*.

Note to Leaders: Draw *x*- and *y*-axes and a steep line going up toward the top right. Explain:

"Instead of seeing your emotions and urges going from 0 to 100 instantaneously, we want you to notice the onset of your emotions and urges here in this 0–10 range [point to the bottom left portion of the steep line]. When you are aware of emotions and urges early, you can make a choice not to act on them and instead to use skills to cope (e.g., distress tolerance, emotion regulation, or mindfully urge surfing)."

---

2. ***Being mindful can reduce your suffering and increase your pleasure.*** A huge advantage of using mindfulness skills is that it can reduce a person's suffering while also increasing his or her ability to experience pleasure and joy. Think about it. If you can learn how to focus fully on the present moment, like on this lesson right now, you are less likely to feel sad about a problem that happened earlier today. You're also less likely to be worried about your upcoming SAT [Scholastic Aptitude Test], job interview, or dance recital.

If you are truly participating in this moment as it is, you can laugh out loud without being self-conscious; play basketball without worrying about people in the stands watching you; have an intense heart-to-heart conversation with a loved one; eat a meal slowly and really notice the taste, smell, and texture of the food; go for a walk outside and literally smell the roses. You will be aware of things you don't typically notice because you are usually thinking about your to-do lists instead. This is one of the only ways to access joy and pleasure; this is *living life* with your eyes wide open in the *present moment*.

DISCUSSION POINT: *Ask if anyone can think of a time in the recent past when he or she was able to be in the present moment fully and able to reduce suffering and/or access a deeper kind of pleasure? Invite several members to share a brief example.*

3. ***Being mindful can help you make important decisions.*** Whenever one is faced with having to make an important decision in life, it is important to make a mindful decision. Have you ever been angry and quickly texted or e-mailed someone without thinking about the consequences? That's a nonmindful response. Have you ever been anxious and avoided a situation or avoided talking about something important, only to make your anxiety worse? That's typically nonmindful and a decision driven purely by emotion.

4. ***Being mindful can help focus your attention and make you more effective and productive.*** When we can stay focused, we can learn more effectively, stay actively engaged in a relationship, play music and sports effectively. When you can remain focused on your goals, you are more likely to reach them (e.g., study for a test and pass the test, finish a task, have an important conversation without getting sidetracked). Uninterrupted focus and attention help improve your performance on reading, learning, and other academic tasks.

5. *Being mindful can increase compassion for yourself and others.* When you practice being aware while being nonjudgmental, your harshest criticisms turn into descriptions of observable facts. This process allows for compassionate acceptance of one's own and others' experiences. For example, instead of calling yourself a "stupid idiot," you could stick to the facts and say, "I performed poorly on my chemistry test after being sick and being out for a week. Now that I'm feeling healthy, I can go for some extra help after school and hopefully get back on track." Notice the contrasting emotional reactions to the two examples.

6. *Being mindful can lessen your pain, tension, and stress* and, in turn, even improve your health. Jon Kabat-Zinn (1990) has written extensively about mindfulness-based stress reduction. This research demonstrates that if you practice mindfulness, you can actually reduce your physical pain, stress, and tension and even improve medical conditions such as psoriasis. It's amazing how much your mind can directly affect your body and your health!

Mindfulness Skills Take Practice, Practice, Practice

To reap any of the advantages of these skills, you need to build up your mindfulness muscles. You don't just snap your fingers and become good at this. Just like any other skill in life, you need to *practice, practice, practice* mindfulness skills to become more proficient in them. If you're just starting to become a runner, we don't expect you to run the 26 miles of a marathon tomorrow. Do not get discouraged by your inability to stay more focused and more aware right away. It takes time and it takes practice. We will start with small practice exercises and build up your muscles and stamina over time.

THREE STATES OF MIND

Refer participants to Mindfulness Handout 3, "Three States of Mind."

To better understand mindfulness skills, it helps to understand three states of mind. At any given time, we might be in Reasonable Mind, in Emotional Mind, or in Wise Mind.

Note to Leaders: Draw the Venn diagram from Mindfulness Handout 3 on the board and label Reasonable Mind and Emotional Mind in their respective circles, and Wise Mind in the center, in the overlapping part of the circles. Explain:

"Reasonable Mind is what you think to be true. It is when you are acting or thinking about something without emotions present. It's logical, planful, rational, 'just-the-facts' kind of thinking. [For younger children, we refer to this as 'calculator mind.'] Emotional Mind is what you feel to be true; it is when you are acting or thinking entirely based on emotion, without planning, using logic, or thinking about consequences. Wise Mind is what you know to be true. It involves an intuitive form of knowing, thinking, or acting, using both logical and emotional information. Let's discuss what each of these states of mind looks like."

Emotional Mind

What is Emotional Mind? Emotional Mind is when your emotion consumes you. It takes over and it's hard to think rationally about consequences.

Note to Leaders: Give a personal example, such as the following example, that captures the essence of Emotional Mind. Name the emotion and the corresponding thoughts, physical sensations, and urges and actions.

"While I was driving on the highway to group tonight, I had to slam on my brakes because someone who was weaving in and out of lanes cut me off. I was scared, since I almost crashed into him and then the guy behind almost rear-ended me. My body was stiff, tense. I was slightly hyperventilating, very alert (in a fight–flight response), and I had the thought, 'That *@#$@ almost killed me. Who the @#%$* does he think he is?' I started accelerating to try to catch him, to see who he was. I wanted to give him the good old 'Bronx cheer,' which is a nasty hand gesture for those of you who don't know what I mean.

"This is Emotional Mind—emotion completely controlled my body, my mind, and my action urges. Luckily for me, I was able to access my Wise Mind in time and then decelerate. I did not give my Bronx cheer, which could have led to road rage, car accidents, or other poor outcomes."

DISCUSSION POINT: *Invite participants to share examples of Emotional Mind. Ask each to name the emotion and what he or she felt an urge to do or what he or she actually did.*

Note to Leaders: As participants give emotion examples (both negative and positive), write the emotions and their potential corresponding urges or actions on the board under the Emotional Mind side of the Venn diagram. For example:

anger → slamming door, screaming at people, self-harming
sad → crying, lying in bed, using drugs/alcohol
guilt → hiding, overapologizing
fear → cutting classes
worry → excessive rumination, overeating
shame → avoiding people/activities, lying, thinking about suicide
very happy and excited → blurting things without thinking, acting impulsively, spending money
love → allowing impulsive unprotected sexual behavior, cutting school and lying about it to spend time with this person

---

- *Emotional Mind is not always a problem, but sometimes it is.* Sometimes allowing yourself to have a good cry over a sad event is an effective thing to do. Emotion-filled dancing at your best friend's wedding, singing at the top of your lungs at a concert with your favorite band, or jumping up and shouting when your team wins a play-off game, might be joy-filled events that you remember for years to come. However, Emotional Mind can sometimes lead people to do more problematic things. Instead of just crying, the sad person may end up staying in bed, not going to school or work, etc. Even positive emotions can sometimes lead to problem behaviors, like doing something impulsive when excited.

Reasonable Mind

What is the polar opposite of Emotional Mind? Reasonable Mind. Given what you have now learned about Emotional Mind, can someone define Reasonable Mind? [*Invite participants to share their ideas.*] Reasonable Mind is when you are acting or thinking about something *without* emotions present or without taking your feelings into account. It may involve problem solving, thinking logically, planning, or thinking about consequences.

> **DISCUSSION POINT**: *Ask for several examples of Reasonable Mind and discuss the thoughts, body sensations, action urges, and actions associated with it; for example, doing simple math problems or balancing a checkbook (unless you're math phobic or have no money in the account to balance); making a grocery list before going to the supermarket—bread, eggs, juice; working with a computer's edit function to cut, copy, and paste words on documents. We all need Reasonable Mind to make effective decisions about day-to-day life.*

> **DISCUSSION POINT**: *Ask*, "What are the disadvantages of making all your decisions or acting only in Reasonable Mind? What about career choice? Because you're good at math, your family thinks you should become an accountant like your mother, even though you love art and writing and you visualize yourself pursuing journalism and graphic arts." *Ask rhetorically*, "Shouldn't that decision be made in Reasonable Mind since having a solid profession is so important?"
>
> "What if you want to buy a new home?" *Ask rhetorically*, "Shouldn't that be decided in Reasonable Mind since you need to consider number of bedrooms, bathrooms, cost of house, school district?"
>
> "How do you decide whom to ask out on a date with someone?" *Ask rhetorically*, "Shouldn't that be decided in Reasonable Mind since you need to consider intelligence, talents (e.g., as athlete or musician), and physical features (e.g., height, hair color)?"
>
> "What if you want to make a decision about college?" *Ask rhetorically*, "Shouldn't that be decided in Reasonable Mind since you want to consider locale, size of school, student–teacher ratio, range of courses that you want to study?"
>
> "What about behaving only from Reasonable Mind? Do you know someone in your life who seems to act only from Reasonable Mind? How do you experience that person?"

Note to Leaders: Many group members will know a partner, parent, or teacher who is highly logical and does not seem to understand his or her emotional experience and thus leaves them feeling invalidated.

- *Both emotion and reason are needed for important decisions.* We would argue that decisions about careers, colleges, a potential new romantic interest, and a new home all need to involve both Reasonable Mind and Emotional Mind. Although there are facts to consider reasonably in each of these scenarios, we believe that emotion should also play a role. When you visit a college, choose a home, or go on a date, you *also* want to notice what you feel to inform your ultimate decision. Otherwise, you might end up miserable! Maybe you choose a college because it is close and affordable, but still not the right fit for you because you ignored your emotional reactions.

However, we don't want you to rely on *only* feelings since you might end up going out with the sexiest person alive but you find out they have little personality and no interests that you share; you may end up choosing to move into the biggest place you can find, but it turns out you can't afford it and it is in a weak school district; you may end up choosing a school based on a single desirable feature (e.g., new athletic center, party school, great college town), but you realize you want to study music, which is their weakest department.

Wise Mind

When you need to make decisions in your life, especially important ones, it is important to get into Wise Mind. Wise Mind is the synthesis (i.e., blend) of Emotional Mind and Reasonable Mind. Wise Mind is what you "know to be true." Rather than just a combination of emotion and reason, when we draw from both we reach a sort of elevated state from which we can make optimal decisions and choices about how to act. The idea is that there is wisdom already within each of us and we need to learn how to access it. Have you ever noticed a "gut feeling" or had a "hunch" or an "intuitive sense"? If that feeling is also informed by factual information, it's probably Wise Mind and not Emotional Mind. For example, say you're in a relationship, and you have ongoing conflicting emotions—love, anger, frustration, disappointment, and hurt—and you realize logically that there are some major differences in interests and values between the two of you. At this point, your Emotional and Reasonable Minds come together and create a gut feeling that tells you it is time to break off a relationship even though you're still attached— that's Wise Mind. It doesn't mean you don't have strong emotions or that it's easy, but that you know it's the right decision, based on your feelings, values, and long-term goals.

Wise Mind is also valuable for choosing the best ways to behave. This might involve *not* acting on impulse and instead practicing a skill when distressed, dysregulated, or noticing strong urges. For example, you have the urge to avoid your therapy session tomorrow because you anticipate a painful discussion; however, Wise Mind tells you to keep the appointment and face the discussion so that you can cope more effectively with your life problems in the long term.

> **DISCUSSION POINT:** *Invite participants to share examples of Wise Mind.*

> **Note to Leaders:** If needed, give one more example to illustrate the input from Emotional Mind and Reasonable Mind in coming to a Wise Mind decision, such as the following:
>
> "How many of you are pet lovers? Imagine you have two dogs at home already, but on your way home from school or work, you stop by the local animal shelter. Immediately as you enter, you see a litter of three golden retriever puppies jumping up and down, wagging their tails, and looking irresistibly cute. Emotion Mind says, 'They are so cute; they're pent up in this little cubicle. I need to rescue them, love them, and therefore adopt them today!'
>
> "Reasonable Mind says, 'I have two dogs already.' It's expensive to care for dogs. They need vaccinations, food, and you won't have enough time to exercise them since you are at school or work and have sports practice most days. So there will be dog-walker expenses. It's not financially feasible to adopt three more dogs. Moreover, you calculate that the house is too small to have more large dogs. In addition, you don't want your older two dogs to feel neglected by having three more dogs join the house.
>
> "Wise Mind says that you cannot adopt them given your Reasonable Mind considerations, but you can do your best to get them adopted by people you know, ASAP. You choose to take pictures of the puppies and e-mail them to all of your friends and family

and let them know how irresistible they are. You hope that your dog-less friends will come and adopt. To sweeten the deal, you offer to loan your friends your crate for house training them and to provide free puppy care advice. By doing this, you are honoring both your Emotion Mind and Reasonable Mind. The Wise Mind decision recognizes your long-term goals and values. You want to be able to continue your schooling and sports activities while giving attention to your existing pets while also trying to find a home for these adorable puppies.

"When we next teach the 'what' and 'how' skills, we will teach you how to access your Wise Mind."

ASSIGNMENT OF HOMEWORK

Assign Mindfulness Handout 4, "Practice Exercise: Observing Yourself in Each State of Mind." Ask participants to observe themselves in each of the three states of mind during the following week: Emotional Mind, Reasonable Mind, and Wise Mind. Ask them to write down the emotion (if any), thought, and behavior that occurred during the example. Ask participants if (1) they are willing to do this practice and (2) whether they have any questions. Note that this handout will need to be copied each time you reteach mindfulness.

Note to Leaders: In our program, the session usually ends at this point with a wind-down exercise (see Chapter 3).

SESSION 2
BRIEF MINDFULNESS EXERCISE

Note to Leaders: At the onset of every skills group session (with the exception of the Orientation session), we introduce a mindfulness practice exercise. Before the practice, the leader tells a story, such as the following, to engage the participants as well as illustrate the relevance of mindfulness to their daily lives and long-term goals.

"The other day, there was a meeting for class parents at my kids' middle school. I showed up there after a long day of work prepared to sit back and listen to the discussion. To my surprise, they started the meeting and put me on the spot by asking my opinion about a school matter of which I had given zero thought. Immediately, I experienced a wave of panic, as all eyes were on me and everyone appeared to be awaiting my eloquent answer. Momentarily in Emotion Mind, I froze. I thought, 'Oh, gosh—I'm not prepared for this!' I had the urge to run out of the room, I began to sweat, and my heart was racing. I then noticed my anxious response and quickly said to myself nonjudgmentally, 'Let me gather myself, take a breath, and then offer a somewhat thoughtful response.' My Reasonable Mind facts about the school matter were actually in my head; I just needed to get my emotions down somewhat so I could access them. Instead of focusing on 'all eyes on me,' I turned my camera lens inward to access the facts and present the relevant information.

"So I needed some mindfulness skills to stay focused and do what the situation called for. Now I'd like to introduce a mindfulness practice exercise that emphasizes the skills of observing and describing. That's what I had to do first to bring myself out of Emotion Mind and into Wise Mind. So what I'd like you to do now is to sit with your feet on the floor, your back upright, your hands in your lap, and when I ring the bell, I would like you to observe your current emotions. You may want to pay attention to any thoughts, body sensations, and action urges you may be having. If your mind wanders to other things, notice it without judgment, and gently bring your attention back to this activity."

Practice this mindfulness exercise for 3–5 minutes, and then invite group members to share their observations for another 3–5 minutes. Leaders need to help participants by shaping their responses to be nonjudgmental and noninterpretive, and instead, to be focused on observable experiences. For example, rather than say, "This was stupid," ask the participant to say, "I noticed I had the thought, 'This is stupid.'"

As the participants become more seasoned, they are invited to lead a mindfulness practice exercise on a rotating basis. Simple mindfulness exercises to start off with for members new to the practice include noticing physical sensations (e.g., feet on floor, back against chair, hands on table), sounds (e.g., breath, cars passing by, the hum of a heater or air conditioner, the rain), focusing on the breath as it enters and leaves the body, or focusing on one external object and nonjudgmentally observing and describing the details (e.g., a penny, a picture in the room, the back of their hand).

HOMEWORK REVIEW
• • • •
BREAK
• • • •

STEPS TO WISE MIND

Mindfulness skills are the way to synthesize Emotional Mind and Reasonable Mind and access Wise Mind. There are three mindfulness "what" skills and three mindfulness "how" skills. To get into Wise Mind, these skills are what you need to do and how you need to do it.

MINDFULNESS "WHAT" SKILLS

Refer participants to Mindfulness Handout 5, "Mindfulness 'What' Skills."
    The three mindfulness "what" skills are *observe*, *describe*, and *participate*.

Observe: What Is It?

• *Watch wordlessly.* Just *notice* your experience in the present moment. Slow yourself down to the "preverbal" level to just notice. Don't rush to describe or act on the experience. This can be very difficult since we're all prone to put words to our experience and make interpretations as a way to make sense of our experience.

• ***Observe outside of yourself: Look at pictures, people passing by, objects, nature.*** Observe both outside yourself using all the five senses: sight, smell, taste, touch, and hearing.

• ***Observe inside yourself.*** Watch your thoughts and feelings come and go, as if they are on a conveyor belt . . . or as if each one is a cloud in the sky passing overhead. Notice a wave of emotion building in your stomach; notice your palms getting sweaty; notice the tightness in your chest; notice any thoughts passing through your mind.

• ***Have a Teflon mind.*** Let experiences come into your mind and slip right out (not holding on), like a Teflon frying pan.

• ***Don't push away your thoughts and feelings.*** Just let them happen, even when they are painful. As if your brain were a popcorn popper, see the thoughts and emotional reactions as just going to pop. And you notice them popping, one after the other, without trying to control them. Or as if your mind were a blanket, spread out to accept every leaf, twig, or raindrop that falls on it.

> **DISCUSSION POINT**: *Say to participants,* "Many of us prefer to focus on the outside world rather than our own inside world, especially when we're uncomfortable with our own feelings and thoughts. The Observe skill is intended for both inside and outside observing with special attention paid to noticing what is happening on the inside."

One way to think about observing is to think about what we do when we go to an aquarium and watch fish in a large tank. We tend to notice what swims in front of us—the features, colors, shapes, sizes of the fish—and maybe the trajectory of their swimming path. As the experience changes moment to moment, we attend to it, but we don't create or control the experience.

EXERCISE: PRACTICE OBSERVING

Orient participants and ring the mindfulness bell three times. Ask participants to observe their thoughts as they pop up, by trying to count each new thought (e.g., by jotting down a hash-mark [/] on a piece of paper as each new thought pops up).

An alternative practice is to explain that to tell the difference between *observing* thoughts and *thinking* thoughts, group members can watch what pops into their minds after certain word cues. A group leader can slowly say a list of words, such as *water, table, air, ice cream, car, green, morning.* When participants notice with curiosity what words, thoughts, or images come into their minds following each word, that is observing. They can then apply this type of mindful observation to their own spontaneous thoughts.

Each time you teach any of the "what" and "how" skills, try to introduce a novel way to practice the skill so that participants can learn from different examples and practices. The end of this chapter contains a list of mindfulness practices emphasizing specific "what" and "how" skills.

Describe: What Is It?

• ***Wordful watching.*** Put what you have observed into words. Label what you have observed—for example, "I feel sad," or "My face feels hot," or "I feel my heart racing," or "I'm having the thought that I can't do this," or "I noticed I had a lot of worry thoughts related to my history test."

• *Describe only what you have observed.* No interpretations—just the facts, Ma'am! Instead of "that person has an attitude," you could describe that person as "rolling his eyes, speaking with a loud voice," etc. [*Refer to the "observe" practice exercise above and highlight how the words group members used to describe what they observed is the "describe" skill.*]

DISCUSSION POINT: *After validating how hard it is for all of us to describe without interpretations and sticking only with the observable facts, ask participants to reflect on why this skill is so important. How might it help us stay out of Emotion Mind?*

EXERCISE

A co-leader should stand at the front of the room with arms crossed, furrowed brow, downward-turned mouth, and intense gaze. Invite participants to observe and then describe the co-leader. Say, "OK, group, what do you see?" Responses often include, "You're angry, you're upset, you're thinking hard about something." The leader should ask participants to describe *only what they see* without interpretation—thus, correct responses include "furrowed brow, downward-turned mouth, arms crossed, eyes fixed in one position." Point out how hard this skill is to apply and why it is so important—because misattributions and interpretations (e.g., she's angry) often trigger or worsen our emotional state. This makes it more difficult to access Wise Mind.

EXERCISE

A related exercise is to cut out pictures of entertainers and politicians, especially those who evoke strong feelings in some people. Randomly pass the pictures out and ask members to practice describing the person on their piece of paper, correcting any interpretations or judgments.

Participate: What Is It?

• *Throw yourself into the present moment.* Try not to worry about tomorrow; don't focus on the upsetting events of "yesterday"; don't distract from now; throw yourself into the present moment fully (e.g., dancing, playing ball, eating, cleaning, taking a test, engaging in a lively conversation with a friend, feeling sad in the moment). This approach allows you to live life to the fullest, experiencing the richness of each life experience, enhancing the capacity for pleasure and joy, allowing yourself to experience even negative emotions without avoiding them, and not just sitting on the sidelines of life—which can leave us feeling empty, disconnected, lonely, bored, and even depressed. [*Many of the teens we work with tend to quickly escape and avoid intense emotions.*]

By not allowing these emotions to register, by not experiencing them fully, you miss the opportunity to use their information to help you make wise decisions. For example, say a teacher embarrasses you in class, and your immediate urge is to change your experience of shame by blurting out a hostile retort and running out of the room. By sitting for a moment with the uncomfortable emotion, however, we can recognize that although uncomfortable, the emotion is tolerable, and that a hostile retort or running out might create greater embarrassment or shame. Thus, instead, you might choose to sit quietly, compose yourself, and calmly talk to the teacher after class.

A second use of the "participate" skill is when you choose to participate fully in a distraction from a current distressing situation as a method of coping. For example, if you are feeling very sad about a conflict with a friend, it isn't effective to be crying and preoccupied in the middle of your gym class. Ideally, you would throw yourself into the volleyball game and have a good cry, if needed, when you get home.

> **DISCUSSION POINT:** *Ask participants to think of a recent time in which they were participating fully, becoming one with whatever they were doing, or being "in the zone," as we say. Elicit an example from all participants and ask them to differentiate that experience from times when they were only half-engaged in an activity, or when they were multitasking.*

- *Experience fully without being self-conscious.* When we are self-conscious, we are evaluating ourselves and are no longer "in the moment." We're outside looking in on our experience. Participation involves letting go of evaluating ourselves and others and just "being," just experiencing what we feel and engaging in this moment as it is. For example, when I am playing music with my band mates, I'm not worried about how I sound or what people are going to think of my voice or my keyboard playing—I'm letting it all "hang out" and feeling the music inside and out.

- *Participating is what life is about.* A participatory life means having a good laugh or a good cry without being self-conscious; it means gardening, talking with a friend without getting distracted, being absorbed in running or dancing, making music by singing a song or playing an instrument by yourself or with others. Anyone who has played in a band knows how the synergistic energy creates a "flow" that is not easy to replicate in other activities in life. This is the challenge—for each of us to find our "flow moments" no matter what we're doing.

EXERCISE

Invite participants to play "Sound Ball" or "Snap, Crackle, and Pop" described in the list of mindfulness practice exercises at the end of this chapter. After the game, invite participants to share observations. Many are self-conscious at first as they engage in this group exercise and, by definition, not participating fully. If time allows, ask them to try the exact same exercise again—this time, trying to participate without being "as self-conscious" and throwing themselves in "more fully." Afterward, ask participants if they noticed any difference between their experiences of the two practice exercises.

- *Experience even negative emotions fully to help your Wise Mind make a decision about what to do (instead of acting impulsively).* If you are distressed, it is important to pay attention to that feeling, to know what you are feeling, so that you can make a Wise Mind choice on what to do about it. If you act impulsively rather than at least briefly sitting with the emotions, you can make your situation worse. For example, if you don't even realize you are highly anxious and just start to do shots of alcohol to relieve it, you don't give yourself a chance to choose other ways of managing your anxiety.

- *Remember to use your "how" skills [which follow] while participating.* [*The following section can be taught after participants have gone through the Mindfulness Skills module at least once and have already been introduced to the "how" skills, or as a segue to introducing the "how" skills.*]

One is able to participate more fully and for longer periods of time when the "how" skills, which we teach next, are being used. Consider this: When you are judgmental, you are evaluating rather than participating. When you are multitasking, you are not doing one thing in the moment and are less likely to be participating fully. And when you are allowing emotions to dictate your behavior, regardless of their impact on your long-term goals, you are not likely to be participating fully in a skillful manner. For example, if you feel slighted by a friend and you choose to curse him or her, you may be participating fully in your emotional tirade—however, it's likely not effective and helpful for you in the long term. If you choose to get yourself into Wise Mind, participating fully while doing what works may involve expressing your hurt and disappointment without letting your anger control the discussion.

So our "how" skills teach us how to do this—how to be nonjudgmental, how to focus on just one thing at a time, and how to do what works effectively.

MINDFULNESS "HOW" SKILLS

Refer participants to Mindfulness Handout 6, "Mindfulness 'How' Skills."
The "how" skills are *how* you observe, describe, or participate. There are three "how" skills: *Don't judge, stay focused*, and *do what works*.

Don't Judge

Notice, but don't evaluate what you notice as good or bad. Stick to the observable facts, using only what is observed with your senses.

• *Acknowledge the harmful and the helpful, but don't judge it.* For example, replace "You're being an idiot" with "I feel mad when you walk away when we're talking."

• *"Judging" is sometimes shorthand for acknowledging what's harmful or helpful.* In all fairness, quickly judging things can *sometimes* be helpful as a shorthand way of moving through the world. Judging has its place, and we all need to do it sometimes. For example, you are about to sit down to eat breakfast. You pour cereal into the bowl, reach for the milk, open it up, and catch a whiff of a foul odor. You look inside and see that it is curdled, and you say to your family, "This milk is bad." Perfect. We don't need more description since we want people to steer clear of that milk and drink something else. At 7:30 A.M., when people are rushing around the house before school and work, they don't need a dissertation about the type of odor, the color of the milk, the curdling process, etc. Our society is built on judgments—just watch *American Idol* and the judges saying, "You're the best one in the competition" or reading *People* magazine's "Worst Dressed/Best Dressed." Americans like to judge. And, it can be useful to judge people or things that can cause us harm.

DISCUSSION POINT: *Ask*, "When does judging others *or* yourself become a problem? Think about this question as it relates to getting yourself into Emotion Mind or keeping yourself stuck in Emotion Mind." *Help participants recognize that judgments (e.g., "You loser!" or "I'm so stupid!") often intensify Emotion Mind, which then often leads to Emotion Mind behaviors such as blurting out in class, yelling at someone, physical aggression, self-harm, and so on.*

 • ***Be more aware of your judgments.*** The more you are aware of and observe your own judgments, the more readily you can access your Wise Mind, make Wise Mind decisions, and reduce your suffering.

EXERCISE 1

First, invite participants to describe, without holding back judgments, for example, a controversial event in the news that elicits strong emotions. Whatever example is chosen, it is important to give sufficient detail so that every member in the group will be adequately prompted to experience strong reactions, including judgments.

Next, invite participants to describe the same even without judgmental language, just sticking to the facts. Discuss observations about how difficult this is to do, *and* how describing nonjudgmentally lessens one's emotional reactions.

EXERCISE 2 (OPTIONAL)

Invite those who identify as Democrats to write down their feelings about a controversial figure from another political party on a piece of paper. Ask Republicans to do the same. No one needs to identify their political affiliation if they do not want to; however, by sharing their examples, they sometimes show it. Ask the other group members to practice listening without judgment. Leaders could also use other opposing groups, such as rival sports teams.

EXERCISE 3 (OPTIONAL)

Ask participants to nonjudgmentally describe a beloved figure in their lives (famous or not) without judgment. Stick just to the observable facts about this person. Ask participants to nonjudgmentally describe a "hated" or loathsome historical figure, or someone recently in the news. *Note:* Ask members to select a person who will *not* dysregulate them! Share observations about how difficult it is to practice thinking, writing, and speaking nonjudgmentally. Ask them to notice, when they are expressing themselves nonjudgmentally, what it does to their emotional state.

 • ***Catch and replace judgments.*** You can't go through life without making judgments; your goal is to catch them and replace them with descriptions so you have more control over your emotions. One way to think about this is to return to the fish tank example at the aquarium, from the above discussion on the skill of describing, rather than judging. When you're staring at fish going around the tank, you'll rarely hear someone say, "That fish is a real jerk!" You might say, "That one has gold, shimmery scales; that blue and orange one swam past the yellow one; or that little one is swimming along the bottom." Think about these examples when trying to restate your judgments with factual descriptions.

 • ***Don't judge your judging.*** Many of us become judgmental; then, when we realize how judgmental we sound, we judge ourselves for that. Again, try to mindfully observe not only your initial judgments but the judgments *about* your initial judgments and try to let those go.

EXERCISE

Find pictures or videos representing fashion and hairstyles from an earlier decade, or of controversial figures in politics or entertainment. Ask participants to describe without judgment.

EXERCISE

Write down unedited recent self-judgments; describe the effects of these self-judgments (e.g., "I'm worthless"; "I look ugly").

How to Let Go of Judging

To let go of initial or secondary judgments, one needs to practice the following:

1. Observe judgment nonjudgmentally.
2. Describe the observable facts about the selected focus. For example, instead of saying "I'm a dummy," you could say, "I got 6 out of 24 math questions wrong; my teacher gave me a 75 on my test. I notice the feeling of embarrassment and anger at myself for doing that poorly, given how hard I studied. I notice myself clenching my jaw and shaking my head when I think about it. I notice having the urge to avoid my math homework this week."
3. Practice again and again (starting now).

Stay Focused (One-Mindfully)

Sometimes when I come home from work, I pick up the mail from the mailbox. As I enter my home, I am opening up some of the mail. I sometimes turn the phone on speakerphone and listen to the voicemail messages while also reviewing the mail. Occasionally the TV news may be on, and I'll also be glancing at that. I might grab an apple from the fridge and take a bite, while listening to the voicemail, reading my mail, watching TV. If my spouse or kids walked by and said, "Hey, how are you?" I don't think I would be aware of the answer given the load of information I was trying to process and how unfocused I was. In fact, I would likely have no idea in that moment.

• ***Do only one thing in the moment.*** To become aware of what one is thinking, feeling, or doing, one needs to try to do *only* one thing in the moment.

Our minds sometimes become like a messy room. They are cluttered, piled high with stuff, disorganized, and it's really hard to find what we're looking for in there. When we do only one thing at a time and really focus the mind, it's like we organized stuff and put it away. We can better pull things out that we need.

• ***Stop multitasking.*** Multitasking is (1) *not* efficient, according to the latest research, and (2) it can cause information overload, be potentially stress inducing, and cloud one's awareness of thoughts, feelings, and urges [*e.g., see Parker-Pope, 2010*].

- *Slow down.* In order to be mindful, it is important to slow yourself down enough to do one thing at a time. Do you ever notice how much time you waste by trying to do two things at once? Think about the last time you were texting a friend while carrying on a conversation with someone else simultaneously. The text takes longer and the conversation needs to be resumed continuously. Not to mention the toll it takes on the relationship itself when you keep saying, "Wait, what did you say—I didn't hear you, I was texting someone else."

> **Note to Leaders:** You can address common challenges to this notion of one-mindfully. Some teens argue that they are masters of multitasking. Below is an example that helps to illustrate the value of doing only one thing at a time, and the perils of multitasking.

DISCUSSION POINT: *Ask,* "How many of you have driven in cars with people who are texting while driving? How about people who are driving and talking on the phone, hands free, in a heated discussion with someone?" *Many teens will say they have, or they have done this themselves, and that it is fine; they can handle it.*

Then ask, "So what if you were in surgery? How many of you would feel comfortable with your surgeon texting with one hand while doing surgery? How about if the surgeon were talking on the phone—hands free, of course—while repairing your aorta? How's that working for you?" *Invite responses. Most teens will say, "No way!" Ask why, which results in* their *now arguing on the side of one-mindful participation in important activities.*

How to Stay Focused

Invite participants to discuss and then review the following points:

1. Do one thing at a time (e.g., observe, describe, or participate).
2. Let go of distractions.
3. Concentrate your mind (the opposite of multitasking) and refocus your attention, again and again, when it drifts.
4. Stay focused so that the past, future, and current distractions do not get in your way.

DISCUSSION POINT: *Say to participants,* "How many of you notice yourself sitting at school or sitting at work and find that your mind is focusing on upsetting past events, worrying about the future, or being grabbed by distractions? If you are not focused on the current moment, you are *not* living in the moment. If you are not living in the current moment, you will *not* be able to access the potential joys of the current moment. In fact, you may only be perpetuating your own misery by living in the past or future.

"This is not to say that you should *never* lament the past or prepare for the future. We are saying only that we think we spend too much time in the past and future and *not enough* time in the present, thereby missing golden opportunities to live in the *now.* Try to *only* focus on your conversation with your friend and *not* text or look at your other screens or electronic gadgets. Try to eat that slice of pizza or eat that piece of chocolate and really taste it. Try to walk outside and notice the blooming flowers, plants, and trees and not focus on what else you have to do afterward. Practice doing only one thing at a time."

EXERCISE

Have participants practice doing only one thing at a time for 2–3 minutes. They can walk around the room and notice the sensations of walking; stare at a penny, snow globe, picture, or kaleidoscope; notice their breath; read a magazine; or engage in a conversation with another group member. What-ever the activity, they should concentrate their minds on it with no distractions, and bring their attention back if they notice it grabbed by something else. After, invite observations.

EXERCISE (FOR ENERGIZING THE GROUP)

Pass out lists of simple addition/subtraction problems, or ask people to start with 100 and subtract backwards by 7s on paper. At the same time as members are completing the math, have the group sing aloud together a well-known song such as "Happy Birthday" or "Row, Row, Row Your Boat." After, ask group members to try focusing *only* on the math or on the singing. Ask group members what they noticed about the contrast between doing two things at once versus focusing one-mindfully on one task at a time. What did they notice about their attention? Their emotions?

Do What Works (Effectiveness)

Focus on what works. Don't let emotions control your behavior; cut the cord between feeling and doing.

- *Acting on feeling usually doesn't work.* Many of you probably act on how you feel, right? The last time you were pissed off at your teacher, you may have had the urge (and maybe even acted on it) to not do your homework. Do you remember the last time you were angry at your parents when they denied your request to go to a party, or wouldn't give you the car keys? Did you yell at them before slamming the door? Do you remember the last time you were worried about a social situation and you decided to avoid it? That is *not* focusing on what works; instead, it's allowing your Emotion Mind to control your behavior. Focusing on what works is doing the following:

- *Play by the rules to meet your goals.* We mean being aware of and following the rules of the specific culture and context you are in (i.e., your family, your school, your team).

- *Act as skillfully as you can.* Use skillful means as opposed to getting what you want through Emotion Mind action.

- *Do what you need to achieve your Wise Mind long-term goals.* This is not always imme-diately evident. For example, one senior in high school was upset when her teacher embar-rassed her in front of her peers by saying, "Elizabeth, you didn't turn in your homework again." Although it was true that Elizabeth had a history of noncompliance in this arena, she was sure she had handed in this assignment. She felt angry and had an urge to "set the record straight" in the moment. Her short-term goals would have been met by relieving her anger and having the teacher know immediately that he'd made a mistake. Yet, her long-term goals would not have been met by acting on the impulse, since this teacher would not have liked being called "wrong" in front of the class. So, Elizabeth decided that "doing what works" meant tolerating her distress until the end of the period and using her DBT interpersonal effectiveness skills (GIVE and DEAR MAN) with her teacher to clarify what appeared to be a misunderstanding.

   • *Let go of negative feelings* (e.g., vengeance and useless anger). They can hurt you and make things worse. (*Refer to the example of Elizabeth above.*)

   • *Let go of "shoulds."* Being flexible is often more effective. Many of us feel as though we need to *prove* a point and let the person know how we *really* feel so that there is no confusion about it. Ask yourself: How do you feel when someone says to you, "You should do this," or "You shouldn't have done that"? Usually bad. So, try not to "should" on yourself or anyone else. Instead say, "It would be helpful if . . ." or "I'd prefer it if . . . ," and so on. This will alleviate the pressure to prove a point and in turn may reduce your emotional distress and help you access your Wise Mind.

HOW TO PRACTICE MINDFULNESS

Refer participants to Mindfulness Handout 7, "Mindfulness Cheat Sheet."

> **Note to Leaders:** Alert participants that the information about how to engage in a mindfulness practice is written down, step by step, on Mindfulness Handout 7. Explain: "This is your basic quick-and-dirty cheat sheet on how to practice mindfulness. We will model it for you at the beginning of every group; however, we'd like you to get used to practicing mindfulness in daily life outside of group, and here are the instructions."
>
> At the end of this chapter is a list of various mindfulness exercises that adolescents and families report finding helpful.

ASSIGNMENT OF HOMEWORK

Assign Mindfulness Handout 8, "Practice Exercise: 'What' and 'How' Skills." Ask participants to commit to practicing one mindfulness "what" skill and one mindfulness "how" skill over the next week. Check on the skills practiced on Handout 8 and briefly describe what, when, and where the skills were practiced and how they affected their thoughts, feelings, or behaviors.

MINDFULNESS EXERCISES FOR ADOLESCENTS[*]

This section presents a sampling of mindfulness exercises that work well with adolescents. Some of these were taken or adapted from standard DBT; we have developed others for this population. Therapists can use still other mindfulness exercises as well, as we do at times. These exercises often allow for practice in all components of mindfulness; thus the descriptions of which aspects of mindfulness are taught refer to those aspects that are particularly emphasized in each exercise.

---

[*]From Miller, Rathus, and Linehan (2007, pp. 275–284). Copyright 2007 by The Guilford Press. Adapted by permission.

General Tips for Conducting Exercises

The group leaders should briefly orient the members to each exercise, including making a link between the exercise and a treatment goal (e.g., "helping us notice our experience more fully," "helping us reduce judgments, so that we can minimize Emotion Mind"), or telling a story to illustrate the utility of a mindfulness practice.

- All group members should participate, including family members.
- For most exercises, members can either close their eyes or focus on a point in front of them that will not be distracting.
- Cell phones and other potential distractors should be turned off, and objects group members are holding (e.g., pens, notebooks) should be put down.
- Most exercises can run for between 2 and 5 minutes. As group members gain more experience with doing exercises, they can run longer.
- Participants can be instructed that if their thinking or attention drifts, they should nonjudgmentally notice the drifting and bring attention back to the exercise.
- Group leaders should allow several minutes for participants to share observations regarding the exercise.
- Leaders can conclude by stating one purpose of the exercise (learning to participate without judgment; observing and describing emotions as the first steps for getting into Wise Mind; getting more information about a situation by taking the time to stop and notice our experiences; etc.).

Exercise 1: What's Different about Me?

Two group members pair off and mindfully observe each other. Then they turn their backs, change three things (e.g., glasses, watch, and hair), and turn back toward each other. Can they notice the changes?

Variant: Whose penny? Every group member takes a penny from a bowl, holds it a moment, and puts it back in the bowl. Then each member takes one again, and *really* studies it (staying focused, doing one thing at a time), and puts it back in the bowl. Finally, each member tries to pick out his or her own penny. Discussion follows: Could they have identified their own pennies the first time? Why not?

Aspect of mindfulness taught: Observing one-mindfully.

Exercise 2: Sound Ball

One group member "throws" a sound across the room to another group member. That member then "catches" the same sound by repeating it exactly and then "throws" a new sound to someone else— and so on, with a new sound each time.

Variant: Word ball. Same as above, using words instead of sounds.

Aspect of mindfulness taught: Observing and participating one-mindfully.

Exercise 3: Snap, Crackle, and Pop

All group members are instructed to say "snap" when they cross their chests with their left or right arm and point immediately either left or right; to say "crackle" when they raise their left or right arm over their heads and point immediately left or right; and to say "pop" when they point at anyone around the circle (who does not need to be immediately left or right). Any one person starts by saying "snap" while simultaneously pointing immediately either left or right. Whoever receives the point says "crackle" while simultaneously pointing immediately left or right. Whoever receives the point says "pop" while pointing at anyone in the circle. That person then starts with "snap" and begins the sequence again. Anyone who misspeaks or misgestures, while trying to maintain a reasonably fast pace, is out of this portion of the exercise. These people then become "distractors" and stand outside of the circle trying to distract their peers (verbally, without physical contact). The "snap–crackle–pop" sequence continues until there are only two people remaining in the circle.

Aspect of mindfulness taught: Observing and participating one-mindfully.

Exercise 4: Observation of Music

Leaders play a piece of music that is typically not a teen favorite and ask group members, while listening quietly, to observe and describe nonjudgmentally while fully letting the experience surround them (their thoughts, emotions, physiological changes, urges). Variants include playing segments of two or three very different pieces (in terms of style, tempo, etc.) and having group members observe changes in the music and in their internal reactions.

Aspect of mindfulness taught: Observing, describing, and participating without judgment.

Exercise 5: Egg Balancing

Several members try to balance an egg upright on a table for 2 minutes.

Aspect of mindfulness taught: Observing one-mindfully, nonjudgmentally, and with effectiveness.

Exercise 6: Hand Exercise

Group members stand around an oval or rectangular table. Each member is instructed to place his or her left hand on the table. Then each member places his or her right hand underneath the left hand of the person to the right. One person starts the sequence by picking the right hand off the table and quickly placing it back down. The person to the right quickly lifts up his or her right hand. The hand movements continue around the circle in sequence—until someone does a double tap. This move reverses the direction of the hand movements, and these continue in the reverse direction until someone does a double tap again. Anyone who picks up a hand too early or too late removes that one hand and leaves the other hand on the table (if the other hand was doing what it was supposed to do). The exercise continues until only a couple of hands are left.

Aspect of mindfulness taught: Observing one-mindfully and nonjudgmentally.

Exercise 7: Mindfully Unwrapping a Hershey's Kiss

Each group member sits in a comfortable position with a Hershey's Kiss in front of him or her. A leader says:

> "After I ring the bell the third time, observe and describe the outside of the Hershey's Kiss to yourself. Feel the differences in the texture between the paper tag and the foil. As you begin to unwrap the chocolate, note how the shape and texture of the foil change in comparison to the paper tag as well as the chocolate. Feel the chocolate and how it changes in your hand. If your mind wanders from the exercise, note the distraction without judgment, and then return your attention to the chocolate."

Aspect of mindfulness taught: Observing and describing one-mindfully.

Exercise 8. Mindfulness PB&J

A leader says:

> "Often when we are engaged in a monotonous activity—something we find boring, unengaging, or even unpleasant (but required)—we find that our minds wander. Rather than attending to what we are doing, our heads fill with thoughts of what we wish we were doing, how we can't stand what we are doing now, how unfair and stupid it is that we have to do this, and so on. Instead of being aware of our thoughts, feelings, and sensations in the present moment, without judging them, we cloud our minds with negative thoughts, feelings, and judgments. By using 'Wise Mind,' we are able to participate fully in the moment, without worry about future concerns or feelings of self-consciousness.
>
> "Imagine that you are on the social committee for a group picnic. Your task is to make peanut butter and jelly sandwiches. Your supplies are arrayed on the table in front of you. I want you to pretend you are making a peanut butter and jelly sandwich. Go through each of the actions that you would need to do in order to make the sandwich. Take two pieces of bread, pick up your knife, and so on. Don't leave out any steps. As you are making your sandwich, concentrate fully on the act of making the sandwich—think about how creamy the peanut butter is, how the consistency of the jelly is different, how you have to handle the bread so as not to damage it. When you are done making your sandwich, put it aside and begin making the next sandwich. Your goal is to concentrate on the act of making the sandwich. If your mind starts to wander, bring your attention back to participating fully in the task."

Aspect of mindfulness taught: Observing, describing, and participating one-mindfully and non-judgmentally.

Exercise 9. Repeating an Activity

A leader says:

> "When the bell rings, sit at the table with your arms resting on the table. Very slowly, reach several inches to pick up a pen. Raise it a few inches and then set it down. Move your hand back to its original position of rest. While you repeat this action throughout the time period, experience each repetition with freshness, as though you have never done it before. You can allow your attention to wander toward different aspects of the movement: watching your hand or feeling the muscles contracting. You can even notice your sense of touch, being aware of the different textures and pressures. Let go of any distractions or judgments you may have. This activity will help you to become mindful of a simple activity that you perform often throughout the day."

Aspect of mindfulness taught: Observing and describing one-mindfully, nonjudgmentally.

Exercise 10: Focusing on Scent

Leaders bring in scented candles. Group members are instructed: "Choose a candle. When the bell rings, sit back in your chair and find a comfortable and relaxed position. Close your eyes and begin to focus on the smell of the candle. Let go of any distractions or judgments. Notice how the smell makes you feel and what images it evokes." Afterward, leaders and participants discuss observations, emotions, thoughts, feelings, and sensations: "How did the scent make you feel? What images came to your mind? Did the smell remind you of anything in particular?"

Aspect of mindfulness taught: Observing one-mindfully and nonjudgmentally.

Exercise 11: Mindfully Eating a Raisin

Group leaders distribute raisins. Group members are each asked to hold a raisin; observe its appearance, texture, and scent; then put it in their mouths and slowly, with awareness, begin eating—noticing the tastes, sensations, and even the sounds of eating. This can also be done with candies (sweet tarts, caramels, fruit chews, fireballs, etc.).

Aspect of mindfulness taught: Observing and describing one-mindfully and nonjudgmentally.

Exercise 12: Switched-Candy Exercise

Leaders bring in a box of assorted chocolates or a bag of assorted treats, and ask group members to carefully select the item they think they would enjoy the most and place it in front of them. Leaders remind the group members to be fully present and nonjudgmental of the experience. Just before they begin, each member is asked to pass the chosen item to the person on his or her left. Members observe their reactions. Now members place their new piece of candy in their mouths; close their eyes; and use all of their senses to observe the smell, texture, and taste of their candy. Leaders remind them to bring their attention back to the selected focus if their minds wander. After a few minutes, group members are instructed to open their eyes, and leaders elicit observations about the experience.

Aspect of mindfulness taught: Radical acceptance; observing and describing one-mindfully and nonjudgmentally.

Exercise 13: Ice Cube Exercise

Each group member holds an ice cube in a hand, lets it melt, and observes/describes the experience.

Aspect of mindfulness taught: Observing and describing one-mindfully and nonjudgmentally.

Exercise 14: Texture Exercise

Group members feel different-textured objects in a bag, and observe/describe these.

Aspect of mindfulness taught: Observing and describing one-mindfully.

Exercise 15: Banging the Drum

Group members are asked to drum a beat on the table. One person starts, then the adjacent person adds to it, and so on, until all are drumming and keeping their beat.

Aspect of mindfulness taught: Participating one-mindfully.

Exercise 16: Walking the Line

Leaders put a line of tape on the floor. Each group member in turn walks on the line, placing one foot directly in front of the other, with full attention to the activity. The members share observations about it (e.g., losing their balance).

Variant: Balancing on one foot. Group members stand up and get behind their chairs. With one hand on the chair to steady themselves, each member lifts one foot and attempts to balance on the other. When able, each person can remove the hand from the chair and balance on the one foot, with full attention to the activity.

Aspect of mindfulness taught: Observing and describing one-mindfully and nonjudgmentally; also, experiential metaphor for maintaining "balance" of Emotion and Reasonable Minds, and of thoughts and actions.

Exercise 17: Wise Mind Charades

Group leaders act out each of three states of mind, one at a time, while role-playing a scenario (e.g., argument with a relative over curfew). Group members try to guess their state of mind. They then discuss how they came to the answer (tone of voice, body language, word choice, etc.). Finally, leaders ask for two group member volunteers to act out a state of mind in their own role play.

    Aspect of mindfulness taught: Observing and describing states of mind: Reasonable Mind, Emotion Mind, and Wise Mind.

Exercise 18: Row Your Boat

Group members are divided into two or three groups and are asked to sing "Row, Row, Row Your Boat" in rounds, starting with the first group. Leaders gesture when each group should start. Members then describe their experiences, including self-consciousness and judgments. Leaders discuss the notion of nonjudgmental participation, and now ask members to try again—this time really "hamming it up" with hand gestures and booming voices, throwing themselves into the experience. Leaders and participants discuss the difference between the first and second times.

    Aspect of mindfulness taught: Participating without judgment.

Exercise 19: Mindful Listening

Leaders ask group members to break into pairs and discuss a topic of importance to them. The listeners are asked *not* to be mindful, and instead to act distracted or bored. Leaders then ask the speakers what it was like to talk to someone who was not being mindful. Now the pairs practice again, with the listeners being mindful, putting all attention into the interaction. Leaders and speakers discuss the difference: What was it like?

    Variant: Mindful listening and speaking. Same as above, except that the first time, speakers act distracted as well. Then, in the second practice, both speakers and listeners are mindful in the interaction. Both then discuss what it was like to interact with someone who was distracted versus mindful.

    Aspect of mindfulness taught: Observing one-mindfully; also, interpersonal effectiveness and Level 1 validation (see Chapter 3).

Exercise 20: What's in a Face?

A leader says:

> "Be mindful of your face. Notice the different parts of your face from your forehead to your chin. Are they relaxed or tensed? Are there other sensations? What is your facial expression? Try to notice without changing your expression or experience." Afterward, leaders and participants discuss observations.

    Variant: Body sensations. Leaders ask group members to be mindful of sensations, tension, position, and so forth, within their bodies, since paying attention to physical sensations is important for learning to identify emotions. Discussion follows.

    Aspect of mindfulness taught: Observing and describing one-mindfully.

Exercise 21: Focusing on the Breath

A leader says:

> "Get into a comfortable position and just notice the experience of your breath going in and out. Pay attention to what each breath feels like coming in through your nose or mouth, and notice how your lungs expand like a balloon. Then notice how it feels when you exhale."

Aspect of mindfulness taught: Observing and describing one-mindfully.

Exercise 22: Observing Emotions

A leader says:

> "Notice the emotions you are experiencing, and try to note how you know you are having those emotions. That is, what labels do you have in mind? What thoughts, what body sensations, and so on, give you information about the emotions? Describe to yourself where you feel the sensations."

Aspect of mindfulness taught: Observing and describing.

Exercise 23: What's My Experience?

A leader says:

> "Focus your mind on your experience this very moment. Be mindful of any thoughts, feelings, body sensations, urges, or anything else you become aware of. Don't judge your experience, or try to push it away or hold onto it. Just let experiences come and go like clouds moving across the sky."

Aspect of mindfulness taught: Observing and describing one-mindfully and nonjudgmentally.

Exercise 24: Noticing Urges

A leader says:

> "Sit very straight in your chair. Throughout this exercise, notice any urges—whether to move, shift positions, scratch an itch, or do something else. Instead of acting on the urge, simply notice it."

Leaders and participants then discuss the experience. Was it possible to have an urge and not act on it?
Aspect of mindfulness taught: Observing and describing one-mindfully; also, distress tolerance (not acting on urges, even when not acting is uncomfortable).

Exercise 25: Observing Thoughts

A leader says:

> "Notice your thoughts as they come and go, as if they were scrolling by on a message board on a marquee, or on the bottom of the screen on CNN. Truly notice your thoughts, as opposed to thinking them, dwelling on them, pushing them away, or changing them. Try not to get stuck on a thought or get caught up in believing or reacting to them. Notice what they are, which are just . . . thoughts."

Aspect of mindfulness taught: Observing one-mindfully and nonjudgmentally.

Exercise 26: Blowing Bubbles

Leaders pass out containers of bubble solution to group members. Members are asked to dip their wands and begin blowing bubbles—focusing all of their attention on this one moment, on the bubbles; noticing their shapes, textures, colors, and so on. If they get distracted by other thoughts, they should gently bring their attention back to the process of bubble blowing.

Aspect of mindfulness taught: Observing one-mindfully and nonjudgmentally.

Exercise 27: Imagery of a Recent Experience

A leader says:

> "Think of a time you were upset recently with a boyfriend, girlfriend, or family member. Take a moment and try to conjure up the experience as though it were happening now—notice your thoughts, feelings, urges, body sensations, and so forth. Observe your experiences, let yourself experience them fully without judging them, and then silently put words on these experiences (e.g., 'Tears are welling up in my eyes,' 'My shoulders feel tense,' 'My thoughts are racing'). Your goal is to practice getting into Wise Mind as if you were in the situation this moment."

Variant: Doing what works. Same as above, except that after 2 minutes of observing experiences, the leader says: "Think of one goal of yours in this situation. Think of something you could do or say to 'do what works.' That is, focus on effectiveness."

Aspect of mindfulness taught: Wise Mind, observing and describing nonjudgmentally and effectively.

Note: Instruct members to choose a scenario that will not dysregulate them!

Exercise 28: Changing One Letter

Group members sit in a comfortable position. When a group leader rings the bell the third time, he or she will start the exercise by saying a three-letter (or four-letter, if leaders would like to make it a bit more complex) word. Then the next person changes any one letter in the word just said by the leader to make a new word, and says it out loud. After that, the next person takes this new word and changes one letter to make a completely new word, and so on. (Sample sequence: *dog, dig, pig*)

Aspect of mindfulness taught: Attending one-mindfully (staying focused).

Exercise 29: Last Letter, First Letter

To begin this exercise, group members sit in a circle. The first person begins by saying a word. Then the individual to the right must say a word that starts with the last letter of the word the first person says. (Sample sequence: *bus, steak, key, yellow*) As you continue around the circle, let go of any distractions. Notice any judgments you may have regarding your ability to think of a word quickly." Afterward, leaders and participants discuss observations.

Aspect of mindfulness taught: Attending one-mindfully and nonjudgmentally.

Exercise 30: Formal Walking Meditation

A leader says:

> "To do the walking meditation, you need a place with enough space for at least 5–10 paces in a straight line. Select an unobstructed area and start at one end. Stand for a moment in an attentive position. Your arms can be held in any way that is comfortable. Then, while breathing in, lift one foot and bring it forward. While breathing out, bring the foot down and touch the floor. Repeat this for the other foot. Walk slowly to the opposite end, then turn around slowly and stand there for a moment before you walk back. Then repeat the process. Keep your eyes open to maintain balance, but don't look at anything in particular. Walk naturally. Place your full attention on this experience of walking. Watch for tensions building in the body; put all of your attention on the sensations coming from the feet and legs. Experience every tiny change in tactile sensation as the feet press against the floor and then lift again, so that the feet become your whole universe. If your mind wanders, note the distraction in the usual way, then return your attention to walking. Don't look at your feet while you are doing all of this, and don't walk back and forth watching a mental picture of your feet and legs."

Aspect of mindfulness taught: Observing one-mindfully.

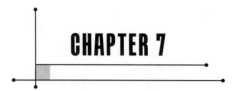

CHAPTER 7

Distress Tolerance

SESSION OUTLINES

Session 1

▶ Brief Mindfulness Exercise

▶ Homework Review

▶ Break

▶ Orientation of Clients to Distress Tolerance Skills and Their Rationale

▶ Crisis Survival Skills

▶ Assignment of Homework

▶ Session Wind-Down

Handouts and Other Materials

▶ Distress Tolerance Handout 1, "Why Bother Tolerating Painful Feelings and Urges?"

▶ Distress Tolerance Handout 2, "Crisis Survival Skills Overview"

▶ Distress Tolerance Handout 3, "Crisis Survival Skills: Distract with 'Wise Mind ACCEPTS'"

▶ Distress Tolerance Handout 4, "Practice Exercise: Distract with 'Wise Mind ACCEPTS'"

▶ Mindfulness bell

▶ Whiteboard or other large writing surface and markers

▶ A selection of materials for "distracting" activities (e.g., games, puzzles, magazines, music)

Session 2

▶ Brief Mindfulness Exercise

▶ Homework Review

▶ Break

- Self-Soothe with Six Senses
- IMPROVE the Moment
- Assignment of Homework
- Session Wind-Down

Handouts and Other Materials

- Materials to use for self-soothing activities (e.g., herbal tea, music, scented candles)
- Distress Tolerance Handout 5, "Crisis Survival Skills: Self-Soothe with Six Senses"
- Distress Tolerance Handout 6, "Practice Exercise: Self-Soothe Skills"
- Distress Tolerance Handout 7, "Crisis Survival Skills: IMPROVE the Moment"
- Distress Tolerance Handout 8, "Practice Exercise: IMPROVE the Moment"
- Mindfulness bell
- Whiteboard or other large writing surface and markers

Session 3

- Brief Mindfulness Exercise
- Homework Review
- Break
- Pros and Cons
- TIPP Skills
- Assignment of Homework
- Session Wind-Down

Handouts and Other Materials

- Distress Tolerance Handout 9, "Crisis Survival Skills: Pros and Cons"
- Distress Tolerance Handout 10, "Practice Exercise: Pros and Cons"
- Distress Tolerance Handout 11, "Crisis Survival Skills: TIPP Skills for Managing Extreme Emotions"
- Distress Tolerance Handout 12, "Practice Exercise: TIPP Skills"
- Mindfulness bell
- Whiteboard or other large writing surface and markers
- Chilled cold compresses, gel eye masks, or 1-pint reclosable plastic bags with ice cubes; paper towels (for TIPP temperature)
- A large clock with a visible second hand (for paced breathing)

Session 4

- Brief Mindfulness Exercise: Half-Smile
- Homework Review

▷ Break

▷ Reality Acceptance Skills

▷ Assignment of Homework

▷ Session Wind-Down

Handouts and Other Materials

▷ Distress Tolerance Handout 13, "Create Your Crisis Survival Kit for Home, School, or Work"

▷ Distress Tolerance Handout 14, "Accepting Reality: Choices We Can Make"

▷ Distress Tolerance Handout 15, "Accepting Reality: Turning the Mind"

▷ Distress Tolerance Handout 16, "Willingness"

▷ Distress Tolerance Handout 17, "Ways to Practice Accepting Reality"

▷ Distress Tolerance Handout 18, "Practice Exercise: Accepting Reality"

▷ Mindfulness bell

▷ Whiteboard or other large writing surface and markers

TEACHING NOTES

Nothing is more desirable than to be released from an affliction, but nothing is more frightening than to be divested of a crutch.
    —JAMES A. BALDWIN

It is our choices . . . that show what we truly are, far more than our abilities.
    —ALBUS DUMBLEDORE (in *Harry Potter and the Chamber of Secrets*, by J. K. Rowling)

ABOUT THIS MODULE

Distress tolerance skills help clients tolerate difficult situations and emotional pain when the problems cannot be solved right away. This module contains two types of distress tolerance skills. Sessions 1–3 cover the first type, the crisis survival skills. They emphasize changing one's experience of the distress by distracting, self-soothing, improving the moment, considering pros and cons of impulsive versus effective action, and "tipping" one's body chemistry to rapidly reduce extreme arousal. These strategies help one survive the crisis without making it worse through impulsive action. Importantly, these skills provide short-term solutions that do not solve the core problem causing the distress and do not necessarily make people feel better. Instead, they help one bear pain skillfully by not engaging in problem behaviors, including substance use, disordered eating, or self-harm.

To teach the distraction and self-soothing skills, skills trainers should bring a number of distracting and soothing materials into the respective sessions. Distracting materials might include word search puzzles, Sudoku, colored markers and paper, and magazines. Showing brief, funny YouTube videos could also work. Self-soothing materials might include lotions, herbal teas, scented candles, small stuffed furry animals, music, photos of sunsets and beaches, silky scarves, chocolates, and so on. To teach TIPP skills, skills trainers should bring in chilled cold packs or ice water in small ziplock bags. In addition to practicing the various distress tolerance skills in the skills training session, the homework for this set of skills includes the creation of a personalized crisis survival kit. We also encourage the creation of a portable, mini-distress tolerance kit for use in school, at work, at camp, or in transit.

The remaining module time is devoted to the second set of distress tolerance skills: reality acceptance skills. These help one learn how to fully accept painful circumstances that cannot be changed, rather than avoiding or fighting them in a way that only increases suffering. Through radical acceptance and a willingness to embrace reality as it is, one can reduce emotional suffering and move forward in a more centered and effective manner. As described in the teaching notes, we suggest that the half-smile be used as a mindfulness exercise at the start of Session 4.

SESSION 1
BRIEF MINDFULNESS EXERCISE
· · · ·
HOMEWORK REVIEW
· · · ·
BREAK
· · · ·

ORIENTATION OF CLIENTS TO DISTRESS TOLERANCE SKILLS AND THEIR RATIONALE

Start by explaining that the next few weeks will be spent on skills for distress tolerance.

*Ask the teens, "What does *distress* mean? What does *tolerance* mean?" Leaders take definitions from the group, noting that tolerance involves putting up with, rather than changing or getting rid of, an unwanted situation. Leaders should then share a personal example, such as the following:*

"Has anyone ever been on a cruise ship or seen one on TV? So, imagine me—I am on this cruise ship leaving New York Harbor. We get out into the Atlantic heading south toward Florida. I am walking around the promenade deck taking in the sights one afternoon when all of a sudden I skid on a banana peel and fall overboard. Now, by the time I land in the water, become submerged, and then rise back up to the surface, the cruise ship has moved quickly past me. In the far distance I see another boat and it looks like it's heading toward me. I cannot see land at all. What do you think I am feeling? What is my urge? What would you do in that moment—seeing your cruise ship moving away?"

DISCUSSION POINT: *Elicit comments. Typically someone suggests swimming to the cruise ship, others say to frantically wave and scream for help. Give everyone a chance to think about it, validating the emotion of fear/panic, validating the action urge to swim and scream. Then offer the Wise Mind distress tolerance solution: to not swim, to not scream, but rather to do what is known as the "survival float" until the other boat arrives. Explain to participants:*

"It requires enormous mindfulness and distress tolerance skills to not act impulsively. If I were to act on my panic, I would most likely make the situation worse and drown. This is what you need to understand about distress tolerance skills. It is not about making yourself feel better. I wasn't feeling good floating in the Atlantic Ocean—I was quite *distressed*! However, I was not doing things impulsively that would make my situation worse; rather, I *tolerated* the situation."

DISCUSSION POINT: *Elicit one or two examples of someone in distress acting impulsively and making the situation worse.*

Why Bother Tolerating Painful Feelings and Urges?

Refer participants to Distress Tolerance Handout 1, "Why Bother Tolerating Painful Feelings and Urges?"

- Everyone has to deal with pain in life; life is not pain-free. (*Invite participants to agree or disagree.*)
- Always trying to avoid pain might lead to more problems than it solves. (*Invite participants to agree or disagree.*)
- Avoiding pain may lead you to act impulsively, and you may end up hurting yourself or not getting what you want. (*Invite participants to agree or disagree.*)

For example, say you are really upset, so you get drunk. Then you get caught, and you get grounded. Now you have even more things to be upset about. Much of our skills training focuses on how to change distressing events and circumstances, such as reducing arguments with people or improving depression. But distressing situations often can't be changed immediately. Therefore:

- You need to have ways of coping with and accepting distress.
- You will learn skills to survive and do well in really tough situations without falling back on old behaviors that will make things worse.

CRISIS SURVIVAL SKILLS

Refer participants to Distress Tolerance Handout 2, "Crisis Survival Skills Overview."

Over the next few sessions, we will teach you crisis survival strategies. These are strategies that help you get through a crisis. What is a crisis? When you are really upset or things are really stressful, it is a short-term situation and you want it resolved now but can't. Perhaps the only solutions you can think of will make it even worse. These skills help you cope with overwhelming emotions or intolerable situations. They aren't supposed to solve your problems, but they will help you survive painful emotions and not act on your urges.

Distract with Wise Mind ACCEPTS

Distraction can be effective in the short term to help cope with distress.

Self-Soothe with Six Senses

Soothing oneself is also a critical crisis survival skill. Some people are better at being soothed when they are not highly distressed and find it more difficult when they are. Practice can help.

IMPROVE the Moment

Introduce the idea that there are ways to improve the moment we are in by managing what we are doing internally, within ourselves.

Pros and Cons

Weighing the advantages and disadvantages of acting impulsively versus acting skillfully (considering Wise Mind goals) is a fourth crisis survival skill we will teach. This skill requires some time and thought and can buy you time before acting impulsively.

TIPP

TIPP skills tip our body chemistry rapidly. These skills can be used when you are so highly distressed that you cannot think clearly and remember other skills to use.

Distress Tolerance Skills Require Mindfulness Skills

All of these skills require individuals to use their mindfulness skills first. You can't possibly make use of your crisis survival skills if you are not aware (i.e., mindful) that you are distressed and need skills in the first place. Thus, your Wise Mind will hopefully indicate the need to use distress tolerance skills.

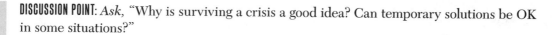 **DISCUSSION POINT:** *Ask*, "Why is surviving a crisis a good idea? Can temporary solutions be OK in some situations?"

Harmful "Coping" Strategies

Let's talk about the ways many people currently get through crises/painful emotions. When stressed, upset, dysregulated, or numb, many people cope by:

Eating too much or too little
Drinking
Using drugs
Smoking cigarettes
Skipping or avoiding school
Cutting themselves
Too much screen time (e.g., TV, computer, tablet, phone)
Risky online behavior
Overexercising
Too much caffeine
Exploding with anger

Social withdrawal
Lying
Working too much
Procrastinating
Spending too much money
Sleeping too much or too little

Raise your hand if you have *ever* used any of these or similar strategies to cope when distressed (*everyone in group is likely to raise their hands*).

The problem with these "coping" strategies is that they often make the original problem even worse or create new problems—that is, they mess you up. Some of these behaviors are fine in moderation; some are always harmful.

One person's effective coping strategy can be another's maladaptive behavior. Even for the same person, a behavior can be a problem, or not, depending on when, how (e.g., impulsively, obsessively), and for what purpose it is used. For example, spending time on Facebook can be socially pleasing, relaxing, and distracting; it can also be addictive and used to avoid and procrastinate. Exercising can be a distress tolerance skill [*e.g., TIPP*] and an emotion regulation skill [*a PLEASE skill*], or a maladaptive behavior when excessive.

In this module, we will learn how to tolerate distress and survive crises so that we can reduce our use of these maladaptive coping strategies.

DISTRACT WITH WISE MIND ACCEPTS

Distracting can reduce distress in the moment by reducing contact with things that cause painful emotions.

EXERCISE:

Ask people to rate their distress levels this very moment from 0 (none) to 100 (maximum). Next, spread out on a table various distracting materials (e.g., word-search puzzles, coffee-table books, cool building blocks, kaleidoscopes, deck of cards, crossword puzzles, Sudoku, colored markers and paper, magazines). Ask each group member to select an activity and then to mindfully participate in that activity for 5 minutes, throwing him- or herself into it completely. At the end of 5 minutes, ask group members to rate their distress levels again. Then ask for comments/observations on the exercise. Did their distress levels change? Did the activity solve all their problems? Was it supposed to?

> *Note to Leaders:* If the mood of the group is down (i.e., flat, low energy, withdrawn), consider using an energizing activity to distract, such as a funny movie clip or YouTube video. If the energy is too high (e.g., hyper, impulsive, disinhibited), consider using an activity such as crossword puzzles, reading, and drawing to downregulate emotions.

- *Some skills help some people some of the time.* One kind of distraction may not work at all, and thus you have to try others to figure out which might be effective for you at that particular time. Furthermore, you may find that some activities can be used for 5–10 minutes and achieve the desired effect; others may need to be used for longer periods of time, and sometimes several different skills need to be used in sequence over several hours to help reduce distress.

If an activity used in the exercise lowered your distress, that effect is useful information for you to note. That activity, and perhaps others like it, can be used next time you're distressed. If you were not distressed in the first place, it is nevertheless helpful to practice this and other activities. Practice makes you more likely to try it next time you are distressed.

> ***Note to Leaders:*** Intermittently remind members of the purpose of crisis survival skills. They are not going to make participants feel good. Their point is to help participants feel less bad so that they do not make their situation worse by acting impulsively.
>
> Refer participants to Distress Tolerance Handout 3, "Crisis Survival Skills: Distract with 'Wise Mind ACCEPTS.'" Go through each item on the handout and elicit examples from group members of what they find helpful. For some items, such as Activities, it is useful to go around asking each group member for an example of one activity that he or she can easily do as a distraction. If group members identify examples not on the list, invite them to write those on the handout.

Activities: Do Something

Invite participants to read the list of activities on the page and ask, "What activities work to distract you?" *Add effective distraction activities not listed on the handout. These need to be activities that members can access quickly in different settings (e.g., home, school, work). Sledding and scuba diving may be wonderful activities for distraction, but they may not be easily accessed.*

Contributing: Do Something Nice for Someone

Invite participants to read from the handout. Some teens have trouble understanding that this doesn't necessarily mean doing something nice for the person with whom they are upset. Give the example of a teenager being annoyed by a younger sibling in the house:

> "Instead of yelling or hitting your annoying younger sibling, you could 'contribute' by helping another, nonoffending sibling with his or her homework or helping your parent prepare for dinner by setting the table. The idea is that doing a "good deed" for someone else may lower your distress. It could be as grand as collecting toys for kids in the hospital, or as simple as holding a door for someone and smiling. Doing for others not only makes the other person feel good but elevates our mood as well. Has anyone ever noticed this?"

Take one or two examples.

Comparisons: Compare Yourself to Those Less Fortunate Than You

This skill always seems to elicit discussion, and it is often misunderstood. People tend to respond that this type of comparison will not work, and often find it invalidating. Group leaders can validate the responses and then give examples of how this skill can be helpful. One of us gives the following example:

"When I was in my early 20s, I developed a condition in my knees that made it difficult to walk up and down stairs in the hospital in which I worked. One day, I was feeling a lot of knee pain and moaning to myself, "Why me? This isn't fair." Then I looked up and noticed patients in wheelchairs and on stretchers who were not able to walk around at all without assistance from others. Although I was in pain, at least I could walk by myself. This perspective helped lessen my distress temporarily."

Another way to use comparisons is to ask group members to think of times when they felt worse or were doing worse than now. Explain: "No one skill will work for everyone! People do not have to use this skill if they do not find it helpful. But everyone should be able to find some skills that work for them!"

Emotions: Create *Different* Emotions

Invite participants to read the handout and to identify one activity listed that creates different emotions than the current one.

How many people listen to dark, depressing music when depressed? [*Wait for a response, then explain:*] That is *not* using this skill. The idea is to select music, movies, TV shows, friends, websites, or other activities that will evoke emotions *different* from the distress. Things that are upbeat, funny, fun, invigorating, energizing, exciting, or calming, may all help bring about different emotional states.

> *Note to Leaders:* We sometimes illustrate the above point by showing a short movie clip in the group. Many teens report that listening to sad music when sad, for example, feels validating, and in so doing, they feel less dysregulated. One could argue that although this choice functions to lessen their distress, it is still not the skill of distracting from current emotions—it may be another skill—for example, the skill of self-soothing or self-validation. The skills trainer can give examples of activities that change emotions: for example, watching a funny TV show on TV/DVD or putting on calming music when feeling irritable/anxious; listening to upbeat songs on an iPod when feeling blue.

PUSHING AWAY: PUSH THE PAINFUL SITUATION OUT OF YOUR MIND TEMPORARILY

Invite participants to read from the handout and think of an example of pushing away. Many teens and parents ask, "Isn't pushing away the opposite of what we're supposed to be doing in therapy?" The leader can say that in the long term, we don't want to push away and continually avoid emotions or tough situations, but in a crisis situation, facing the painful situation isn't necessarily helpful. Examples are useful here. One of us then gives the following example:

"My father was ill in the hospital. If I allowed myself to think of him lying in a hospital bed in acute pain while I was at work, I'd be very sad, anxious, and unable to pay attention to my clients. *Pushing away* was a way to put it all on the sidelines temporarily while I focused on my work; upon returning home, I allowed myself to experience the full range of emotions and think about my father."

Optional example:

"A client told a story about a female peer who was apparently trying to provoke a fight with her in school. Instead of the client staring at the other girl during class (which would inevitably get the client angrier and more unable to focus), the client pretended that she had "horse blinders" on her head and could only look straight ahead and not to the side where the other girl sat. This allowed her to finish her last few weeks of school without engaging in a fight that might have resulted in a school suspension or even expulsion."

Some group leaders do exercises to help people symbolically or physically push away, such as decorating a small box in which they place slips of paper on which they have written their painful emotions, thoughts, and images. The slips of paper can be taken out at a later time.

Thoughts: Replace Your Thoughts

Invite participants to read from the handout and think of an example of replacing thoughts. Some teens and family members might say that "counting to 10 or noticing colors in a poster in one's room" is silly and ineffective. The leader needs to make two points here:

• *If it doesn't work, try another.* Some of the skills help some of the people some of the time. If this one truly doesn't work for you, then find another one.

• *But to work, it must be done mindfully.* This skill, like most others, requires the participant to practice mindfully. This means trying to fully participate in the distraction exercise, such as mindfully repeating the lyrics to a song in your mind or counting the different shades of blue in the poster. When your mind drifts back to the distressing situation, notice it and gently bring attention back to the specific alternative thought.

One of us uses the following example:

"I have a hard time getting blood drawn for checkups or getting an IV that has been necessary for some procedures. I used to count ceiling or floor tiles to distract my mind, or count backwards from 100 by 3s. I've also taken a copy of the *New York Times* and thrown myself into reading a good article while they were feeling for veins in my arm. I do this until it is done. Occupying my mind in this manner works wonders for being able to tolerate the distress."

Sensations: Intensify Other Sensations

Invite a participant to read from the handout and think of an example of intensifying other sensations. For some teens, doing sit-ups and push-ups until exhaustion works. For others, tightly hugging one's mattress or pillow may serve this function. Make a point of explaining how to use this skill without hurting oneself! Snapping a rubber band on one's arm may involve a stinging sensation, but it is not considered "hurting oneself" if there is no bruising or tissue damage. From a shaping or harm reduction perspective, the stinging rubber band is better than cutting oneself, in which tissue damage and even scarring may occur. The leader can point out that eventually, the participant may not require the stinging sensation to effectively distract him- or herself. This skill can also involve intensifying sensations of temperature (e.g., an icy drink or a hot shower, though not to the degree of burning), hearing (e.g., listening to loud music in one's room), taste (e.g., sour pickles or spicy salsa), and so on.

A Brief Quiz

Tell participants to turn over their handouts and then quiz them about what the acronym ACCEPTS stands for. For example, "OK, who can tell me what A stands for? What does the first C refer to?" And so on. Make sure everyone is able to recite the meaning of at least one or two letters, demonstrating some degree of accurate recall. Tell them that they may need to use this skill in the middle of the night, in the middle of a school day, or in the middle of the Atlantic Ocean (so to speak), when they cannot necessarily access their skills handouts. They need to have these skills committed to memory.

ASSIGNMENT OF HOMEWORK

Assign Distress Tolerance Handout 4, "Practice Exercise: Distract with 'Wise Mind ACCEPTS.'" Ask each member to commit now to using two specific distraction skills when faced with even mild distress during the week. They should write their selections on the handout.

TEACHING CHALLENGES FOR CRISIS SURVIVAL SKILLS

When assigning homework, leaders can anticipate some of the challenges that might come up. Note that these apply to not only Distract with "Wise Mind ACCEPTS" skills but with other crisis survival skills as well. Group members may say, "Distress tolerance skills didn't work for me." Or, "When my friends all ditch me, listening to music just isn't going to make it better." Leaders can respond by saying, "Try to vary your skills practice enough to find the ones that do work."

    Some members may say, during the skills lesson or next week's homework review, "Distress tolerance doesn't make me feel better" or "It didn't last long enough." Leaders can respond by saying, "These skills are not intended to necessarily make you feel better or to solve your problem, but rather to prevent you from making the situation even worse. If you don't do a harmful or risky behavior when really upset, then it worked." As for it not lasting long enough, leaders can say, "You may need to string several distress tolerance skills together to ride out the highest levels of distress sufficiently."

SESSION 2
BRIEF MINDFULNESS EXERCISE
. . . .
HOMEWORK REVIEW
. . . .

BREAK

During the break, skills trainers can place self-soothing items brought to the session on a table.

SELF-SOOTHE WITH SIX SENSES

Orientation of Clients to the Self-Soothe Skills and Their Rationale

Self-soothing is a form of self-care during a crisis. Each of the five senses can be used to soothe yourself, and you can also use movement (i.e., the kinesthetic sense). Some people find it difficult to even think about doing anything "self-soothing" when they are upset. Although it may not feel natural at first, self-soothing skills can become extremely useful if you give yourselves a chance to practice.

EXERCISE

Invite participants to rate their distress (0–100) and then ask them to engage in some form of self-soothing by using one of the materials on the table (e.g., soothing music CD, herbal teas, freshly baked chocolate chip cookies, aromatic lotions, scented candles, large photos of soothing scenes such as sunsets and beaches, stuffed animals, cozy scarves). Participants can also use movement and stretching to self-soothe. Have group members participate fully in the experience for about 5 minutes. Then ask them to rate their distress again and to share their observations.

Note to Leaders: Some members might not find the selected self-soothe activities to be particularly soothing for them in that moment. Leaders can normalize this response and state that it is important to try different self-soothe objects to figure out what works most effectively for each individual. Sometimes people will need to employ multiple activities that engage multiple senses to obtain the desired reduction in distress. Also, some self-soothe activities could create negative emotions or become maladaptive behaviors if done in excess (e.g., eating too much ice cream, doing too much exercise, drinking too much coffee).

Remind participants that the point of distraction and self-soothing skills is not necessarily to make themselves feel better; it is to prevent themselves from feeling worse and engaging in a maladaptive coping strategy. Members should think of these activities as a sort of emotional tourniquet. If you are in a lot of distress and pain, a tourniquet does not necessarily help you feel better or fix the source of the problem, but it does save your life.

Review Distress Tolerance Handout 5, "Crisis Survival Skills: Self-Soothe with Six Senses"

A good way to remember these skills is to think of soothing six different senses. Self-soothe with vision, hearing, smell, taste, touch, and one we might not always think about—movement.

Discuss each of the six senses on the handout, eliciting examples from all group members of activities they use or would find soothing. It is also helpful for leaders to share their personal favorites among the strategies as an ice breaker and model. Also ask participants to consider which of the self-soothe exercises can be accessed immediately (e.g., if one loves the beach but is in school, perhaps stare at a picture of the beach on one's phone).

IMPROVE THE MOMENT

A benefit of IMPROVE the Moment skills [*Handout 7*] is that you need no props like many of the distraction and self-soothing skills entail. Some IMPROVE strategies involve changing the way you think about yourself or the situation (e.g., from despair to encouragement, finding meaning). Others involve changing the way your body has responded to events (e.g., from tense to relaxing), and still others involve focusing your mind in a helpful way (e.g., on imagery, prayer, one thing in the moment, vacation).

Note to Leaders: Ask participants to read each IMPROVE skill aloud and identify which of these they have used or may consider useful.

Imagery

Using imagery means visualizing a relaxing, comforting, or confidence-boosting scene in your mind. It can be used to distract, soothe, build confidence and courage, or make goals more motivating and achievable by picturing them (e.g., like a runner visualizing victoriously crossing the finish line).

Meaning

It can help to find meaning or purpose in the pain, although this is not always possible to do. Not every problem has a silver lining, and this is not about trivializing a painful situation. However, handling the care of a sickly, elderly relative, for example, can sometimes bring estranged siblings together; focusing on the newly reestablished relationship is a way of making meaning. Teens or young adults who have experienced hardships or emotional pain sometimes choose a career in mental health to use their insights to help others, thereby making meaning of their suffering. Making meaning could involve a situation as simple as getting a bad test grade, going to a teacher's extra help session, and realizing that the grade has led to an hour of support from a nurturing teacher. The point is, sometimes we have to work to actively create meaning—to make lemonade out of lemons, as the saying goes. We can find ways to learn from mistakes, find valued others to connect with when there has been loss or distress, and transform pain into acts of kindness.

Prayer

Have any of you ever used prayer to cope with distress? If so, have you found it helpful? Participants who are not religious can turn to their own Wise Mind or meditate on a situation for which they are seeking greater clarity. Ask for strength and acceptance of the pain, rather than for the crisis to be taken away.

Relaxation

The purpose of relaxation is to change how your body responds to stress. Often people hold tension throughout their bodies, as if that could change the situation. Acceptance of the situation by the body, demonstrated through a generally relaxed posture, can help with acceptance by the mind. What do you all do to relax? [*Take examples.*]

One Thing in the Moment

This skill involves focusing only on what you are experiencing *this moment*. We often suffer more than is needed by focusing on past suffering, anticipating future suffering, or distracting ourselves from potentially positive experiences in the present. If preoccupied with past, future, or negatives about the present, we can miss the neutral or even pleasant features of this moment. For example, you might be riding on a train ruminating about an argument you had that morning, or irritated abut the people talking loudly nearby, rather than one-mindfully noticing the pretty scenery.

Vacation

We all need a vacation from the stresses of life sometimes. We don't mean that you have to fly to a Caribbean Island. Just take a few hours or even minutes for yourself. Stop dealing with the situation for a short period of time and take care of yourself or let someone else take care of you. Go to Starbucks for a latte. Read a book for pleasure for an hour. Unplug from all electronic devices for a period of time. Take a walk outside or go to the gym. Get your nails done and pay attention as they massage your hand.

Example of using the skill of vacation: I flew down to Florida to help move my beloved grandmother out of her home into an assisted-living facility when she could no longer live independently. It was a stressful and emotional couple of days, and so at one point I removed myself from the situation. I drove to the nearby beach, parked, took off my shoes, and walked by the water in the sunshine. After a half hour, I returned, calmer and refreshed to continue the difficult tasks at hand.

Encouragement

Are you often your own harshest critic? Do you say things to yourself like, "I never do anything right," "I'm gonna fail this test," or "I'm so fat." Encouragement requires that you talk to yourself as you would talk to someone you care about, or as you would like someone to talk to you. What have you said to support others? What have supportive others said to you when you were going through tough times?

> *Note to Leaders:* Members might generate comments such as "There are plenty of things you do well." "If you study hard enough, you can pass the test." Or "You are beautiful as you are." Group leaders can also model encouraging statements, such as "This is hard, and I believe in you," and "I can get through this if I break it down, one step at a time." Elicit some more examples from members; cheerlead members' using them on themselves.

ASSIGNMENT OF HOMEWORK

Assign Distress Tolerance Handout 6, "Practice Exercise: Self-Soothe Skills." Ask each member now to commit to using two self-soothing activities when faced with even mild distress during the week. They should write their selections on the handouts in advance, if possible.

Assign Distress Tolerance Handout 8, "Practice Exercise: IMPROVE the Moment." Ask each member now to commit to using two IMPROVE activities when faced with even mild distress during the week. They should write their selections on the handouts in advance, if possible.

SESSION 3
BRIEF MINDFULNESS EXERCISE
• • • •
REVIEW HOMEWORK
• • • •
BREAK
• • • •

PROS AND CONS

Why Bother with Pros and Cons?

The skill of considering pros and cons allows people to see that coping skillfully with pain and impulsive urges leads to better results than acting impulsively and rejecting reality. We basically use this skill any time we do something we'd rather not do, such as going to a doctor's appointment, or getting out of bed for school or work rather than turning off the alarm and staying under the covers. As such, it is a central skill for changing mood-dependent behaviors.

How to Do Pros and Cons

Have you guys ever made pros and cons lists before? Maybe lists about whether you should date that guy, or break up with that girl, or go to that dance? Well, we're going to teach you how to do that a little differently and in a way that can help you cope with distress.

EXERCISE

Write an example of a maladaptive behavior that messes you up on the board, such as binge drinking, perhaps caused by an argument with a friend who won't communicate. You can also take one from the group that will be relevant but not too triggering. Then write PROS and CONS on the board with a line down the middle to make two columns. Go through the group, eliciting from them the pros of the impulsive behavior and then the cons of the impulsive behavior. Next, draw a horizontal line under the items in both columns. Then ask for the pros of not acting impulsively and the cons of not acting impulsively. See Figure 7.1 for an example.

Listing the pros and cons of both *doing* the problem behavior and *not doing* the behavior gives you additional information. Consider the following points.

• *Consider what the problem behavior does for you.* The *pros of doing* the impulsive behavior and *cons of not doing* it tell you what the behavior does for you! This is important because you can then think of more skillful ways to achieve the same things. For example, if yelling gets you your way in an argument (pro for yelling), and the absence of yelling will make you feel weak (con for not yelling), think about more effective ways to get your way and not feel weak. For example, the DEAR MAN skills from the Interpersonal Effectiveness Skills module might get your way for you *and* make you feel effective and powerful.

• *Consider all of the pitfalls of the behavior.* The *cons of doing* the behavior and the *pros of not doing it* highlight the natural consequences of the behavior. In other words, there are basic pitfalls with continuing to rely on this behavior.

	Pros	Cons
Old way: acting impulsively (binge drinking)	• Distraction (ST) • Pain goes away (ST) • Get buzzed/feel good (ST) • Something to do, including more social (ST) • Fun (ST) • Feel courage/strength (ST)	• Feel pain more intensely • Getting sick (ST) • Feeling more guilt/shame (ST/LT) • Could lead to other risky behaviors (ST/LT) • Reality returns, with a headache (ST/LT) • You miss an opportunity to practice new skills (ST/LT)
New way: tolerating distress (refraining from drinking; choose a skill)	• Less chance of making a mistake, hurting yourself or others (ST/LT) • Better chance to resolve the problem (ST/LT) • By using skills, feel more mastery, empowered, and more in control, and can increase self-respect (ST/LT) • Developing the habit of tolerating distress and living more skillfully (LT)	• You don't escape the feelings, and it doesn't relieve the distress as quickly (ST/LT) • Requires more effort and thus more difficult (ST)

FIGURE 7.1. Sample pros and cons of binge drinking. ST, short-term; LT, long-term.

• *Consider whether each pro and con has a long-term or short-term effect or both.* For example, cursing out your boyfriend might release your tension in the short term while also having potential short-term and long-term negative consequences on your relationship. Now let's go through each pro and con again, this time looking at whether each is a short-term or long-term pro and con. [*The leader can write* ST *or* LT *next to each pro and con, ideally in a different color marker. See Figure 7.1 for an example.*] For example, the pro of yelling to get your way tends to be short term, but a con of yelling is hurting the relationship, and it may be a long-term effect.

• *Identify the pattern.* Often engaging in maladaptive behavior has more short-term than long-term benefits, and refraining from engaging in the maladaptive behavior (i.e., using DBT skills) has more long-term benefits. When all pros and cons are labeled as either short term or long term, there tends to be a pattern. Do you see that pattern in your own life? The pros of behaving impulsively and the cons of not behaving impulsively (i.e., what the behavior does for you) are mostly short-term benefits. However, the pros of *not* engaging in the impulsive behavior and the cons of engaging in it tend to provide a greater number of long-term benefits along with some short-term benefits.

• *Build a life for the long term by considering the pros and cons and choosing to tolerate distress.* If you want to build a fulfilling life, there are good reasons to work on stopping the coping strategies that mess you up and replacing them with effective coping strategies. The pros of tolerating distress skillfully generally outweigh the cons.

EXERCISE

Invite each member to take 5 minutes to think about a recent distressing event in which he or she engaged in a maladaptive behavior, or had an urge to do so. Ask members to write down their examples on the top of the Pros and Cons handout (Distress Tolerance Handout 9), and fill each of the four cells, rating whether each pro and con has short-term and/or long-term effects. Depending on time, invite one or two participants to share their examples on the whiteboard and discuss with the group.

When to Use Pros and Cons

Fill out a Pros and Cons handout ahead of time (alone or with your individual therapist) about a typical target or addictive behavior. It can then be used in the moment of distress to review the pros and cons of acting and not acting on an urge. In this way, it can remind you of your long-term goals and the advantages of tolerating distress in the short term. Even if you don't have the handout with you at that moment, quickly reviewing pros and cons in your mind can help you choose to cope effectively with an urge rather than relying on a harmful behavior.

When filled out in advance, the handout can also be used to remind you about what functions a target behavior fills; it can serve as a guide to replacing them (e.g., replacing alcohol with an IMPROVE skill of doing something else to relax if you find that alcohol relaxes you). In other words, this skill could be part of a "cope-ahead practice" when you are at risk for engaging in a certain problem behavior.

REDUCE EXTREME EMOTIONAL AROUSAL QUICKLY WITH TIPP SKILLS

Why Bother with TIPP Skills?

Extreme emotional arousal can make it impossible to use most skills. Have any of you been in situations where you are so upset that nothing you try seems to work, you can't think straight, and you can't even remember the skills you learned? [*Usually most people will nod emphatically.*] When this happens, you've entered the "red zone" of emotional distress, and you might even start to panic at this point. We call this the "fight-or-flight" response when you are too aroused to practice skills. This might happen when you find out that your boyfriend or girlfriend has cheated on you, that your friends ditched you on your birthday and posted about it online, or that you failed a test you needed to pass. Whatever it is, your emotions get really amped up, in Emotion Mind, in the red zone.

We hear this all the time: "I was too upset to use my skills." What we are trying to do here is teach you ways of being skillful when you are the *most* upset (e.g., higher than 75 out of 100, if 100 is most distressed ever). Most of you probably didn't come to therapy just to learn how to cope when you are feeling a little bit annoyed! TIPP skills are for those times when you feel too upset, too emotionally dysregulated, to remember, let alone implement, other skills you may already know. When you are in a crisis, when you are overwhelmed, when you are caught in Emotion Mind and can't get out and other crisis survival strategies or skills don't work, these are the times to use the TIPP skills. They reduce the intensity of your emotions quickly. Note that the effects of these skills usually last only about 5–20 minutes, so they are not a long-term solution! They will calm you down just enough to buy you time so you can determine which skills to use next.

TIPP skills are a way to quickly "tip" your body chemistry when you're really upset. Some of you have relied on maladaptive behaviors to take the edge off of your distress. Others may have medication (i.e., a "PRN") to ease your agitation or anxiety. We recommend that you try a TIPP skill to bring down your distress just enough so that you can think of other skills to try.

Reasons to use TIPP skills include:

- TIPP skills change your body chemistry to reduce arousal.
- TIPP skills work very fast, within seconds to minutes, to bring down arousal.

- TIPP skills are as effective as dysfunctional behaviors (e.g., drinking, using drugs, eating, self-harm) at reducing painful emotions but without the negative short- and long-term results.
- TIPP skills work like fast-acting medications but without the cost of medications or the aftereffects that some medications cause.
- TIPP skills are easy to use and don't require a lot of thinking.
- Some TIPP skills (paced breathing, some parts of progressive relaxation) can be used in public without others knowing that you are using the skill.

How TIPP Skills Work

For emotions such as anger, anxiety, or fear, we usually want to reduce our physical arousal level. TIPP skills work by triggering the body system that calms our arousal levels.

Sympathetic Nervous System

When we are stressed, threatened, or upset, the body's sympathetic nervous system (SNS) activates. This is the body's fight-or-flight system we've mentioned before. When the SNS is activated, our heart rate, blood pressure, and saliva production increase; our pupils become dilated; and our digestion slows. The body prepares for action.

Parasympathetic Nervous System

The parasympathetic nervous system (PNS) helps us to rest and slow down. It is the opposite of fight or flight, and it regulates our emotions. When the PNS is activated, our heart rate, blood pressure, and saliva production decrease; our pupils constrict; and our digestion increases.

TIPP Skills Activate the Parasympathic Nervous System

TIPP skills activate our PNS for about 5–20 minutes so that our emotions decrease quickly, and we can think about what other skills we can use. When we can quickly decrease the intensity of our emotions, we are less likely to act impulsively. The body's physiological reactions are an important component of emotions; changing any part of the emotion system affects the entire system.

For example, say you step out into the street and suddenly realize a speeding car is heading right toward you. What happens in your body? [*Allow responses.*] Your SNS, with its fight-or-flight response, has activated to get you quickly to safety—which is helpful in this situation. Now imagine that your friend texts you and tells you that another friend said something about you that really upsets you. What's happening in your body, and what are your urges? [*Allow responses.*] You are likely becoming very hurt and angry, and may have urges to call up the other friend and start yelling, text some nasty accusatory words, or do other things that can cause more problems for you. This is a good time to calm the fight-or-flight response by using a TIPP skill.

> *Note to Leaders:* If members protest that they shouldn't have to just "take it," point out that using TIPP skills to regulate emotions does not mean that you are passively accepting the upsetting comments. Using a TIPP skill simply buys us time—and a clearer state of mind—in which to select a skillful rather than an impulsive response, such as selecting

helpful interpersonal effectiveness skills to speak to the friend or crisis survival skills to get us through until we see the friend the next day to speak in person.

Refer participants to Distress Tolerance Handout 11, "TIPP Skills for Managing Extreme Emotions."

There are four TIPP skills. Remember them with the acronym *TIPP*:

- <u>T</u>ip the temperature of your face with very cold water.
- <u>I</u>ntense aerobic exercise
- <u>P</u>aced breathing
- <u>P</u>rogressive muscle relaxation

Temperature: Tip the Temperature of Your Face

We can quickly activate our PNS and calm down by exposing our faces to cold water or cold temperatures. When we put cold water on our faces, it activates the *dive reflex*. This reflex is the tendency in humans (and other mammals) for the heart to slow to below resting heart rate when the person is immersed in very cold water without oxygen. This effect is due to increased activation of the PNS.

> **CAUTION:** It is important to alert group members that using cold water to induce the dive reflex can reduce heart rate very rapidly. Individuals with any heart disorder, a heart rate below their normal baseline due to medications, other medical problems, or anorexia or bulimia should use this procedure only with permission of their medical providers. Anyone with an allergy to cold should not participate in the ice water exercise unless cleared by their physician. In general, it is a good idea to recommend that members check with their medical providers before using the procedure. Adolescents should seek parental permission as well!

One way to use this skill is to bend over, hold your breath, and place your face—up to the temples—in a bowl of very cold water for 10–20 seconds, or shorter if you can't hold your breath that long. Then lift your face, breathe, and repeat the process up to three times. The longer the immersion and the colder the water, the better it works. However, *do not make the water too cold*. Water below 50 degrees may cause facial pain during immersion.

You can substitute this immersion approach with alternatives: by sitting in a chair and putting an ice pack, refrigerated gel eye mask, ziplock bag of ice with water, cold wet compress, or cold beverage can to your cheek bones just below your eyes. If an ice pack or other item is too cold, wrap it in a cloth or paper towel. Wet the side touching your face. Holding your breath at the same time appears to increase the effect when the face is not in water. For some individuals, simply bending over a sink and splashing cold water on the forehead, eyes, and cheeks may even be sufficient.

Cold water or cold packs can be helpful in the following types of situations: high emotional arousal, panic and/or skills breakdown due to feeling overwhelmed; anxiety interfering with tasks requiring concentration; inability to sleep due to ruminating or anxiety; dissociation, including dissociation during therapy or skills training sessions; high anger, other intense emotions, or inability to let go of intense emotion-inducing ruminations; a strong urge to engage in a problem behavior.

Short-Lived Effects

The physical effects of the cold water are actually very short-lived. Thus, if not careful it is easy to get the out-of-control emotion going again. If you continue to focus on the emotional trigger or urge, the emotion is likely to be set off again. So, once extreme arousal is down, it can be important to practice a different set of skills, such as self-soothing or distracting. If you are triggered by a situation that needs attention right away, then after intense emotional arousal is reduced, you can focus on problem solving.

EXERCISE

You will have brought to this session ziplock plastic bags with ice cubes or chilled gel eye masks for each participant. *Screen participants for medical issues.* To each of those not ruled out for medical reasons, distribute a cold pack wrapped in a wet paper towel. Explain:

> "We are going to practice using frozen ice packs. For the next minute, think of someone or something you hate or feel anger toward, noticing your emotions and any urges to act on the emotion. *Do not select people or things that will dysregulate you!* After 1 minute, I will tell you to put the ice pack wrapped in paper towel on your face. You'll want to make sure it is at least touching your cheekbones just under your eyes. While you hold the ice pack on your face, notice any changes that occur within your body or any changes to the emotion. Hold the ice pack on your face about 30 seconds or longer if you can."

Ask participants for observations regarding any changes they noticed in their body sensations, emotions, and urges from putting the ice pack on their faces. Alternatively, they can take their pulse before and after practicing. Make it very clear that participation in the practice in class is optional and that the exercise is in no way an endurance contest.

Intense Aerobic Exercise

As we will learn in the Emotion Regulation Skills module, emotions organize the body for action. For example, anger prepares us to attack, fear to run, and so on. When the body is prepared for action and highly aroused, it can be difficult to not act. So, rather than acting impulsively on our emotional urge, we can intensely exercise to re-regulate the body, reduce our emotional intensity, and gain control over our behavior.

Aerobic exercise for 10–20 minutes or so can have a rapid effect on mood, decreasing negative mood and increasing positive mood after exercising. Examples can include going for a run, swimming, jumping rope, or working out with a high-intensity weight circuit. If you don't have access to a gym or particular props, you might try running in place or around the block, dropping to the floor and doing push-ups and sit-ups, jumping jacks, power walking, or putting on music and dancing around one's room. The key is to do it intensely.

> *Note to Leaders:* At the same time, caution group members that one can overdo exercise; thus, it must be done to a safe degree. Exercise should be intense but relatively brief— minutes, not hours—and should not exceed one's fitness level. Use proper medically informed judgment regarding degree and duration of exercise, as with exposure to cold temperatures.

Once the exercise stops, the PNS becomes activated and brings down your body's arousal for about 20 minutes. Have you ever had this experience of your body slowing down after intense exercise, like after running a race, walking up many flights of stairs, running to catch a bus, or after playing an athletic game like soccer, tennis, or basketball? What did that feel like? These feelings are the effects of activation of your PNS.

Wouldn't it be helpful to bring about that feeling if you were experiencing intense emotions and needed to bring them down quickly? During this time of slowing down, you are more able to consider what other skills can be used to maintain control over your behavior. We want to mindfully participate in the exercise and then think about what other skills we might use. If we keep focusing on whatever it was that triggered the intense emotion, it will get the emotion going again, and it will be harder to bring it down.

Paced Breathing

Paced breathing entails slowing our breathing and making our exhale longer than our inhale. Pacing our breathing by slowing it down has been found by researchers to quickly bring down emotional dysregulation by activating the PNS. In turn, we can think more clearly about what to do next. This strategy can be used anywhere, any time because we always have access to our breath, which may not be the case with ice packs or intense exercise.

Paced breathing can change sympathetic and parasympathetic activity. Slowing breathing to approximately five or six breath cycles per minute (one complete breath cycle of inhale and exhale lasting 10–12 seconds) is effective at reducing emotional arousal by activating the parasympathetic nervous system.

EXERCISE

Position a large clock with a second hand facing toward group members. Instruct group members as follows:

"1. Place one hand on your abdomen and notice the rise and fall with each deep breath. This is the type of breathing you want to do, not shallow breaths only from your chest.
"2. Count your complete breath cycles for 1 minute. A complete breath cycle is the entire in-breath and out-breath. I will time you for 1 minute. [*Teens average about 12–16 complete breaths per minute.*]
"3. [*After 1 minute*] Now, we will begin to practice paced breathing. You can use the clock or a watch to count your breaths, or you can count in your head. Slow your breaths so that out-breaths are longer than in-breaths. Try breathing in for about 4 seconds and exhaling for longer—about 6–8 seconds, or about 10–12 seconds per breath cycle. We will do this for 1 minute. Our heart rate increases slightly during inhalation, and decreases slightly during exhalation; thus, we want to lengthen the exhalations to promote the slowing-down effect and activate the PNS.

"For a set of breathing pacers that will help you track your breathing in and breathing out, go to *www.dbtsandiego.com/current_clients.html*, a website designed by Milton Brown at the DBT Center of San Diego. You can also find smartphone apps for paced breathing—for example, both iPhones and android phones have breath pacer apps), and breath pacers are available on YouTube."

Some clients might say that longer exhales are uncomfortable for them. Leaders can suggest more practice. When clients continue to express not being able to elongate their exhales, they can still receive some relaxation effect by practicing slowing and deepening their breath, breathing in for about 5 seconds and out for about 5 seconds for a total of 10 seconds per breath cycle (Brown, 2012). Ask for observations regarding the paced breathing.

Progressive Muscle Relaxation

Progressive muscle relaxation offers another way to slow down the body and regulate emotions. This relaxation technique can be taught in the group with a full progressive muscle relaxation script or demonstrated with just a few muscle groups and no repetitions if leaders are short on time. Allow at least 15 minutes for this exercise. If time allows, or if practiced at home, this exercise can be longer (up to 30 minutes). Members can be invited to record the exercise so that they can listen to the recording at home. After repeated practice, the relaxation induction can be abbreviated and completed much more quickly (e.g., 5 minutes) because merely beginning the exercise cues a state of relaxation. Group members may eventually be able to cue a relaxed state in themselves without the muscle-tensing component. Note that when doing this at home, members should find a quiet place and time when they will not be interrupted. Members will need to practice progressive muscle relaxation daily for about 1 month to achieve the full benefits of the skill.

Progressive Muscle Relaxation Script

First orient members to the fact that they will be relaxing their bodies by systematically focusing on their muscles from head to toe. Members should get in a comfortable position (when at home, they can either sit in a comfortable chair or lie down). Noticing muscle sensations also involves practice in mindfully observing body sensations. Participants should close their eyes as you begin to speak:

"Notice your forehead and eye area, and squeeze your forehead and eyes so that they are as tense as possible, squeezing your brows together, wrinkling your forehead, and shutting your eyes tightly. Hold that tension [*for about 10 seconds*]. Now release, trying to relax those muscles fully [*for about 10 seconds*]. Notice the sensations of tension flowing out of those muscles, and notice the difference between the tension and the relaxation in those muscles. [*Then repeat with same muscle group.*]

"Next, tighten the muscles in your cheeks, nose, mouth, and jaw. Scrunch up nose, bring cheeks and upper lips up toward eyes. Hold for 10 seconds, as tightly as possible. Then, release and fully relax those muscles for 10 more seconds, noticing the difference between sensations in those muscles when tense versus when relaxed. [*Repeat, using same muscle group.*]"

Note to Leaders: Continue this format, repeating each step using the same muscle group before moving on. Take your time, allowing pauses between each step so participants can fully take in the relaxed sensations that follow from releasing each muscle group and releasing the tensed position. Progress through the following muscle groups:

- Neck and shoulders (tighten neck and raise shoulders high)
- Back (arch back, bring shoulder blades together)
- Chest (take deep breath and hold it; let go when becomes difficult)
- Arms (make fists and bend both arms up to touch shoulders)
- Hands (into tight fists)
- Abdomen (hold stomach in tightly)
- Buttocks (squeeze butt)
- Legs and thighs (legs extended and flex the feet toward body to tense the calves, tense thighs)
- Ankles and feet (legs extended with toes curled under and pointed inward, heels out)
- Now have participants tense all of the muscle groups in the body together, squeezing as tightly as they can, and holding for 10 seconds. Release, fully relaxing all of the muscle groups for 10 seconds and noticing the difference between the tensed and relaxed state. Repeat this full-body tensing and relaxing process again.
- Lastly: "Scan your body's muscle groups for any remaining tension and let that tension go. Now allow your body to remain in a relaxed state and focus your attention on your breath as you slowly breathe in and slowly breathe out. Continue this for 1 minute."

Invite group members to share their observations of progressive muscle relaxation, including whether their arousal went down, stayed the same, or went up. Many tend to notice a decrease in emotional arousal, even when practiced in the group for only 5–10 minutes.

CAUTION: Some people may experience "relaxation-induced panic" in reaction to not meeting the expectation that they will relax. To prevent this unwanted response, caution members that tensing and relaxing muscles may not result in relaxation; the important part of the exercise is to become aware of their body tension. They should also feel free to stop at any time during practice. Allow those who are self-conscious when practicing to simply observe the demonstration and/or face the wall during practice.

Brief Relaxation in a Crisis

In a crisis or when you have very little time, it can help to simply tense and then relax a few sets of muscles that are not visible to others—for example, stomach, buttocks, and chest muscles. Another version of this brief relaxation practice is *paired muscle relaxation*. Tense every muscle in your body, and then let all the muscle tension go, saying the word *relax* in your mind. Practicing this pairs the word *relax* with full muscle relaxation. The aim is to eventually cue full muscle relaxation with the word *relax*.

ASSIGNMENT OF HOMEWORK

Assign Distress Tolerance Handout 10, "Practice Exercise: Pros and Cons." Invite participants to complete their practice exercise handout of pros and cons during the week when feeling at least mildly distressed.

Assign Distress Tolerance Handout 12, "Practice Exercise: TIPP Skills." Next, invite participants to practice their TIPP skills at least one time during the week as well and complete this handout. If in-group practice involved temperature, paced breathing, and progressive muscle relaxation, leaders should ask participants to try intense exercise for homework.

Assign Distress Tolerance Handout 13, "Crisis Survival Kit for Home, School, or Work." Ask members to put together a personalized crisis survival kit to use at home. It should include a total of 5–10 items selected from Distract with "Wise Mind ACCEPTS," Self-Soothe with Six Senses, IMPROVE the Moment, Pros and Cons, and TIPP. The kit can be housed in a shoebox, sturdy bag, or basket and may include distracting games, a favorite soothing playlist of music, body lotion, pictures of pets, inspiring poems, a small furry stuffed animal, a schedule of gym classes, a letter from a loved one, or herbal teas.

For IMPROVE the Moment skills such as making meaning or giving self-encouragement, participants can list what they could say to themselves on a card and place the card in the kit. Participants can also include their lists containing their pros and cons of engaging in a harmful behavior. Ask them to bring in their kits next week for a "show and tell." The idea is that when participants become dysregulated, they can go right to their kits, and they do not have to give much thought to what to use to help them tolerate their distress right away.

Portable Survival Kit for School or Work (Optional)

Many of the teens in our programs have found it helpful to construct a smaller, portable, crisis survival kit specifically for use in school (and parents can create one for work). For those kids who are going through the skills modules a second time, or for those who experience much distress in school or work, we recommend considering making a specialized kit that includes distress tolerance skills that are appropriate for a classroom (or work) setting, such as multicolored rubber bands to manipulate in various ways; paper and pens for doodling; a mini-pack of Play-Doh, a squeeze ball, silly putty; a list of visual stimuli in the classrooms the student can use to distract him- or herself; extra snacks to self-soothe; a list of friends, teachers, or counselors to approach after class or at lunch time. This portable kit can also be used in transit or taken to camp or on vacation.

SESSION 4
MINDFULNESS EXERCISE: THE HALF-SMILE

> **Note to Leaders:** For this week's mindfulness exercise, we recommend teaching and then practicing the half-smile skill as an introduction to the notion of reality acceptance.

Facial expression and body posture influence your emotional state, just as your emotions influence your facial expression and posture. A more accepting physical stance can help persuade your brain to accept, rather than fight, the reality of a painful situation. One way to assume a more accepting physical stance is through your facial expression, as your facial muscles communicate with the emotion center of your brain. If you are hunched over and grimacing, your brain interprets danger or distress. If you are sitting upright, comfortable, with your facial muscles relaxed, then your brain interprets and communicates greater physical calm and emotional contentment. You can use this skill when contemplating a distressing reality that you cannot change, at least in the short term.

For today's mindfulness exercise, we are going to practice the half-smile skill. We first ask you turn your chairs around and face away from one another, so as not to be distracted. In your mind rate your current distress level, from 0 to 100, for the next 5 seconds. Now we ask you to relax your facial muscles, from your forehead to your jaw. Pay special attention to your mouth, and gently and slightly upturn the corners of your mouth into a subtle smile, so that others might not even be able to detect it, but you can feel it. That is the half-smile. Mindfully sit with this expression for the next minute.

[*After 1 minute*] Now, silently rate your level of distress again, on that scale from 0 to 100. Notice if there is any difference in your pre- and postrating.

> **DISCUSSION POINT**: *Invite observations and discussion. The skill of the half-smile often creates skepticism and questions in the group. For example, a group member might protest, "So you're saying I should just put on a happy face when I am upset? That's what my dad always told me. That feels invalidating!" It is important to validate how the half-smile could seem that way and then point out how it is different. Leaders can demonstrate the difference between a full, fake, smile, which increases distress, and the subtle, relaxed-face, half-smile, which alleviates distress.*

HOMEWORK REVIEW

> **Note to Leaders:** This homework review is unique in that it involves a "show and tell" of members' personal crisis survival kits in addition to the assigned handouts on skills practice. (If there is no time to also review the Pros and Cons and TIPP homework sheets, members can mention which aspects of those skills they included, or could include, in their kits.) Typically, group members have fun reviewing the kits because they can share a more personal side of themselves, and get inspired from seeing others' creative ideas. For the sake of time, leaders instruct group members to take out five of their favorite items. In turn, they are told to describe each one briefly and to say what skill or skills it represents. For example, one group member might take out a lavender soap and explain that it represents the self-soothe skill of smell, or take out a favorite book and explain how it can serve as a Distract with "Wise Mind ACCEPTS" activity, as another emotion, or as other thoughts. Note that an item can function as multiple skills; for example, playing with a pet could be both a distracting activity and a self-soothe skill.

BREAK
· · · ·

REALITY ACCEPTANCE SKILLS

Refer participants to Distress Tolerance Handout 14, "Accepting Reality: Choices We Can Make."

Radical Acceptance

Leaders should start by sharing a personal example of something difficult to radically accept. One of us tells the following story:

"About 20 years ago, my right knee swelled up to the size of a grapefruit. The doctor told me to get an MRI [magnetic resonance imaging]. The results indicated that I had a torn meniscus and torn ligament that would require major knee surgery and rehabilitation. My college roommate had had that surgery and I remembered how awful that was. I started to accept the diagnosis and then get myself mentally prepared for the procedure and potentially 9 months of rehab.

"Over the next few weeks, before the surgery, my left knee swelled to the same size as the right. What could this be? The doctors reexamined me and sent me for more tests. Now they told me, 'It's not a torn ligament—you have psoriatic arthritis.' What!? Yes, one-third of those who have the skin disorder, psoriasis, also develop arthritis. In addition to skin flare-ups, you also can develop joint inflammation—any joint at any time. Oh my goodness! Why me? How can this be? I'm only in my 20s and I'm walking around like an 80-year-old man. This isn't fair.

"I got angry, then depressed. The doctors now told me that there was no surgery for this problem. I was prescribed physical therapy and anti-inflammatory medications. Did I follow their recommendations? No! I was not willing to accept the facts. I avoided the doctor, avoided the treatment, and just felt sorry for myself for a few months. My condition worsened, as did my mental state. Finally I said to myself, *wait a second*. Although it is true that I have this medical condition—psoriatic arthritis—it doesn't have to destroy my life. What if I saw this condition for what it was, tried to accept it radically, deeply, and then willingly followed the doctor's treatment recommendations?

"I did just that—took the meds, went to physical therapy, and you know what?—it gradually began to help my condition. Equally importantly was the improvement in my mood, my outlook on life, and the quality of life. Although I still have this chronic condition with flare-ups from time to time, by seeing reality as it is, I could begin to take some steps to ease my physical discomfort and in turn, embrace my reality and no longer fight it, which had been perpetuating my own suffering. Acceptance of problems we cannot immediately change reduces suffering, and helps us to cope more effectively."

Optional Additional Teaching Point

Consider the following situation: You're worried after having an argument with a family member; you called him or her a nasty name. What to do? There are five possible responses. [*Leaders can write the five possible responses on the board.*]

1. Solve the problem.
2. Change how you feel about the problem.
3. Accept it.
4. Stay miserable.
5. Make it worse.

DISCUSSION POINT: *Ask the group what each of the five above responses might look like.*

If you can change the source of the pain (*solve problem*; change the situation), by all means, do it! Perhaps you can repair the conflict. (But your family member has just left town on a trip and you cannot solve the problem right away.)

If you can change the painful emotion (*change how you feel*), by all means, work on doing that! For example, you might try to think about it differently and tell yourself, "It's not worth worrying about; he'll get over it." (But you cannot find a way to feel differently about it now; it does not work because you know how much it hurt him.) You also might try to use IMPROVE the Moment skills—for example, by using imagery and imagining yourself repairing the transgression and it working out well, finding meaning in the pain, or relaxing your body. If these still don't work in changing your painful emotions, you might try acceptance of the situation.

We will talk about *accepting it* because what is the alternative?

One could *stay miserable*—screaming, crying, cursing, and complaining to your other family members about how that relative did you wrong, and remaining angry, worried, and repeating out loud that "This isn't fair! He always blames me!" And, we could *make it worse*. [*Ask the group how the situation could be made worse than it already is. Examples include by breaking things, driving recklessly, using drugs, impulsively texting the family member nastier sentiments, and being unable to focus on anything else.*]

So back to *accepting reality*. What would that look like? Perhaps e-mailing your family member an apology immediately, accepting the consequences gracefully, asking the family member what could be done to repair the relationship damage, and committing to communicating your feelings more effectively, without name-calling, in the future, and following through on it. Accepting the situation means that you deal with what actually is happening and figure out what the situation calls for.

> **DISCUSSION POINT:** *It can be helpful to lead a discussion about immediate and long-term problems that may be hard to accept (and that you may not be able to change right now). Group members can use the following examples or ones of their own to discuss what nonacceptance (including maybe making it worse) versus acceptance might look like in these situations. Note in the examples below that it can be hard to accept life-altering realities as well as minor annoyances.*
>
> - *Loud people get on the train when you want to read.*
> - *You are a runner or dancer and you injure your knee.*
> - *You didn't get your favorite teacher and are stuck with the one you have.*
> - *You feel left out when you discover that a group of friends is getting together tonight without you.*
> - *You were planning on watching a favorite movie that you'd taped and found that it accidentally got erased.*
> - *You don't have enough money to go on a trip with your friends, or to buy the same kind of clothes.*
> - *A friend is moving away.*
> - *Your romantic relationship breaks up.*
> - *There are family problems such as divorce, conflict, or a relative who is always letting you down.*
> - *You know that you will have to see a difficult relative at the upcoming holiday get-together.*
> - *You lost your cell phone.*
> - *You lose your summer job.*

Why Bother Accepting Reality?

When you avoid all contact with things that cause you discomfort, the more they come back to haunt you. Facing and accepting distress head-on reduces suffering. You cannot always deal with painful situations immediately; sometimes you have to tolerate and accept painful feelings that you cannot change, at least for the time being.

What Is Radical Acceptance?

Sometimes there is nothing you can do to change or improve a bad situation. *Radical acceptance* is the skill of accepting the things you can't change. Acceptance helps you cope effectively with your emotions and move on rather than suffering with bitterness.

DISCUSSION POINT: *Ask*, "How many of you have something you have to accept, that is hard to accept? Take a few minutes to think of what that might be—perhaps the death of a family member (including a pet), or you or a family member was diagnosed with a mental disorder or a major medical condition, or you have a learning disability, or you just moved to a new home and school. Think about whether you have been able to accept that situation yet. If so, take a moment to reflect about the difference between before and after you accepted. Denial of the facts does not change the facts."

Ask each person, if willing, to briefly share an example. If there are no takers, offer an example to the group. One of us provided this example:

"One teen's parents got divorced, but the father couldn't accept it. He moved to another house, but said how he felt it was not a "home" without his full family there, even though his kids visited regularly. Because he could not accept the reality of his divorce, he did not fully furnish the house—only the bare minimum—and he hung no pictures on the walls. Finally, he realized his divorce was real. It was actually happening to him. He decided to get real furniture and hang pictures. His house then felt more home-like, and the kids felt much more at home there, too. Did it remove the pain of the divorce? No, but it allowed him to move forward and have a life. It reduced the additional suffering he was causing himself by living in stark surroundings. Nonacceptance gets you stuck and you cannot move forward or be effective."

Turning the Mind

Refer members to Distress Tolerance Handout 15, "Accepting Reality: Turning the Mind." Leaders can ask group members to read from the handout. Explain: Acceptance is a choice. *Turning the mind* refers to making the choice to accept a situation, sometimes over and over again. Acceptance is a process rather than a one-time decision, and we may have to repeatedly turn our minds to go down the acceptance road when we find ourselves not accepting with reality. Two factors that can interfere with our acceptance are beliefs and emotions that we hold.

Beliefs

For example, you believe that if you accept your painful situation, you will become weak and just give up (or give in), approve of reality, or accept a life of pain.

Emotions

You feel intense anger at the person or group that caused the painful event; you feel unbearable sadness at the loss; guilt about your own behavior; shame over something about yourself; rage about the injustice of the world.

Remember, acceptance does not mean approval!

> **DISCUSSION POINT:** *Some members may ask, "Are you implying that I'm supposed to just 'accept' the abuse [or the bullying, etc.]?" Leaders can respond by saying:*
>
> "Acceptance does not mean approval. However, seeing reality for what it is can convert pain you cannot cope with—that is, suffering—into pain you can cope with—that is, expressing your feelings in a moderated way, getting needed social support or professional help, or progressing in your life instead of staying stuck and spinning your wheels."

Willingness versus Willfulness

Refer participants to Distress Tolerance Handout 16, "Willingness."

Willingness is doing exactly what a situation calls for. It is being effective. *Willfulness* is the opposite: It is not facing reality, not doing what's needed or what the situation calls for. An example one of us uses follows.

> "My daughter was too tired to finish studying for a test. So she went to bed, setting her alarm for 6:15 A.M., when she planned to finish studying. Instead, she slept through her alarm. She woke up and got immediately very dysregulated, yelling at us, 'Why didn't you wake me up??!! I can't believe it! It can't be 6:45 already!' She started to cry and pace hurriedly from room to room with no particular aim, continuing to protest, all costing her more time. This was willfulness. What would willingness look like?
>
> "I tried to coach her at the time, but it didn't really work. I spoke to her later, at a calmer moment, about how she was cutting off her nose to spite her face. Things she might have done instead to be more effective could have included expressing her frustration briefly, taking a 3-minute shower, and then quickly getting ready so she could still have some time to study and be on time for school. That behavior would exemplify willingness. She still would have had less time to study than she'd planned for, *and* she still could have done something to prepare instead of nothing. In other words, willingness is doing what is needed within the given context. Replace willfulness with willingness!"

> **DISCUSSION POINT:** *Referring to the handout on willingness, ask group members to describe a situation when they noticed themselves being* willful *and one when they were* willing. *Ask them to describe the associated thoughts, feelings, behaviors, and outcomes. Consider the emotional tenor of the group. If the group is high energy, have them do a quiet, solitary writing exercise on willingness versus willfulness. If the group is downregulated, break into triads and have members share their examples with one another.*

Ways to Practice Accepting Reality

Refer participants to Distress Tolerance Handout 17, "Ways to Practice Accepting Reality." Read through items 1–6 with group members, which summarize the points taught so far. Answer any questions.

ASSIGNMENT OF HOMEWORK

Assign Distress Tolerance Handout 18, "Practice Exercise: Accepting Reality." Ask group members to describe a situation during the week when they were distressed and could not change the situation right away. They should use this handout to describe the situation and whether they tried to radically accept it.

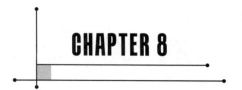

CHAPTER 8

Walking the Middle Path

SESSION OUTLINES

Session 1

▷ Goals of the Module
▷ Dialectics
▷ Assignment of Homework
▷ Session Wind-Down

Handouts and Other Materials

▷ Walking the Middle Path Handout 1, "Dialectics: What Is It?"
▷ Walking the Middle Path Handout 2, "Dialectics 'How-to' Guide"
▷ Walking the Middle Path Handout 3, "Thinking Mistakes"
▷ Walking the Middle Path Handout 4, "Dialectical Dilemmas"
▷ Walking the Middle Path Handout 5, "Dialectical Dilemmas: How Does the Dilemma Apply to You?"
▷ Walking the Middle Path Handout 6, "What's Typical for Adolescents and What's Cause for Concern?"
▷ Walking the Middle Path Handout 7, "Practice Exercise: Thinking and Acting Dialectically"
▷ Mindfulness bell
▷ Whiteboard and markers

Session 2

▶ Validation

▶ Assignment of Homework

▶ Session Wind-Down

Handouts and Other Materials

▶ Walking the Middle Path Handout 8, "Validation"

▶ Walking the Middle Path Handout 9, "How Can We Validate Others?"

▶ Walking the Middle Path Handout 10, "How Can We Validate Ourselves?"

▶ Walking the Middle Path Handout 11, "Practice Exercise: Validation of Self and Others"

▶ Mindfulness bell

▶ Whiteboard and markers

Session 3

▶ Behavior Change: Ways to Increase Behaviors

▶ Assignment of Homework

▶ Session Wind-Down

Handouts and Other Materials

▶ Walking the Middle Path Handout 12, "Behavior Change"

▶ Walking the Middle Path Handout 13, "Ways to Increase Behaviors"

▶ Walking the Middle Path Handout 14, "Practice Exercise: Positive Reinforcement"

▶ Mindfulness bell

▶ Whiteboard and markers

Session 4

▶ Behavior Change: Ways to Decrease or Stop Behaviors (38)

▶ Assignment of Homework

▶ Session Wind-Down

Handouts and Other Materials

▶ Walking the Middle Path Handout 15, "Ways to Decrease or Stop Behaviors"

▶ Walking the Middle Path Handout 16, "Practice Exercise: Extinction and Punishment"

▶ Mindfulness bell

▶ Whiteboard and markers

TEACHING NOTES

It really boils down to this: that all life is inter-related. We are all caught in an inescapable network of mutuality, tied into a single garment of destiny.
—MARTIN LUTHER KING, JR.

The wave cannot exist for itself, but is ever a part of the heaving surface of the ocean.
—ALBERT SCHWEITZER

This sounds simple and it is, but it's not easy.
—JON KABAT-ZINN

ABOUT THIS MODULE

We developed the Walking the Middle Path module specifically for teens and families (Miller, Rathus, & Linehan, 2007; Rathus & Miller, 2002; see Rathus, Campbell, & Miller, in press, for findings of the module's acceptability to teens and parents). It addresses several issues that arise repeatedly with this population, including polarized, nondialectical thinking and behavioral patterns experienced by families with emotionally dysregulated adolescents; a greater need for a focus on validation; and the explicit application of learning principles to self and others. These learning principles also overlap substantially with the major behavioral parenting treatment protocols. The module emphasizes the dialectical view that opposites can both be true, and that there is more than one way to see a situation or solve a problem. This perspective allows clients to work on changing painful or difficult thoughts, feelings, or circumstances while at the same time accepting themselves, others, and circumstances as they are in the moment.

The description of the "middle path" in parenting complements the work of Baumrind (1991), who discusses authoritative parenting as most linked to healthy adjustment in children. Authoritative parenting involves firm discipline with clear rules and follow-through, with a flexible, democratic style whereby discussion and negotiation are allowed, within reason. Most evidence-based parenting programs follow this approach. This module also helps familiarize families with developmentally normative adolescent behaviors, which helps them find a middle path to their parenting dilemmas.

A common pitfall when teaching dialectical dilemmas is to spend too much time engaging parents on their parenting dilemmas and so losing the kids' attention. Remember to continually ask teens what they think and how the ideas impact them. One way we accomplish this is to have each family create a family tableau based on each dialectical dilemma. We ask each teen to stand up and position him- or herself and the caregiver against a wall, where one corner of the wall represents one pole of the dilemma and the other corner represents the other pole. We then ask each caregiver to position self and teen from his or her own point of view. This exercise generates much discussion.

The explicit focus on validation forms a critical part of this module and relates to the bio-social theory; that is, it aims to increase validating responses in a possibly invalidating family context. It also teaches teens to validate parents, however, and teaches all group members validation as a skill to improve communication and reduce relationship conflict in general. Some points in this section are derived from Linehan (1997) and Fruzzetti (2006).

Note that the material on dialectics, validation, and behavior change may be more than can be covered in a typical skills training group. (Note also the handout on self-validation [*Walking the Middle Path Handout 10*]. This has not been used in research but may be a helpful addition for kids who struggle with validating themselves.) Multiple examples and teaching scenarios are provided to facilitate group leaders' understanding of the concepts and to offer group members multiple examples if they need more practice; many of the examples are optional. As in teaching all DBT skills, remember to make lecture points succinct, provide frequent examples, and elicit examples from group members. Any material not covered in the group can be used in family sessions or in supplemental parenting sessions.

SESSION 1
BRIEF MINDFULNESS EXERCISE
••••
HOMEWORK REVIEW
••••
BREAK
••••

ORIENTATION OF CLIENTS TO THE WALKING THE MIDDLE PATH SKILLS AND THEIR RATIONALE

Goals of the Walking the Middle Path Module

In this module, we look at adolescent–family conflict and the ways that families get polarized, don't see eye to eye, and find themselves escalating or shutting down. We then teach ways of deescalating and resolving conflict through walking the middle path between acceptance and change. This module has three parts:

- Dialectics: Balancing acceptance and change by "walking the middle path."
- Validation: Working on acceptance.
- Behavior change: Working on change.

DIALECTICS

Orientation of Clients to Dialectics

Think of some words to describe yourselves. Do you see yourselves as outgoing or shy? Organized or disorganized? Do you pick words that represent extremes? Could it be possible that you actually have elements of both qualities? This section of the skills training teaches us to think about the possibility that multiple views can be true, even if they seem like polar opposites.

[*Next, leaders draw a deep ravine on the blackboard, with the figure of an adolescent on the top of one side and the figure of a parent on top of the other, as demonstrated in Figure 8.1. The skills trainer then asks:*]

What are the issues that polarize teenagers and parents? When do you find yourselves on opposite sides? How about curfew? Grades, computer time, friends, dating, body piercings, smoking cigarettes, drinking alcohol, driving? Do you find yourselves getting stuck and unable to find a middle path between you? On what issues do you find *yourself* flipping back and forth from one position to another? For example, do you ever feel you have been too lax with yourself (or your child), and then jump to the other side and become overly strict?

We can address these extreme positions through dialectical thinking and acting. The skills in this module help people consider alternative points of view and how to "walk the middle path" behaviorally.

The problem is that when in Emotion Mind, many people act in extreme black-or-white, all-or-nothing ways. For example, a teenager comes home repeatedly after curfew and the parent tells him or her, "You're grounded for the rest of the school year." [*Elicit other examples of extreme behavioral responses from participants at this point.*]

DISCUSSION POINT: Consider the dilemma of a teen wanting to extend the curfew to 2:00 A.M. and the caregiver pulling back and insisting on 10:00 P.M., given recent concerns about the adolescent's behavior. Dialectically speaking, if we are going to find a middle path, we need to "honor the truth" in the other's perspective. *Ask parents,* "What are the kernels of truth in the teen's perspective of wanting to stay out past midnight?" *Ask teens,* "What are the kernels of truth in the caregiver's perspective of wanting you home by 10:00 P.M.?"

Note to Leaders: With the discussion point above, acknowledge that both the caregivers and teens in the group might have a hard time volunteering the answers to the questions out of fear that doing so will undercut their arguments. It is important to note that "honoring the truth" and thereby validating the valid actually helps with negotiations. The common "truths" are that the teens want to stay out later to have more fun, to be with their friends, to feel more autonomous and mature. The common "truths" for caregivers are their concerns about their teens staying safe; not getting involved in drugs, sex, or drunk driving; and as the hour gets later, more trouble tends to arise. Once these truths are expressed and then validated, it is useful to consider how to honor both positions and find the middle path. In this example, is splitting the difference between 10 and 2 and making midnight the curfew the middle path? Not necessarily. In this example, the teen might say, "Given your concerns about my whereabouts as the night goes on, I commit to call or text you every 30 minutes to verify where I am and who I am with. If I do that, can I stay out until 1:00 A.M.?" The caregiver might say, "Given your wish to spend more time with your friends and have more fun, while also recognizing my own anxiety about some recent events with you and your friends, I'd like you to text me every 30 minutes. We'll start with an 11:00 P.M. curfew and extend it later if this goes well."

Dialectics: What Is It?

Refer participants to Walking the Middle Path Handout 1, "Dialectics: What Is It?"

People who get stuck viewing a situation only one way find that family conflict increases. When we get stuck in our own viewpoint, how do we get unstuck? A dialectical approach can help us get unstuck. This approach takes into account our current viewpoint *and* an opposing viewpoint, which leads to a synthesis of both perspectives— and change occurs.

For example, one mother was concerned about her teenage daughter's romantic relationship with an older boy. She was afraid that they were having sex and that her daughter might get pregnant. She wanted to break up the relationship. But taking that extreme action would alienate her daughter, and that increased her distress. So she started to avoid the topic of the relationship completely in order to avoid her distress—the opposite extreme of trying to break up the relationship. Finally, rather than opting for one of these extreme positions, she learned to consider both. This led her to a "middle path" synthesis: to speak calmly to her daughter about appropriate birth control methods.

Dialectics teach us a number of important life points. For example:

 1. ***There is always more than one way to see a situation and more than one way to solve a problem***. The idea here is that *there is no absolute truth*, as is consistent with the DBT assumption we discussed in our orientation session. Instead, truth evolves over time. [*Use examples of rules or positions that are no longer true but used to be correct when the adolescent was a child, or when the parents were not divorced, or when they were less experienced as parents.*]

 2. ***Each person has unique qualities, and different people have different points of view***. *According to dialectics, we are all interconnected and influencing one another in our transactions. Thus, one person's extreme stance can push another to the opposite extreme.* Since we are all connected, treat others as you would like them to treat you. Remember, your moods and behaviors influence other people, just as theirs influence you (try and notice these effects). If you act in a way that is harsh, critical, or invalidating, you'll likely receive the same treatment in return. Rather than seeing differences as cause for conflict, this point normalizes differences among people's attitudes and behaviors. Some people believe that anything deviating from their point of view is wrong. For example, a parent insists that the teen begin his homework immediately after school. The teen insists on watching TV to unwind from a long day. The parent's perspective is that the teen does not begin his homework until after dinner and then stays up past bedtime to complete the work. This results in being overtired and less focused the next day. The adolescent's perspective is that he is mentally fatigued and requires a break before beginning his homework.

 3. ***Change is the only constant***. When you feel hopeless and think that nothing will ever change, remember that a dialectical philosophy argues that change occurs continually. So on any given day, things are never the same as the moment before or the moment after. Regarding relationships, allow those you care about to grow and change over time. Practice radical acceptance when people or relationships change in ways you wish they wouldn't.

 4. ***Two things that seem like opposites can both be true***. We can gain wisdom from examining the truth in opposing perspectives. Looking at our first handout [*Walking the Middle Path Handout 1, "Dialectics: What Is It?"*], let's consider these examples of opposing points of view that are nonetheless equally true: "You are doing the best you can *and* you need to do better, try harder, and be more motivated to change." "You are tough *and* you are gentle."

 5. ***Honor the truth on both sides of a conflict.*** This does not mean giving up your values or "selling out," and it does not necessarily mean compromising in the middle. To honor the truth is to validate the truth verbally and behaviorally as described before in the curfew example. [*Leaders can refer again to the example of the teen wanting a 2:00 A.M. curfew and the caregiver saying 10:00 P.M.; the middle path is not necessarily midnight. Review all the examples of dialectics in the first handout.*]

Dialectics can help pave the way toward the middle path by helping you:

- Expand your thoughts and ways of considering life situations.
- "Unstick" standoffs and conflicts.
- Be more flexible and approachable.
- Avoid assumptions and blaming.

How to Think and Act Dialectically

Refer participants to Walking the Middle Path Handout 2, "Dialectics 'How-to' Guide."
 How can we use these ideas?

1. *Move to "both–and" thinking*. Move away from either/or or all-or-nothing thinking. This means acknowledging, mentally and verbally, that "both this is true *and* this is true too." Avoid extreme words such as *always, never, you make me. . . .* Instead, be descriptive. For example: Say, "Sometimes I am treated fairly *and* at other times, I am treated unfairly" instead of saying "Everyone always treats me unfairly."

2. *Practice looking at all sides of a situation and all points of view*. Find the kernel of truth in every side by asking yourself what is being left out ("What am I missing here?"). Be generous and dig deep as you consider others' points of view. Example: Why does my mom want me to be home at 10:00 P.M.? Why does my daughter want to stay out until 2:00 P.M.?

3. *Remember:* No one *has the absolute truth*. Be open to alternatives.

4. *Use "I feel . . ." statements* instead of "You are . . .," "You should . . .," or "That's just the way it is" statements. For example: Say, "I feel angry when you say I can't stay out later just because you said so" instead of saying "You never listen and you are always unfair to me."

5. *Accept that different opinions can be valid*, even if you do not agree with them: "I can see your point of view even though I do not agree with it."

6. *Check your assumptions*. Do not assume that you know what others are thinking. "What did you mean when you said . . . ?"

7. *Do not expect others to know what you are thinking*. "What I am trying to say is. . . ."

EXERCISE

Have group members read the "Practice" examples at the bottom of Walking the Middle Path Handout 2, "Dialectics 'How-to' Guide," and circle the statements that reflect a dialectical viewpoint. Next, discuss members' answers and check their understanding of the both–and concept. For example, a parent says to her adolescent, "I want you to rely more on yourself and less on me when it comes to making decisions, and you must ask me before you make plans to go to the city with your friends." Discuss how the preceding "both–and" statement makes sense and may promote change.

Group members might find additional examples of both–and dialectical thinking helpful:

- "I am working to accept my situation *and* change it."
- "You're doing the best you can *and* you need to do better."
- "The teacher is really strict *and* really nice."
- "Your point of view makes sense *and* my point of view makes sense."
- "I am glad you are speaking calmly and behaving appropriately now, *and* you still don't get your iPad back after hitting your sister with it."
- "I can be athletic *and* feminine."
- "I can be rational *and* emotional."

How We Can Get to Extremes

Sometimes, in our own positions, we go from one extreme response to another. This can happen because of strong emotions. A parent might say, "I let the little things go and don't react, but then they build up until I explode."

We can flip to the other extreme when one position has failed. For example: "I stayed on top of her homework each night, but all we would do is get into screaming battles, so I gave up and I now leave her alone."

Sometimes, we take one extreme position and our family member takes another. Examples of nondialectical statements include these:

- "It's all my parent's fault [kid's fault/spouse's fault]!"
- "I'm either going to ignore my kid's messy room or go throw everything out."
- "In our house, it's either yelling and fighting or avoiding conflict and retreating."
- "It's either bingeing on candy or starving myself."

DISCUSSION POINTS: *Use one or more of the examples below to discuss the validity of perspectives from multiple sides. Extreme positions are often problematic, and it becomes a matter of acknowledging that and finding a middle path. There is no single right answer. The point is to come up with a response that acknowledges the validity of both sides. Ask, "What might a middle path solution be to these scenarios?"*

- *Scenario 1.* A teen asks her father whether all her friends can hang out at their house that Friday night. Dad says, "No, I don't want all of those kids over at the house. They are loud and they make a mess." The teen says, "But you've said you don't want us hanging out in the park at night; it gets dangerous. We want to just hang out together, and we don't want to sneak into a bar or anything like that. We don't want to get in trouble on the street. My friends' parents said no."

Which side is right? How would you handle this? Can both the father and daughter be "right" at the same time? What can they do?

[*The teen might agree to have only two friends over, promise to stay in her room, and clean up after, or the father might agree to give her money for bowling or a movie, so they won't be on the street but also will not be home.*]

- *Scenario 2*. A teen has been telling his father that they don't spend enough time together, and he wishes his father would make time for him. One week, the dad purchases a used car for his son, who is starting driver's education. The dad excitedly spends a whole Saturday detailing the car by hand for his son, a labor of love, happily anticipating his son's reaction when he surprises him with it. Upon presenting the car and explaining how he scrubbed, waxed, and polished it by hand for him, the son looked hurt and said, "I would have loved to spend the day doing that with you! That's a perfect father–son activity, and I've told you we never spend time together! You just don't get it, do you?" The dad felt confused and angry, not understanding how his son could not see his obvious caring and effort.

Which side is right? Can the father and son both have a kernel of truth? How would you handle this?

[*The father can acknowledge his son's hurt feelings and commit to making more of an effort to spending time together, while the son could express his hurt and gratefully acknowledge his father's way of showing caring, even though it is not his preferred way.*]

- *Scenario 3.* A mother agreed to let her daughter stay out past curfew to go to a 9:00 P.M. movie with a friend, if she called when the movie got out and told her when she'd be on her way home. She did indeed call when the movie got out, but found her mother really anxious and upset with her. This was because the movie ran 3 hours and 15 minutes, and neither the mother nor the daughter knew this ahead of time. The mother had been expecting a call at 11:00 P.M.

The daughter was outraged that the mom was upset when she called, considering she had done exactly as promised. [*The daughter did what she promised,* and *the mom was still really mad and frightened.*]

THINKING MISTAKES

One of the reasons we can get highly emotional and polarized is because we can misinterpret situations. We call these "thinking mistakes." They include all-or-none thinking, jumping to conclusions, labeling, and "shoulds," and they often push us toward extreme thinking and Emotion Mind. [*Review Walking the Middle Path Handout 3, "Thinking Mistakes," and ask participants to share examples of how each thinking mistake applies to them presently or in the past.*]

Adolescent–Family Dialectical Dilemmas

Refer participants to Walking the Middle Path Handout 4, "Dialectical Dilemmas."
    As we've described earlier, there are times when you find that you're going along with a certain way of thinking and acting, and then something hits you and you swing to the other extreme. For example, parents let their kids do what they want, such as coming in late, slacking off on homework or being disrespectful, and then one day they say, "That's it! I've had it! No going out and no TV for the rest of the school year!" Does that work? Is that usually an effective way of changing a teen's behavior?
    From our experience, and from the research literature, the answer is "no." And as you may know from your experience, teens do not respond, and then you revert to your old ways. Teens can also swing from one extreme to the other in trying to manage their own emotions and behaviors—for example, have you ever lamented: "I keep spending too much money when I go out with my friends; I'm not going out any more this year!"
    Parents and their teens also get stuck on opposite sides of polarized positions. For instance, parents say, "Come home early!" and teens say, "I'm coming home late!" One of the goals of this module is to help you find the middle path within yourself and in your relationships to achieve your goals. If you find yourself at one extreme or the other, you are unlikely to be able to maintain that position. Even if you are, it is likely to be ineffective in the long term.
    When the polarized positions occur, we call them *dialectical dilemmas* because they pose a dilemma about how to proceed and get unstuck. They can take place within a person or between two people. Three dialectical dilemmas commonly occur within families:

1. Being too loose versus too strict
2. Making light of problem behaviors versus making too much of typical adolescent behaviors
3. Forcing independence versus fostering dependence

> *Note to Leaders:* Note that for each of the dilemmas on this fourth handout, the wording was simplified for use in skills training from the original: excessive leniency versus authoritarian control, normalizing pathological behaviors versus pathologizing normative behaviors, and forcing autonomy versus fostering dependence, respectively (Rathus & Miller, 2000). Define each dilemma, as described below, and then explain that the aim is to notice when these arise and work toward synthesis.

Too Loose versus Too Strict

Being *too loose* refers to being overly permissive with your teen or with yourself (teens, that is) with too few demands, limits, or consequences. This can also refer to too little monitoring—you don't know where your teen is, whom he or she is with, or what he or she is doing much of the time. The other extreme, being *too strict* with your teen or with yourself, refers to imposing too many demands and limits, or too much monitoring, while being inflexible. For example:

- A 15-year-old girl insists on getting body piercings, staying up past midnight video-chatting with friends, and sleeping at her boyfriend's house. The parent insists that she not have a boyfriend or any body piercings until she turns 18, and that she has to be in bed by 10:00 P.M.
- A high-achieving, perfectionistic teenage boy has been avoiding doing homework for the past several weeks, for a variety of reasons. The teen then gets a poor report card, which propels him into dismissing all social plans and leisure activities and focusing exclusively on homework.

DISCUSSION POINT: What might the problem be with either extreme in these two examples? [*Some group members might endorse one of the responses in the above examples. If so, ask:*] What are the potential consequences of holding one of these extreme positions in the long run?

Offer other examples of too loose and too strict behavior.

- ***"Too loose" parenting examples.*** No standard mealtime; no requirements regarding school or general behavior; kids' stuff piled all over house; the kids have no responsibilities; kids go out with no curfew and parents don't know where they are; little or no supervision.

- ***"Too loose" teen examples***. No bedtime, texting nightly until the early morning hours; eating what you want when you want; spending all your money the minute you get it; putting off school assignments until the last minute or not doing them at all. [*The problems with "too loose" include the teen's possibly being irresponsible, living a chaotic life that increases emotional vulnerability, getting into trouble, or taking risks that leave him or her unsafe.*]

- ***"Too strict" parenting examples***. Often or permanently removing TV, Internet, phone, or socializing (i.e., overuse of punishment); perfectionist standards regarding the teen's performance in school, sports, or other activities; no privacy; spying on teen's texts and e-mails and going through teen's drawers and schoolbag.

- ***"Too strict" teen examples***. Excessive studying—not balancing schoolwork with some pleasurable activities or with self-care activities such as sleep and physical activity; dieting to the point of deprivation; perfectionist standards regarding school, sports, appearance, or other activities. [*The problems with "too strict" are that the rules are hard to enforce or maintain, and they are demoralizing to the teen. The overly strict approach can kill motivation, add to depression, and lead to resentment. It might lead to the teen's participation in the restricted behaviors anyway, but also lead to either becoming better at hiding them or alternating them with the other extremes, such as giving up a night's sleep to perfect a school assignment and then sleeping all weekend, or restricting calories and then bingeing.*]

EXERCISE: DOES THE DILEMMA APPLY TO YOU?

Refer participants to Walking the Middle Path Handout 5, "Dialectical Dilemmas: How Does the Dilemma Apply to You?" Explain that they are each to determine where they fall along the "too loose versus too strict" dilemma continuum and where their family members fall: "Place an *X* on the line to mark where you are right now. Place a *Y* to mark where your family member is. If there's a second family member in the room, mark his or her place with a *Z*."

After allowing members time to mark their sheets, invite each family up one at a time to show where they placed each family member on the dialectical dilemma continuum, including themselves. Explain that two corners of the room represent the poles with the middle of the wall representing the middle path fulcrum seen in the diagram on the handout. Ask family members to physically place themselves and the other family members on the continuum as they see it.

> *Note to Leaders:* Family members often ask, "What if we disagree with where our teen sees us?" The answer is that these observations and considerations can be discussed in a forthcoming family session if this discrepancy is a problem. If a mother and father are on opposite poles, they should consider what steps are necessary to find a middle path for themselves to effectively co-parent. Although there isn't sufficient time in the group session for each family to further discuss each dilemma in detail, the point is to raise awareness of these extreme positions.

• *A middle path between too loose and too strict*. The following dialectical synthesis could help you: Have clear rules and enforce them consistently, *and at the same time*, be willing to negotiate on some issues. This firm yet flexible style strikes a balance in which parents are neither feared nor ignored, and teens feel they have some input (rather than all or none) in their lives. Teens can apply this middle path to themselves, by keeping focused on goals while being flexible enough to also enjoy life.

For example, remember the 15-year-old girl who insisted on body piercings, sleeping over at her boyfriend's house, and chatting with friends past midnight? The parent was willing to negotiate on some issues while not bending on others. For example, sleeping over at the boyfriend's house would not be permissible, but she could spend time with the boyfriend during the day. Furthermore, she could earn the privilege of staying up until 11:00 P.M. and chatting online with friends if she completes her homework and abides by her weekend curfew. However, for this parent, body piercings beyond one in each ear were non-negotiable.

• *A middle path between undermonitoring (too loose) and overmonitoring (too strict)*. Discipline is definitely more challenging in the teenage years as kids struggle to gain more independence. Research actually shows that punishments with teens don't have much impact. There was an article in the *New York Times* several years ago in which the author said this: "In several studies of youth drinking, drug use, and early sex, the best predictor for good behavior wasn't punishment, but parental monitoring and involvement. The best methods of keeping teenagers out of trouble are knowing where they are, knowing who is with them, and spending time with them regularly" [*Parker-Pope, 2010, p. H5*].

So monitor your teens, be involved with their school life, know their friends, and spend time with them. But don't *automatically* go through their private belongings, read their journals, or spy on their e-mails and texts. Teens deserve a certain amount of privacy, and this is normative for their age. On the other hand, if you are concerned that there may be a drug problem, that they are being bullied, or that some type of risky behaviors/communications are occurring, then close monitoring (e.g., knowing all of their whereabouts and activities, reading their posts and viewing their photos on Facebook) is essential. Allow them to earn back their privacy when their behavior and functioning have improved for a consistent period of time.

> **DISCUSSION POINT**: You catch your teen lying about plans. She says she will be studying at a friend's house, and you find that she is making plans to go to a party. Which of the following sounds like a middle path?
>
> 1. Accept the transgression and let her go. After all, kids are kids.
> 2. Install spyware and monitor all e-mails, websites, and text messages.
> 3. Do not allow her to attend this party. Explain your concern about the lie and your ability to trust her, and ask for more accountability. Explain that additional lying will have to lead to decreased freedom.

OPTIONAL EXAMPLES FOR DISCUSSION

Elicit other examples from teens and parents. The following additional examples can be used for discussion, if needed. Leaders can read an example and after each ask the group: What are potential problems with this position? What would a middle path look like?

• *Parenting.* A 16-year-old girl violates her parents' wishes about attending a midnight party and goes anyway. The parents say, "How could we stop her? We can't physically prevent her from leaving." Dad later has a "heart to heart" with her and "understands"— she was depressed and thought staying home and moping would be bad for her. This makes sense to him, so he applies no consequence despite her violation of a limit. He also was afraid that "she'd become suicidal again if I kept her in or took away her iPhone, since it is her lifeline."

• *Interteen.* A 17-year-old boy says, "Because I've been feeling so distressed, can we let my girlfriend sleep over in my room tonight, just this once?"

• *Intrateen.* A teen thinks, "Last time I thought I could pass science without studying, but I didn't! So this time, I am going to study all weekend and not take any breaks."

Making Light of Problem Behaviors versus Making Too Much of Typical Adolescent Behaviors

Making light of problem behaviors refers to minimizing the seriousness of behaviors that could be maladaptive or harmful. *Making too much of typical adolescent behaviors* refers to overreacting to behaviors that are developmentally normative.

MAKING LIGHT OF PROBLEM BEHAVIORS

Example: For a long period of time, let's say, a well-meaning caregiver ignores an adolescent's failing grades, time spent with a drug-using peer group, and greater irritability at home. The parent gives the teen the benefit of the doubt, believing this stage will pass. After the teen gets suspended from school for a fight and makes a suicide attempt, the parent flips to the other extreme, and watches the teen like a hawk, and interprets even minor mood changes or requests for privacy as signs of impending danger.

Example: A teen downplays the fact that she spends 8 hours a day on the computer, regularly meets people online and discloses intimate information, lies to her parents, and sneaks off to parties, saying, "Everyone my age does this stuff." One night she takes five of her prescribed pills at once, comes home drunk, and blacks out. She tells her therapist, "It's no big deal; I was just a little tired."

DISCUSSION POINT: *Ask*, "What might the problems be with either example?"

MAKING TOO MUCH OF TYPICAL BEHAVIORS

Example (parenting): A teen is texting three or four friends every day, wants to sleep over at friends' houses every couple of weeks, and likes to spend an hour or 2 alone in her room each night. The parent tries to put a stop to these behaviors, saying, "You are too focused on your friends and you should spend more time with the family."

Example (intrateen): A teen tells her therapist, "I know I'm supposed to get up early and study all weekend for my finals, but I feel like I want to sleep late since it's the only time I can, and get out and see my friends, at least for a couple of hours. I feel like there's something wrong with me because I'm not motivated enough. Maybe I'm not cut out for becoming a doctor."

DISCUSSION POINT: *Ask*, "What might the problems be with either example?"

WHAT'S TYPICAL FOR TEENS AND WHAT'S CAUSE FOR CONCERN?

Refer participants to Walking the Middle Path Handout 6, "What's Typical for Adolescents and What's Cause for Concern?"

Note to Leaders: Walking the Middle Path Handout 6 offers examples of normative adolescent behaviors, as well as those that should raise a red flag for concern. Leaders can distribute and discuss this handout in the group, or it can be reserved for family or parenting sessions. Not every possible behavior of concern is listed here, and cultural differences might result in varied expectations about what is normative and what is not.

An individual teen's vulnerabilities also come into play. For example, one teen might be able to do homework while listening to music; for another, this may be a distraction. When parents are unsure which behaviors cross the line, they should consult with a professional or an objective friend or family member.

And, ultimately, we recognize that families have their own values that understandably influence decision making. Beware of getting sidetracked with a discussion over what's normative and what's not; the handout is intended as a guideline to help familiarize families with the idea that certain behaviors reflect normal adolescent development and may not be cause for alarm, whereas others may need clinical attention. Note that simply because a behavior might be typical (i.e., it's happening out there among teens) does not necessarily make it desirable.

DISCUSSION POINT: *Using Walking the Middle Path Handout 5, "Dialectical Dilemmas: How Does the Dilemma Apply to You?," as a starting point, elicit examples of teen behaviors from group members and discuss what is and is not typical. For example, a teen answers a cell phone call for 2 minutes. A parent then asks, "Who was that? Why are you always talking on the phone?" The teen looks irritated and leaves the room. Although this example depends on context and tone, it is normal for a teen to want privacy and be able to speak for 2 minutes on the phone without having to account for it.*

EXERCISE: DOES THE DILEMMA APPLY TO YOU?

Instruct everyone to again look at Walking the Middle Path Handout 5, "Dialectical Dilemmas: How Does the Dilemma Apply to You?" Group members will now determine where they fall along this behavior pattern. Explain:

"Place an *X* on the line to mark where you are right now, and a *Y* to mark where your family member is. If there's a second family member in the room, mark his or her place with a *Z*."

Invite each family member up one at a time. One family member physically positions him- or herself and the other family members on the continuum as he or she sees it. As before, use two corners of the room to represent the poles; the middle of the wall between the corners can represent the middle path fulcrum in the diagram on the handout.

• *A middle path between making too light and making too much.* The following dialectical synthesis could help you: A middle path would involve recognizing when a behavior "crosses the line" into a cause for concern and trying to get help for that behavior, *and at the same time*, recognizing which behaviors are part of typical adolescent development.

Example (parenting): A college-bound, straight-A student starts receiving some B's and a C and doing less work. His mother tells him that he is failing and will end up stocking shelves in a store. The teen yells, "It's nothing; I'm doing just fine! Get off my back! I don't need help."

In this example, each polarizes the other. The middle path could be for the parent to recognize the pattern of deteriorating behaviors, genuinely inquire about them, and proactively intervene. The mother's putting down of her son for the grades and likely overreaction to his normal irritation and request for autonomy in response will only escalate their conflict and deflect from the problem.

Example (intrateen): The teen in a previous example took pills, drank too much, and blacked out, but then made light of the situation by telling her therapist it was no big deal. Her middle path might be to say to her therapist: "I love my computer time, and I even meet some nice people online who understand me and go through similar things, and I like to have a drink sometimes at a party. But, lately, I feel like it's all been getting out of control, to the extreme. I feel like I could use some help managing the computer stuff, the pills, and the drinking before something really bad happens." This statement acknowledges the normative yet recognizes what might be crossing the line and becoming a concern.

Forcing Independence versus Fostering Dependence

The third dialectical dilemma is called "forcing independence versus fostering dependence." *Forcing independence* refers to cutting the strings prematurely. *Fostering dependence* refers to restricting moves toward independence. Some refer to those who hold too tightly to their children as "helicopter parents." These parents hover nearby, actively solving problems for their teens before the teens have a chance to do it themselves. This kind of parenting fosters overdependence on the caregiver.

Example (*parenting*): Parents of a 17-year-old daughter had spent the past several years rescuing and protecting her from any negative consequences of her actions (e.g., problems with school, peers, after-school jobs). Then when the daughter became pregnant and insisted on keeping the baby, they switched to the other extreme and demanded that she move out of the house immediately and find a way to support herself.

Example (*teen*): The same pregnant, 17-year-old daughter argues with her parents, packs a bag, and leaves, yelling, "Fine—I don't need you! I'll handle this on my own!"

Example (*between parents*): A high school senior wants to apply to college across the country. One parent says "No way," out of concern she'll be too far away, won't be able to return home frequently, and won't be able to get their help when problems arise. The other parent says, "Let her go! She has to learn to become an independent young woman who follows her own path." Is one parent correct? These parents might polarize each other if they don't each consider the validity in each side of the argument.

> **DISCUSSION POINT:** *Ask*, "What is the problem with pushing away too soon?"

EXAMPLES OF FORCING INDEPENDENCE

Parents provide no help with school or social problems and withdraw communication, time, or attention, saying, "You're on your own—get out of the house," or "Figure it out yourself."

A teen says that he is leaving, or that he'll handle all his problems himself.

In both cases, the teen is likely to flounder; it oversimplifies problem solving and, if anything, will increase problems.

> **DISCUSSION POINT:** *Ask*, "What is the problem with fostering dependence?"

EXAMPLES OF FOSTERING DEPENDENCE

Micromanaging, doing everything for your teen, doing everything with your teen, blocking the teen's movement toward greater autonomy—all foster excessive dependence. Specific examples include organizing the teen's room without the teen even being there, calling the teacher to change a grade, hovering while the teen has friends over, or calling your teen's friend to try to solve an argument.

The teen repeatedly asks a parent's help with basic daily responsibilities, decisions, or problem solving, or seeks a parent's company almost exclusively, at the expense of making friends (e.g., for movies, concerts, and other leisure activities). This teen will not learn responsibility, problem-solving skills, self-sufficiency, or develop a range of social support. He or she will likely fare worse when greater independent functioning is required in high school, college, and beyond. The parents might also come to feel burned out.

EXERCISE: DOES THE DILEMMA APPLY TO YOU?

Instruct members to again look at Walking the Middle Path Handout 5, "Dialectical Dilemmas: How Does the Dilemma Apply to You?" and determine where they fall between the poles of this dilemma.

"Place an *X* on the line to mark where you are right now, and a *Y* where your family member is right now. Can anyone share if you found yourself on one pole or the other?"

Again, invite each family member up one at a time. One family member then physically positions him- or herself and the other family members along a wall representing the continuum between the two poles.

A MIDDLE PATH BETWEEN FORCING INDEPENDENCE AND FOSTERING DEPENDENCE

The middle path for this dialectical dilemma is "holding on while letting go." The following dialectical synthesis could help you. Give your adolescents guidance, support, and rules to help them figure out how to be responsible for their lives; allow an appropriate amount of reliance on others, *and at the same time,* slowly give them greater amounts of freedom and independence.

You can monitor your teens, offer them guidance, and coach them through difficult situations, while encouraging them and allowing them to take more steps toward independence. Should teens strive to be completely autonomous? No. Remember, even world-class athletes have coaches and trainers! That's why part of growing independent involves learning when it is appropriate to seek help.

Example (parenting): Ideally, a middle path for the parents of the pregnant 17-year-old would have been to hold her more accountable for her actions earlier in her life. Now that she is pregnant, they could begin to wean her from their problem solving and decision making gradually and encourage her to take on greater responsibility for herself. At the same time, they could coach her on important issues and help her become more independent while emotionally supporting her.

Example (between parents): A middle path for the parents discussing their teen's college choices might be to allow her to apply across the country and be prepared to become experts at Skype, texting, twitter, and other online forums for communicating regularly. Another middle path might be to say no to schools thousands of miles away, but, if financially feasible, allow the teen to choose from a range of schools that are hours away by car, to honor the desire to live away from home and freely select a school, while still remaining within reach.

> **DISCUSSION POINTS**: *Elicit examples of this dilemma from group members. The following additional examples can also be used if needed. After each example, the leader should ask the group: What would a middle path look like?*

- *Parenting.* An 18-year-old college freshman receives an F. The mother wants to call the school and try to "fix it" by getting it changed to a C based on his mild ADHD. Is this reasonable, given that the F on the transcript could hurt him in the long run? Could the parent's efforts be harmful? [*Let group members comment. Perhaps it is harmful because it teaches the teen that there are no serious consequences, and that parents will step in and solve all his problems. He might not have motivation to work harder.*] What is a middle path?

- *Teen–parent.* A teen with C's and F's feels her parents are micromanaging her schoolwork and grades and says, "Leave me alone! I'll deal with it!" The parents say, "How can we stand by passively as she flounders?" A middle path is to help her less intrusively. Ask *how* can we help her, rather than telling her what to do and trying to fix everything. Don't start by going to the teachers because that embarrasses her. Help her to help herself; for example, coach her on study skills, encourage her to go for extra help at school, provide a tutor, take a look together at her schedule, etc.

• *Parenting.* An 18-year-old enrolls in a class in the city and needs to take the train there. She's phobic about taking the train, so Mom spends the first 3 months accompanying her—that is, holding on too tightly. Finally, the Mom says, "I've had enough of this; you should be able to do this. You're on your own," pushing her daughter into independence too soon. What do you think the daughter's reaction would be to the mother cutting off her support abruptly like this? What would be a middle path for the mother?

A middle path for the mother would be to coach the daughter on how to get the information about the train, guiding her to the website and walking her through the steps. The mother could then take the train with her the first week; in the second week the mother could ride the whole way but in the next car. Then the daughter could take the whole trip alone, but the mother could wait for her at the last stop, and so on, progressing toward independence.

• *Intrateen.* A teen who was always the caretaker of her younger siblings finds she needs help herself, but doesn't ask, believing that she is the "strong one." The middle path would be for her to realize: "I can take care of others *and* ask for help when I need it."

DISCUSSION POINT: *Ask,* "A teen comes home upset and tells her parents that she was treated unfairly by a teacher. Which of the following parent responses would be a middle path?

- Telling the teen to "grow up" and accept that life isn't fair (pushing away).
- Immediately making an appointment with the teacher to solve the problem (holding on too tightly).
- Talking to the teen about how she might skillfully communicate to the teacher about the problem."

> *Note to Leaders:* There are other (non)dialectical behavior patterns that may arise in your interactions with families, such as overindulging versus withholding/depriving, overly intrusive versus overly distancing, and so on. Should you note such patterns in discussions with clients, you can similarly point out the extremes in each position and ask group members to help generate a synthesis.

ASSIGNMENT OF HOMEWORK

Assign Walking the Middle Path Handout 7, "Practice Exercise: Thinking and Acting Dialectically." Ask group members to use this handout to record one personal example of not *thinking or acting dialectically (i.e., getting stuck at one pole of a dialectical dilemma), and one personal example of thinking or acting dialectically.*

SESSION 2
BRIEF MINDFULNESS EXERCISE
· · · ·
HOMEWORK REVIEW
· · · ·
BREAK
· · · ·

VALIDATION

Orientation of Clients to the Skill of Validation and Its Rationale

As we saw, dialectics teaches that multiple perspectives can be true. The skill of validation is one way to handle differing perspectives. We can show acceptance or understanding of how another person sees a situation, even if we don't agree. It is important to *honor* the kernel of truth in the other's perspective. Why? Validation lowers the emotional intensity of the person with whom we are interacting and increases the chance that he or she will remain in the conversation. When emotional intensity decreases, the person's communication reflects a more accurate and effective expression of his or her emotions, and it becomes even easier to validate him or her, resulting in a positive cycle (cf. Fruzzetti, 2006). It also strengthens the relationship.

Note to Leaders: Tell a personal vignette about feeling invalidated by someone or about being invalidating to someone else, but do not describe it using those terms. Highlight the consequences. Alternatively, share the following vignette illustrating invalidation:

"Johnny is sitting in class, trying to pay attention, and he accidentally knocks his notebook off his desk, making a loud noise on the floor. The peers next to him chuckle. The teacher scolds, 'There you go again, Johnny, disrupting the class, trying to get attention. I am really getting tired of this behavior!' Johnny feels extremely embarrassed, hurt, and angry, since he'd been making a true effort to focus. He later goes home and recounts the story to his mother, who replies, 'Why do you keep doing this to yourself? You're never going to get into college at this rate. You'd better shape up!'"

DISCUSSION POINT: *Ask group members what they think Johnny must have felt after his mother's response. Why were his teacher's and mother's responses so hurtful? What was missing from their responses?*

Validation: What Is It?

Refer members to Walking the Middle Path Handout 8, "What Is Validation?" Invite a group member to read the definition of validation:

"Validation communicates to another person that his or her feelings, thoughts, and actions make sense and are understandable to you in a particular situation." With validation, we are making sure not to trivialize the other's feelings or make them seem silly, unimportant, or exaggerated. Rather, we want to convey that we understand a person's emotion or experience, that, "Of course! How could it be otherwise?"

Invalidation, in contrast, communicates through words or actions that another person's feelings, thoughts, and actions in a situation make *no* sense, are manipulative or "stupid," or an overreaction, or not worthy of your time, interest, or respect.

Why Validate?

Ask someone to read this section aloud:
Validation improves relationships. It can deescalate conflict and intense emotions. Validation can show that:

- We are listening.
- We understand.
- We are being nonjudgmental.
- We care about the relationship.
- We can disagree without having a big conflict.

In addition, validation can result in a communication partner who is calmer, less angry, and more receptive to what you have to say.

> **DISCUSSION POINT:** *Ask,* "Can you all think of a time when you felt invalidated and contrast that to another time when you felt understood? How was it different? How did it affect their behavior each time?"

EXERCISE (NONVERBAL INVALIDATION)

Pair off group members into dyads for this exercise or conduct it with the whole group, as follows. Invite one member to practice talking to the group about something and have the rest of the group pay close attention. Then, on cue from the leaders, the group members should act completely uninterested. Ask the speaker for observations of his or her experience. What typically happens is that people speak coherently when being listened to and become incoherent when they are ignored or rebuked.

What to Validate?

Ask someone to read this section of the handout aloud: "We can validate feelings, thoughts, and behaviors in ourselves and other people." *Leaders or group members can provide examples of each or use the previous example of Johnny, as discussed next.*

> **DISCUSSION POINT:** *Ask what would have been a validating action that Johnny's teacher could have said or done when Johnny's notebook fell on the floor? A reasonable response here would be for the teacher to have simply ignored the dropping of the notebook, since ignoring it implies it was insignificant and nondeliberate.*
>
> *Ask what would be a validating response the mother could have given? If group members have trouble answering, then offer an example, such as, "Oh, Johnny, that must have been so upsetting and frustrating for you, especially since you were really trying your best to pay attention and behave appropriately." If teens say this sounds too "sappy," encourage them to put into words a validating response they would welcome from their own parents.*

Validation Is Not Agreement

Remember, validation does not equal agreement. Validation does not necessarily mean that you like or agree with what the other person is doing, saying, or feeling. It means you understand where he or she is coming from. A therapist might validate the adolescent client's desire to get high with his friends by saying, "I do understand that it makes you feel good to spend time with your friends, including when you are getting high. Frankly, however, I don't think it is a good idea for you to get high right now, given your recent depression and the difficulties with focusing on schoolwork."

Validate the Valid, Not the Invalid

You can validate the emotion without validating the behavior. For example, a teen is feeling angry about her low grade on a test even though the parent knows she didn't study for it. The parent can validate the feeling of anger but should not validate the lack of studying that led to the low grade.

How to Validate

Introduce Walking the Middle Path Handout 9, "How Can We Validate Others?"

Emphasize that these points are not listed in order of importance or in order of how types of validation should be carried out. Rather, when people are familiar with various forms of validation, they have a choice of which they can use in each situation. Read the first point on "How can we validate others?"

1. *Actively listen; make eye contact and stay focused*. *After reading this point, leaders might pause and leave a moment of silence, which will result in group members looking up expectantly at the leader. The leader can say:* "This is step 1 in validation. You are doing it. I can tell you are looking and listening right now." *Note that one has to consider culture with regard to this point, as in some cultures (e.g., certain Hispanic subgroups and Asian cultures), maintaining eye contact may be considered disrespectful and thus invalidating. Ask group members to read the subsequent points.*

2. *Be mindful of your verbal and nonverbal reactions in order to avoid invalidation* *(e.g., rolling eyes, sucking teeth, walking away, heavy sighing, saying "That's stupid, don't be sad," or "Whatever," or "I don't care what you say"). As a member reads this point, leaders can illustrate by sighing and rolling their eyes while the participant is reading. Then ask the reader what the experience was like. Say:* "The main point here is, if you are trying to validate someone, be careful to avoid invalidating with verbal and nonverbal behaviors."

3. *Observe what the other person is feeling in the moment. Look for a word that describes the feeling*. For example, you can say, "I see that you are disappointed."

4. *Reflect the feeling back without judgment.* The goal is to communicate that you understand how the other person feels. You might say, "It makes sense that you are angry" or "I understand that you are having a tough time right now." For self-validation, you could say, "I have a right to feel sad right now."

5. *Show tolerance!* Look for how the feelings, thoughts, and actions make sense, given the other's (or your own) history *or* current situation, even if you don't approve of the behaviors or emotions. For example, a teenager might report her unwillingness to attend this treatment because none of her prior therapy experiences were helpful. One validating response based on past experiences might be, "I don't blame you for feeling hopeless about this, given your past experience." Another validating response in terms of the current situation might be, "I don't blame you for being a little uncertain about committing to DBT, given that we're asking you to come to a weekly 2-hour skills group that involves homework and practice done outside of group. That's a big commitment that requires some thought." [*Leaders should use a relevant example generated within the group whenever possible.*]

This type of validation is at the heart of DBT. Validating in terms of the *current* situation means looking for how the person's behavior makes sense because it is a reasonable or normative response to a current situation.

Example: Sharon is sometimes shy in groups. Now, she is attending the DBT multifamily skills training group with her mother, and when she occasionally speaks up in the group, another girl on the other side of the table gives her an angry, threatening look. On the way home, Sharon says to her mom: "That kid across the table was really mean to me. I don't want to sit near her next time." A response that would validate Sharon in terms of what actually happened would be, "Boy, I really understand, and I wouldn't want to sit near her either. She gave you quite a look when you spoke up." A perhaps equally honest but invalidating response would be for Sharon's mother to say, "I know you're shy, and it's hard for you to speak up in group with strangers." When a behavior is supported by current events, implying that it is caused by a quality or attribute demonstrated in the past can be invalidating.

6. *Respond in a way that shows that you are taking the person seriously (with or without words)*. Sometimes words are not necessary to convey validation. For example, if someone is crying, give a tissue or a hug. Imagine a fireman who arrives on the scene and sees someone hanging out the window, yelling, "I'm burning, save me!" and the fireman says, "I see that you are in great pain." A validating response is to jump on a ladder and save the person. So, if a person says, "I'm thirsty," giving them a glass of water communicates validation. Or if a friend or family member says, "I have a serious problem," listening may be sufficient validation. It may also pay to ask, "How can I be most helpful to you? Do you want me to help solve this problem, or do you just want me to hear you out?"

How Do You Validate without Agreeing?

Many people get confused on this point. For example, most parents struggle with how to validate their teen who asks for a later curfew when they don't agree with a later time and so they simply say "No!"

> **DISCUSSION POINT**: *Ask*, "Is there a way to validate a teen's desire for a later curfew without agreeing with the teen?" *If group members cannot generate examples, leaders can provide one, such as saying,* "'I get that you want to stay out later, since you're having fun with your friends. Yet, we agreed this would be your curfew time until you got back on track with your schoolwork.' A teen can also validate the caregiver by saying, 'I know you don't want me staying out later since I haven't been keeping my word with my schoolwork, *and* I am really disappointed with your decision.'"

How Do You Validate If You Don't Understand?

Some group members may raise the point that they do not see how they can validate when they simply do not understand the other point of view—that is, the other person's feelings or behaviors make no sense to them at all. For example, some parents might say that they cannot understand their adolescent's maladaptive behaviors or extreme emotional intensity. The leader can take this as an opportunity to model validation to such a parent by saying, "I can understand how that might be difficult for you to understand." The leader can then offer an explanation, such as, "The teen is in much pain and cannot see a way out of it other than her maladaptive behavior. The behavior seems logical to her in that moment."

If a parent still does not "get" the teen's behavior, a leader can suggest validating the teen's emotional experience: "Even though you don't understand your teen's choice of engaging in this maladaptive behavior as a solution, could you say to her, as a first step, 'I can see that you are obviously in a lot of pain.'" In this case, leaders can explain, the parent is validating the emotion, though not the behavioral urge. This is important because the teen will then feel the parent understands at least one aspect of his or her experience.

An alternative strategy is to say, "I know you want me to understand this and, believe me, I want to understand this, but I just can't get it. Let's keep talking so I can try to understand."

Similarly, teens may think it is sometimes impossible to understand their parents' feelings or decisions. Try having the teens in the room role-play asking questions, using a gentle tone, such as, "Mom, I am really trying to understand your decision not to allow me to drive my friends to the party, and I still don't get it. Can you please explain your reasoning one more time?"

This type of communication, presented in a nonjudgmental way, communicates that the parent's or teen's lack of understanding is the problem in this conversation, not the validity of the other's emotions or behavior. It also communicates deeper interest in the other's difficulties.

Validating Ourselves

Refer participants to Walking the Middle Path Handout 10, "How Can We Validate Ourselves?"

Many emotionally dysregulated adolescents tend to invalidate themselves. They are judgmental toward their own experience. Examples of self-invalidation are thoughts and statements like these: "I shouldn't feel sad about this," or "It's stupid that I got that upset," or "This shouldn't be so hard." Sometimes the self-invalidation comes from modeling the responses of an invalidating environment. Sometimes it comes from looking at the world through the lens of a person who is depressed.

It is important to learn how to validate yourself. Self-validation involves nonjudgmental observation, description, and acceptance of your own emotions. It involves acknowledging that your feelings, thoughts, and actions are accurate and make sense in a particular situation. Self-validation also relates to other-validation. Parents can help their adolescents self-validate, particularly if their adolescents are constantly asking their parents for reassurance.

Why Self-Validate?

Validating ourselves helps us reduce emotional and physical arousal (i.e., it is calming), reduces vulnerability to Emotion Mind and thus helps us access Wise Mind, and helps in processing information—which, in turn, enhances our ability to access and select effective responses.

Let's return to the example of Johnny. After his teacher accuses him of deliberately causing a distraction and trying to get attention, he gets angry, but then he second-guesses his own good intention to pay attention and behave well. As he feels his eyes well up with tears, he thinks,

"This isn't such a big deal. Why am I getting so upset?" This further invalidation intensifies his negative emotion, and impairs his ability to stay focused during the remaining class time.

> **DISCUSSION POINT**: *Ask*, "What could Johnny have said to validate himself?" *If needed, leaders can say*, "Johnny could have said to himself: 'I know this was not intentional. I know I'm trying to pay attention, and I'm doing the best I can. But she didn't see that—no wonder I feel so upset! I'll keep paying attention and talk to the teacher after class to explain this.'"

The following exercises allow group members to practice validating themselves and others.

EXERCISE (SELF-VALIDATION)

Ask group members to offer one quick example of self-validation based on events of the past day.

EXERCISE (OTHER-VALIDATION)

A group leader goes around and makes a statement to each group member; each member is to generate a validating response. An alternative is to have caregivers validate teens, teens validate caregivers, or peers can validate peers. The statements listed below can be used for this practice; leaders or group members can generate others as needed. Leaders can say the statements out loud or they can be written on slips of paper with group members picking one out of a bowl and reading it aloud. Note that it is *critical* for leaders to "drag out" (see Chapter 3) validation skills in the group by listening to members' attempts to offer validating responses and supplying coaching and shaping as needed. Always have members try again after offering feedback. Otherwise, they might think that they've understood validation but not have acquired the skill, and this is one of the most centrally important skills for families in DBT.

Statements by caregivers that teens can validate:
- "I worry about your friends driving you home from the party because I know there is usually a lot of drinking at these parties."
- "Your loud music is really distracting me because I'm trying to get some work done!"
- "I'm really upset about this!"
- "I can't take you now because I have to help your brother with his homework."

Statements by teens that caregivers can validate:
- "I used all of my allowance to buy my friend's birthday present and now I have no money left [*starts crying*]."
- "I'm in a bad mood today because I had a fight with my friend."
- "I have the earliest curfew of all my friends—it's really embarrassing!"
- "It's vacation. I really don't feel like doing my homework!"
- "I miss my friends from camp (*crying*)."

Statements by teens that peers can validate:
- "I can't come out with you because I still have too much studying to do or I'm going to fail my test."
- "I had a really bad time at the party. I felt like people were mean to me."

- "I'm really upset because my parents are not sending me back to my camp."
- "I don't feel like partying tonight because I got in trouble for doing that last weekend."

Statements by anyone that anyone can validate:
- "It took us forever to get here; we were stuck in traffic."
- "I hate dogs—they totally freak me out."
- "I spilled my drink on my keyboard!"
- "I'm really stressed; my friends are coming over and my place is a mess."

EXERCISE (OTHER-VALIDATION)

Another practice exercise can involve asking the group to generate both invalidating and validating responses to the scenario described below. Alternatively, group leaders can use the scenario for a role play to illustrate use of the skill. Co-leaders can play the two roles in the script.

Scenario: A teen joined the soccer team, and her parents warned her about the commitment and hard work. The second week of practice, she had to miss a party because of it. She started complaining, "It's not fair! Why do I have to go practice? And anyway, they make you run so many laps, I'm getting home late, I have no time for homework and it's exhausting!"

Question for group: What would be some invalidating responses?

Examples: "You knew it was going to be like this—we told you!" "You made a commitment—you have to go!" "Fine, you can quit—but that's it for sports. Don't ask us about any more teams!"

Questions for the group: Where is this approach likely to lead? What would a validating response be? Can you be both validating and dialectical? Here's an example: "It sounds really tough, and that is a lot of pressure. At the same time, you made a commitment and we'd like you to stick to your commitment."

Leaders' Role Play without Validation

TEEN: I don't care! I hate it!

PARENT: Well, that's too bad! You wanted us to sign you up, and we already spent all that money on soccer equipment, took you for tryouts . . .

TEEN: Well, I'm not going.

PARENT: Don't you think you're being a little dramatic here?

TEEN: I hate you! (*Runs out of the room crying.*)

Leaders' Role Play with Validation

TEEN: I'm so upset! Talia's party is this Thursday and I have to miss it because of soccer practice! All my friends are gonna be there!"

PARENT: Oh boy—that's really tough!

TEEN: Yeah, and I don't even like going to practice! They make you run so many laps and we stay so late, and I have no time to do homework, and I'm getting home late—it's exhausting! I don't get to do anything!

PARENT: Oh—that does sound hard. It's a lot of pressure on you, isn't it?

TEEN: *So* much pressure!

PARENT: I know. And even though you really wanted to make the team, it's hard when all the hard work and commitment actually comes . . .

TEEN: (*calming down*) Yeah, I mean, I guess I'm still glad I'm doing it in a way. And I'm proud to be on the team and everything. It's just really hard.

PARENT: It is really hard. It's the biggest commitment you've ever made to something, really.

TEEN: Well, I guess my soccer friends are all going through the same thing, and it's kind of cool to be part of a team.

PARENT: Yeah, that does seem cool. We'll figure this out, and you'll get through it. It'll be an adjustment, though, learning how to manage your time and learning to live with the sacrifices, but we'll figure it all out.

TEEN: Yeah, I know we'll figure it out. Thanks, Mom (*starts getting ready for practice*).

DISCUSSION POINTS: *Ask,* "What was different? Why do you think the outcome was different? What happened to the teen's emotion in the first case when she was not validated, and what happened in the second case, when she was? In the first role play, she just escalated her emotion and position. In the second, she calmed down and seemed to access her Wise Mind. Note that even if the teen ultimately wants to quit the team, it would not have been an impulsive decision with parent–teen conflict, as in the first role play."

Challenges in Teaching Validation

Some of the same challenges in teaching validation that arise here will also be relevant in the context of teaching the GIVE skills (see Chapter 10, Interpersonal Effectiveness). Watch for these pitfalls as members role-play validating comments in the group and report on their validation homework during the next skills training session. Point out the misuse of validation and correct.

• *Parents will ask, "Doesn't validation weaken my message and excuse or condone a problem?"* Validation neither weakens parents' message nor indicates agreement. In the soccer team example above, when the parent validated the teen's emotion, it actually strengthened the parent's position since the teen was then able to consider another way of looking at the situation, and the parent could convey understanding of the teen's emotional reaction without agreeing with her desire to quit the team.

• *Members will often confuse validation with reassurance, compliments, or praise.* For example, a teen says, "I'm sure I failed the test—it was so hard!" A reassuring response might be, "I doubt it, but even if you did, this test counts as only 10% of the grade." A praising response might be: "I'm sure you did fine—you always do—you're so smart!" Reassurance or praise can be supportive at times, but at other times it can actually be invalidating and lead the person to escalate the communication. In contrast, a validating response could be, "You must be really upset if you think you failed."

• *People often try to show they understand by talking about their own experience.* For example, someone says, "I had a terrible day! My teacher yelled at me for asking the kid next to me what the homework was when I was just trying to be responsible!" The listener says:

"I've had lots of days like that too, like that day my boss yelled at me last month about those spreadsheets!" Although the second person means well, it deflects the attention onto him or her instead of acknowledging the experience of the speaker. Or even harsher, a teen says, "I'm so upset about that C in English" and a parent replies, "*You're* upset—what about *us*?" This response is likely to slam the door on the teen's communication about a problem. A more validating response might be, "I know—that sucks. So what happened?"

   • *Responder tries to teach logical thinking instead of validating the emotion.* For example, a teen says, tearfully, "I'm so sad because I miss being on our vacation in Florida!" and a parent replies, "That's ridiculous! We spent a whole week there—should we not bother taking you next time because it just makes you upset later?" The remark will likely escalate the emotion, and the communication effort gets punished and may inhibit the teen's reaching out later. The parent misses an opportunity to connect with the teen regarding a positive vacation experience. A validating response might be: "It *is* hard to come home after such a great vacation; I know you miss being there."

   • *Responder focuses on the problem relayed in the communication rather than on the emotions*. A person says, "I feel so guilty and down that Jake's still mad at me 'cus I took a ride with a friend and left him waiting there." The listener responds: "So next time just remember to text him."

ASSIGNMENT OF HOMEWORK

Assign Walking the Middle Path Handout 11, "Practice Exercise: Validation of Self and Others."
   List one invalidating and two validating statements each for self and others. Before one can effectively validate oneself and others, one must catch oneself thinking or stating invalidating remarks. Thus, we'd like group members to self-monitor and notice any invalidating statements that might come to mind. Then, please commit to generating validating statements by using validation skills with someone else or alone in one situation during the week and record the skills use on the handout.

SESSION 3
BRIEF MINDFULNESS EXERCISE
. . . .
HOMEWORK REVIEW
. . . .
BREAK
. . . .

BEHAVIOR CHANGE

Orientation of Clients to the Behavior Change Skills and Their Rationale

When you get frustrated with a family member, do you resort to overtalking things, nagging, repeating yourself, criticizing, getting overly emotional, or yelling? Does that work for you? Do you end up getting the other person to do what you want? Lecturing, getting overly emotional, or yelling are ineffective because they tend not to teach new behaviors; instead, they model being out of control, and they often lead to escalations of emotions and conflict. In this session, we're going to learn more effective ways to change behavior in yourself and in other people.

Ask a group member to read the definition of behavior change skills on Walking the Middle Path Handout 12, "Behavior Change": "Strategies used to increase behaviors we do want and reduce behaviors we don't want (in ourselves or others)." Gently ask the participant to read the statement again a little louder "so everyone can hear." As soon as it is reread, toss a small piece of candy to the reader while saying, "Nice job for projecting your voice while you read."

Assuming our reader likes candy, what I did just then was to *positively reinforce* (reward) the louder reading. This is one of the most effective ways to change another's behavior in the ways you want.

What Behaviors Would You Like to Change?

DISCUSSION POINT: *Ask the group members if there are behaviors they would like to change in themselves or others. If so, what are some of these? Elicit two or three brief examples, especially of what people want to change in themselves. Some examples might include getting someone to nag less, listen more, clean up his or her room more often, give more privileges, or do homework more often. For oneself, these might include exercising more, eating less, yelling less, listening more, engaging in more pleasurable activities (music, sports, etc.), or procrastinating less.*

Make sure the behavior you want to change is specific and measurable. For example, instead of saying, "I want to increase happiness," think about what specific activities, events, or circumstances tend to make you happy and state your desire to increase those—for example, play more basketball, play more piano, see friends more often, and so on.

With behavior change skills, you will:

- Learn how to use positive reinforcement to increase behaviors you want.
- Learn about shaping—that is, reinforcing small steps in the direction of changes you want.
- Learn when to reduce behaviors by ignoring them.
- Learn how to reduce behaviors by effective use of consequences.

Positive Parenting Strategies

The best way for parents to increase behaviors they want to see in their teens is to notice what they're doing right and give them positive feedback about that. In addition, spend positive, enjoyable, or relaxing time with your teens and actively listen to them. These *positive parenting* strategies will be more effective than relying on negative feedback or punishments for what teens do wrong. [*Remind members who have been through the Emotion Regulation Skills module about Emotion Regulation Handout 10, "Pleasant Activities List."*]

DISCUSSION POINT: *Ask, "Teens and parents, would you like to spend more positive time together and hear more positive feedback? Have your interactions become mostly negative?" Many members will agree that by the time they have been referred for DBT, their interactions have gotten more negative. Explain that the following skills can help.*

Ways to Increase Behaviors: Reinforcement

Refer participants to Walking the Middle Path Handout 13, "Ways to Increase Behaviors."

An effective way to increase behavior is to provide reinforcement. A *reinforcer* is any consequence that increases a behavior. Reinforcers tend to be things that are liked and valued—like the candy I tossed earlier. A reinforcer tells the other person (or yourself) that he or she did what you wanted.

- *Reinforce immediately.* Timing is important. The reinforcer needs to follow the desired behavior immediately. If you wait too long, the reinforcer won't be connected with the behavior. For example, say you are trying to improve your backhand in tennis and your coach is observing 30 swings. Would you rather your coach tell you, "That's the swing! Nice job!" immediately after you use the right form, or would you rather he or she wait until you are done and then say "Your 14th swing—I liked that one."

- *Reinforcers must be motivating.* Reinforcers need to be things that you or the other person will work to get. A fresh plate of broccoli normally won't do it for most people. Examples of motivating reinforcers might include a nice dinner in a special restaurant or downloading some new music after the completion of a major project.

- *Two types of reinforcement.* There are two types of reinforcement. Both are used to increase behaviors. Positive reinforcement works by adding a rewarding consequence—giving a reward. Negative reinforcement works by removing something unpleasant—providing relief as a consequence.

Positive Reinforcement

Positive reinforcement increases a behavior by adding a reward. For example, you give a dog a biscuit when he sits, and he is more likely to sit again on command. You say "good job" when your young child says "please" or "thank you" and she is more likely to do it again. Reinforcers can motivate behaviors and so should be used with behaviors we want to increase in others. Ask your family members what kinds of things are motivating to them.

HOW TO POSITIVELY REINFORCE

Positive reinforcement should be (1) short and simple so it seems genuine; (2) immediate, not delayed; and (3) not combined with criticism. Don't forget to reinforce good behavior. We often ignore others when they are doing what they are supposed to do and only give them our attention when they get out of line!

> **DISCUSSION POINT:** *Say,* "Different things are reinforcing for different people, and at different times. How many people find coffee reinforcing? Now, for those coffee lovers in the room, do you find coffee equally reinforcing at every hour of the day? How about if you've just had two full cups? How about at bedtime?" *Allow for a quick discussion and recognition that not everyone loves coffee, and even coffee drinkers find it more appealing at some times than others.* "Be sure the reinforcer you choose is actually motivating for the person you are trying to reinforce!"

EXAMPLES OF POSITIVE REINFORCERS

Here are some ideas of what you can use to reinforce others [*Barkley, Edwards, & Robins, 1999*]. Although the examples focus on teens and parents, you can reinforce pretty much anyone.

Reinforcers for teens:
- Privileges (e.g., 1 hour of electronics, purchasing sporting goods, use of car, going out with friends)
- Praise (e.g., "I like the way you helped your sister study for her math test"; "I'm proud of you for working so hard at your piano practice"; "Thanks for helping out!")
- Money (e.g., for extra chores or a small amount toward desired purchase)
- Time and attention (e.g., time helping teen with a project, playing a game of his or her choice, shopping, or just "hanging out" or listening)

Reinforcers for parents:
- Praise (e.g., "You did a good job not freaking out, Mom")
- Acknowledgment (e.g., "Thanks for picking me up")
- Time and attention
- Help around the house (e.g., doing the dishes, or help cleaning the kitchen)
- Affection

EXERCISE

Go around and ask each group member to state one thing that he or she finds positively reinforcing. Examples might include praise, attention, money, affection, TV, time off, new clothes, makeup, accessories, sporting goods, certain foods or coffee, or the outcome of a goal itself (e.g., good grade, a cleaned room)

WHAT TO REINFORCE

- ***Examples of behaviors to reinforce in your teen.*** Expressing anger calmly without screaming or slamming things, spending time with parent, getting places on time, coming to parent with a problem rather than waiting until it gets bigger, hard work, pitching in around the house, texting parent to let him or her know of whereabouts, and sticking to curfew or following other rules.

- ***Examples of behaviors to reinforce in your parent.*** Note that reinforcement is not only for parents to use with kids! Verbally expressing anger without screaming or slamming things, spending time with you, helping you work out a problem, listening to you and validating you, bringing you places and picking you up, being on time for picking you up, buying you things you need, being involved in your life, not getting stressed out, and giving you increased freedom/trusting you.

WHEN TO WITHHOLD POSITIVE REINFORCEMENT

Reinforce *only* those behaviors that you want to increase. Sometimes it is important to withhold positive reinforcement. In particular, don't reinforce an escalation of maladaptive behaviors. For example, when someone escalates a self-harm behavior, it is important to respond with monitoring, giving serious attention to harm level and risk. Do what is needed, such as locking up sharp objects or pills or obtaining medical attention. But do *not* offer more warm attention and time than usual, give a special dessert, or buy something special—these things could reinforce—and increase—the self-harm.

> **DISCUSSION POINTS**: *Ask,* "What would be a positive reinforcer for the behavior you would like to increase in yourself? What would make you likely to do it?"
>
> *Guide group members in their responses to keep reinforcers small, realistic, safe, and age-appropriate. For example, teens should not choose cars, large amounts of money, drinking alcohol, or staying out all night with friends. Also, search for meaningful reinforcers beyond just money, such as time spent with a parent. In addition, discuss the concept of* satiation: *something that is reinforcing once or twice may not be a reinforcer when given too much, and it may even become aversive. For example, food is not a reinforcer after a really big meal, affection is not a reinforcer if one receives plenty of that, etc. Something is only a reinforcer if it is given in appropriate doses. This is also true with praise. Elicit examples, particularly from adolescents.*

Negative Reinforcement

Negative reinforcement also increases behaviors but in a different way. The best way to remember what negative reinforcement means is to associate it with the word *relief*. Negative reinforcement increases the frequency of a behavior by removing something aversive or unpleasant.

- *Examples of negative reinforcement.* Taking aspirin gets rid of a headache, cleaning your room stops Mom from nagging you, cutting yourself decreases negative feeling, buying something your child wants stops the tantrum. Doing these things will increase the behaviors—from taking an aspirin to cutting to giving in to tantrums—if they provide relief.

- *Negative reinforcers that are harmful.* As you can see, harmful coping strategies such as a self-injurious behavior can be negatively reinforcing. Often people use risky or dangerous behaviors to provide relief from emotional or physical pain. This is usually because the risky behaviors work quickly, are easy to use, or the person hasn't found something else that works as well. Examples include smoking, drinking, posting feelings or inappropriate pictures on Facebook, spending excessive amounts of money, skipping school, or self-injuring.

> **DISCUSSION POINT**: *Ask,* "Can anyone think of more skillful coping strategies that people can use or have used for relief (negative reinforcement) of pain?" *Allow group to respond. Examples of things to try for relief include distress tolerance skills, mindfulness practice, or emotion regulation skills such as short-term pleasant activities.*

DISCUSSION POINT: *Leaders can first share an example of an annoyance, discomfort, or pain and how they found relief, such as having back pain and getting relief by receiving a massage. The reduction in pain increased the likelihood of seeking a massage in the future. Next, leaders ask group members to identify a source of discomfort that they would like relieved or removed, for example, a parent nagging too much. What new behavior might help reduce this discomfort? For instance, if a teen's cleaning of his room led to a reduction in a parent's nagging, the teen would be more likely to clean his room again. Elicit one or two examples from group.*

- **Reinforcers can be helpful or harmful.** Positive and negative reinforcement can be applied in adaptive or maladaptive ways. For example, one can positively reinforce oneself with downloading some new music versus getting drunk. Or, one can get relief from emotional pain by the negative reinforcement of taking a long bath versus binge eating.

Shaping

When the change you want takes time, takes work, or requires multiple steps (e.g., completing a research paper, changing a habit), positive reinforcement at the very end of the process doesn't work very well. It's hard to make a big change and it doesn't happen all at once. If we expect immediate success of ourselves or others, we're setting ourselves up for disappointment and potential failure. This is when we use shaping.

Shaping is reinforcing small steps toward a larger goal or desired behavior. We normally use rewards—positive reinforcements—for shaping behaviors. For example, we might praise ourselves (or our teens) for small steps toward getting a big project done, like making an outline, writing the first section, and so on, rather than withholding a reward until the project is completed. Each small step toward one's goal needs to be reinforced to increase the chances of continuing to work toward that goal.

DISCUSSION POINT: *Ask,* "Parents, have you ever been frustrated with your child for starting a large school project the night before it was due? Teens, have you ever been frustrated with yourselves for this? How could you use shaping?" *Group member examples might include approaches such as saying,* "Why don't you sit down and outline the paper the week before the due date? Once that's done, you can go watch TV." *Step 2 would then be to write the introduction and provide a small reinforcement for that, and so on.*

EXERCISE (OPTIONAL)

Break members into groups by family. Ask them to identify one goal of one family member that can be broken down into smaller pieces, such as a teen improving in school or a parent increasing his or her exercise. Advise them not to choose a hot-button topic, one that any family member can refuse to discuss. They should identify some small steps toward the goal and brainstorm what might be reinforcing to the person as he or she takes those small steps. It's useful if the teen identifies a goal and says what he or she needs from the parents. For example, the teen might say, "It could help if you reinforce my attempts to study, instead of telling me 'that's not enough.'" The exercise can also be useful when targeting a parent's goal. The objective is for everyone to see that behavior change can be broken into small steps that benefit from reinforcement.

Examples of multistep behaviors that lend themselves to shaping include getting to bed earlier, exercising more, improving work or study habits, developing healthier eating habits, or increasing social interaction with others.

Self-Reinforcement

It is important to use reinforcement on yourself! Don't forget to reward yourself for steps toward finishing projects, working toward goals, etc. You can reinforce by allowing yourself a break, some time with a friend, going for a run, treating yourself to a piece of candy, or watching a TV show.

ASSIGNMENT OF HOMEWORK

Assign Walking the Middle Path Handout 14, "Practice Exercise: Positive Reinforcement."

1. Each of you can write down something positive about a family member's behavior that you can report in the group the next week. This exercise will help you identify behaviors that you can reinforce with praise or attention. Try to say at least one positive thing to one another every day.

2. In addition, identify a specific behavior that you want to increase in yourself and a behavior to increase in someone else. Then consider the specific reinforcers you will use for yourself and the other person ahead of time.

SESSION 4
BRIEF MINDFULNESS EXERCISE
· · · ·
HOMEWORK REVIEW
· · · ·
BREAK
· · · ·

WAYS TO DECREASE OR STOP BEHAVIORS

Refer participants to Walking the Middle Path Handout 15, "Ways to Decrease or Stop Behaviors."

The skills we are now going to discuss are for reducing or stopping behaviors you do not want in yourself or others. They are extinction and punishment.

Extinction

We often pay attention to other people when they are doing something we don't like. For example, when our kids are misbehaving, we put down our newspaper or get off the phone and we pay attention to them—it's negative attention, but any kind of attention can actually be a reinforcer. We don't mean it, but we may be inadvertently increasing the behavior we don't want when we pay attention to it.

We can reduce a behavior by withholding the reinforcer we've been giving it. This strategy is called *extinction*. So, if you've been reinforcing misbehavior by paying attention to it, you stop paying attention and ignore the misbehavior. However, to make extinction work, there are two other important pieces.

Reinforce an Alternative Behavior and Ride Out the Behavioral Burst

First, to extinguish a behavior, have in mind a more desirable replacement behavior and reinforce that replacement behavior.

Second, you need to expect, and ride out, the behavioral burst. When you stop reinforcing a behavior, that behavior initially escalates—that's the behavioral burst. It gets worse before it then fades away. For example, if a child begins to throw a tantrum in the supermarket because he or she wants a candy bar, a parent is likely to give in to stop the tantrum. This giving in, however, reinforces the tantrum and makes it more likely to occur during the next visit to the supermarket. However, if the parent withholds reinforcement by not buying the candy bar, the tantrum is likely to escalate (making everyone unhappy). This is the behavioral burst, and it can continue to happen during subsequent shopping trips. But if the parent holds the line by not giving in, then the tantrum behavior is likely to extinguish, or go away, over time. The parent can say to the child, "If you get through this trip without a tantrum, I will let you ride the toy train outside when we leave!" This sets up reinforcement for the replacement behavior, for not having a tantrum, and makes the extinguished behavior more likely to stay away.

Beware of Intermittent Reinforcement

Let's suppose the parent sticks to no candy bar during three supermarket trips but the fourth time gives in and buys the candy bar. This is called *intermittent reinforcement*. The parent might be thinking, "It's just this one time." However, the parent now has an even bigger problem because intermittently reinforced behaviors are the most difficult to stop or change.

Tips for Effective Use of Extinction

Withholding reinforcement doesn't mean being angry or rude. Remain neutral and seemingly unaffected by the behavior. When a more desirable behavior shows up, then warm up and reinforce that immediately!

Give your attention when the person is doing what he or she is supposed to be doing, and withdraw your attention when the person is not. This is how time out works with younger kids; you remove reinforcing activities and attention from them. One might use extinction by ignoring tantrums, escalations of conflict, rudeness, interruptions, protests, and snickering.

- Don't give up in the face of the behavioral burst—you have to ride it out.
- Don't hesitate to tell the person that you are beginning to work on extinguishing the behavior so that it does not seem arbitrary or punitive. For example, "I will not respond to you when you speak to me like that."
- Don't forget to reinforce alternative, adaptive behaviors. We don't want to ignore those or they can extinguish!
- Try not to ignore small, effective requests for help or attention. If ignored, these will tend to escalate and become less effective!

Punishment

Punishment is a consequence that decreases a behavior by adding something negative or removing something positive.

CAUTION: Many parents overuse punishment or use it ineffectively with their emotionally dysregulated and impulsive teens. Punishment comes with risks and can have negative effects:

- One can overdo it.
- It can lead to hiding the behaviors rather than stopping them.
- It can be demoralizing to kids and increase their hopelessness, depression, and anger.
- It does not teach new behavior.
- It does not motivate.
- It may lead to self-punishment.

Put your energy into preventing the need for punishment. Use punishment sparingly.

Effective Use of Punishment

These are important things to know about using punishment effectively:

- First, reinforce desired behaviors to prevent undesired ones.
- Communicate clear rules and expectations.
- Have a menu of possible punishments ready in advance.
- Pair negative consequences with reinforcement of desired behavior.
- Use measured (moderate) consequences related to the "crime" with follow-through.
- Apply consequences immediately.
- Allow natural consequences.

• *Reinforce desired behaviors to prevent undesired ones.* You can prevent the need for punishment by increasing positive parenting strategies such as spending positive time together, becoming involved in your kids' lives, and using reinforcement, shaping, and extinction. For example, it is usually more effective to praise a teen for waking up a little earlier and build on that, than to punish oversleeping.

• *Communicate clear rules and expectations.* Make sure you are communicating clear rules and expectations. This clarity can prevent the need for punishment because teens can take responsibility for earning freedoms and privileges. It is also important to be able to say "no." We notice that some parents are afraid to upset their kids, or fear that their teens won't like them if they assert their parental authority and say "no" at times. Saying "no" and sticking to it helps clarify the rules that can decrease behavior problems and the need for consequences. It also helps kids learn to tolerate distress.

• *Pair punishment with reinforcement of a desired behavior.* Punishment may be necessary at times but will work much better if you reinforce an alternate behavior. Extinction, however, can work to decrease a behavior even if you don't reinforce another behavior.

DISCUSSION POINT: *Elicit examples from teens and parents of behaviors that appear necessary to "punish" versus extinguish. For example, parents may feel they have to punish lying or coming home late for curfew, but that they can ignore siblings' fits of giggling or minor arguing during homework time.*

• *Have a menu of possible punishments ready in advance.* In order not to punish impulsively, from Emotion Mind, or skip a needed consequence because you cannot think of one, it is useful to develop a menu of possible consequences that are rated as more to less severe. Then you can decide how severe an offense is and select one from the list.

> *Note to Leaders:* Many parents have told us that they have no idea what consequences they can apply to their adolescents. They state that their teens are too old for a time out, which might work with younger kids. And, they are physically grown and independent, so parents say they cannot physically stop them from doing certain things, such as leaving the house. Some parents report that when they try to enforce consequences, such as taking away computer or phone time, their teens escalate to physical tactics to assert their access to their property. Thus, it can be useful to have a set of consequences ready to apply, and to explain that a violation of a consequence will lead to another or a larger one. (Remember, it is important to balance this with reinforcements, such as saying, "If you do get to bed on time 4 days in a row, you may stay up an extra 30 minutes on the fifth night.")
>
> Examples of consequences for teens include the following ideas [from Phelan, 1998]: Removing material things (e.g., phone, car access, reduced allowance), removing time spent on activities (e.g., Internet use, videogame time), removing privileges (shopping trip, curfew), removal of attention of family or friends, and grounding (make it short, usually part of a day to 2 days, with a maximum of 2 weeks). Alternatively, parents, you can add aversives such as extra chores or educational activity (e.g., writing a one-page essay on why the offense was harmful).

• *Use specific, time-limited consequences related to the crime, and follow through.* Be specific, moderate, time limited, and make the "punishment fit the crime." In other words, the punishment should match the severity of the "offense" and ideally, it should be related to the offense. For example, if a teen comes home 1 hour late for curfew, a consequence might be a 1-hour-earlier curfew next time, rather than mowing the lawn for the whole summer, which seems more extreme than the violation and is unrelated. Be sure to follow through, so that you are taken seriously, or you will teach your teen that consequences are just empty threats. It is preferable to err on the side of a minor consequence where you follow through, than a major one that you do not follow through.

Often, it is preferable to take away a privilege than to add an aversive. Many parents will "punish" teens with yelling, put-downs, and name-calling ("You're self-centered!"; "You're lazy!"), criticisms ("You're inconsiderate—what's wrong with you?"), and blaming ("You always do this to your sister—it's *your* fault!"). These comments hurt the relationship, increase negative emotions such as anger and sadness, and do not motivate or teach new behaviors. They should be avoided. Ask yourself: Is Wise Mind dictating the consequences and your response?

• *Apply punishing consequences immediately.* Do not delay consequences.

• *Allow natural consequences.* Undesirable behaviors are sometimes followed by their own naturally punishing consequences. For example, a teen doesn't study enough and fails the exam. You don't eat and you feel light-headed during an important job interview. You oversleep, miss the bus, and have to walk to school. When this happens, it can be most effective to let the natural consequence occur and not apply an additional punishment. Parents who hold on too tightly (one extreme of a dialectical dilemma) can interfere with natural consequences or demoralize their teen by inflicting too much punishment.

ASSIGNMENT OF HOMEWORK

Assign Walking the Middle Path Handout 16, "Practice Exercise: Extinction and Punishment."
    Select annoying behaviors of others that you can ignore to practice putting behaviors on an extinction schedule. What is the result? Parents, think of several measured consequences you can use with your teens, so you have them ready in the heat of the moment.

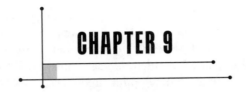

CHAPTER 9

Emotion Regulation Skills

SESSION OUTLINES

Session 1

- ▶ Brief Mindfulness Exercise
- ▶ Homework Review
- ▶ Break
- ▶ Orientation of Clients to Emotion Regulation Skills and Their Rationale
- ▶ Goals of Emotion Regulation Training
- ▶ The Functions of Emotions: What Good Are Emotions?
- ▶ A Model of Emotions
- ▶ Assignment of Homework
- ▶ Session Wind-Down

Handouts and Other Materials

- ▶ Emotion Regulation Handout 1, "Taking Charge of Your Emotions: Why Bother?"
- ▶ Emotion Regulation Handout 2, "Goals of Emotion Regulation Skills Training"
- ▶ Emotion Regulation Handout 3, "Short List of Emotions"
- ▶ Emotion Regulation Handout 4, "What Good Are Emotions?"
- ▶ Emotion Regulation Handout 5, "A Model of Emotions"
- ▶ Emotion Regulation Handout 6, "A Model of Emotions with Skills"
- ▶ Emotion Regulation Handout 7, "Practice Exercise: Observe and Describe an Emotion"
- ▶ Whiteboard or other writing surface and markers
- ▶ Mindfulness bell

Session 2

▶ Brief Mindfulness Exercise
▶ Homework Review
▶ Break
▶ Orientation of Clients to ABC PLEASE Skills
▶ Accumulating Positive Experiences—Short Term
▶ Accumulating Positive Experiences—Long Term
▶ Assignment of Homework
▶ Challenges in Teaching Accumulating Positives
▶ Session Wind-Down

Handouts and Other Materials

▶ Emotion Regulation Handout 8, "ABC PLEASE Overview"
▶ Emotion Regulation Handout 9, "ACCUMULATING Positive Experiences—Short Term"
▶ Emotion Regulation Handout 10, "Pleasant Activities List"
▶ Emotion Regulation Handout 11, "Parent–Teen Shared Pleasant Activities List"
▶ Emotion Regulation Handout 12, "ACCUMULATING Positive Experiences—Long Term"
▶ Emotion Regulation Handout 13, "Wise Mind Values and Priorities List"
▶ Emotion Regulation Handout 14, "Practice Exercise: ACCUMULATING Positive Experiences in the Short and Long Term"
▶ Whiteboard or other writing surface and markers
▶ Mindfulness bell

Session 3

▶ Brief Mindfulness Exercise
▶ Homework Review
▶ Break
▶ Building Mastery
▶ Coping Ahead
▶ PLEASE Skills
▶ Assignment of Homework
▶ Session Wind-Down

Handouts and Other Materials

▶ Emotion Regulation Handout 15, "Building Mastery and Coping Ahead"
▶ Emotion Regulation Handout 16, "PLEASE Skills"

▶ Emotion Regulation Optional Handout 16a, "FOOD and Your MOOD"

▶ Emotion Regulation Optional Handout 16b, "BEST Ways to Get REST: 12 Tips for Better Sleep"

▶ Emotion Regulation Handout 17, "Practice Exercise: Build Mastery, Cope Ahead, and PLEASE Skills"

▶ Whiteboard or other writing surface and markers

▶ Mindfulness bell

Session 4

▶ Brief Mindfulness Exercise

▶ Homework Review

▶ Break

▶ Check the Facts and Problem Solving

▶ Opposite Action

▶ Assignment of Homework

▶ Session Wind-Down

Handouts and Other Materials

▶ Emotion Regulation Handout 18, "The Wave Skill: Mindfulness of Current Emotions"

▶ Emotion Regulation Handout 19, "Check the Facts and Problem Solving"

▶ Emotion Regulation Handout 20, "Opposite Action to Change Emotions"

▶ Emotion Regulation Handout 21, "Practice Exercise: Opposite Action"

▶ Index cards with opposite action role-play scenarios

▶ Whiteboard or other writing surface and markers

▶ Mindfulness bell

TEACHING NOTES

I am not at all in a humour for writing; I must write on till I am.
—JANE AUSTEN

You can't stop the waves, but you can learn to surf.
—JOHN KABAT-ZINN

ABOUT THIS MODULE

This module on emotion regulation skills addresses the biological vulnerability to emotion dysregulation described in DBT's biosocial theory. The theory holds that people with chronic, significant problems regulating emotion have a constitutional emotional sensitivity, high reactivity, and slow return to baseline mood, and lack capacities for regulating emotions. When this emotional vulnerability occurs in the context of a pervasively invalidating environment, the emotional intensity and the environment transact over time to exacerbate each other. The Walking the Middle Path Skills and Interpersonal Effectiveness Skills modules both address the environmental side by teaching validation, reinforcement, and other skills. This emotion regulation module primarily addresses the individual, temperamental factors identified in the theory. Thus, the skills herein teach participants ways to minimize emotional vulnerability and reactivity and to recover more quickly from extreme mood states. These skills involve labeling and understanding emotions, reducing vulnerability to Emotion Mind, creating more positive emotions, preventing negative emotions, and lowering the intensity of negative emotions that have already "fired." Many of the skills derive from established, evidence-based behavioral interventions, such as behavioral activation treatment for depression (short-term pleasant activities and building mastery) and exposure treatment for anxiety and other painful, avoided emotions (opposite action).

One of the most common refrains we hear from members new to DBT skills training is, "I was too upset to use my skills." Leaders can remind members that this treatment was not developed for people who are only a tiny bit upset, but for the real thing—intense and chronic emotional distress. Thus, being very upset is just the time to try a skill, or multiple skills. Mindfulness of current emotions and urges while fully participating in the emotion and doing nothing else (instead of a maladaptive behavior) should come first, even if only briefly. Then, members might choose the opposite action skill to throw themselves into an activity or situation, even when they don't feel like it. This skill will have to be practiced over and over to break the vicious cycle of mood-dependent behaviors that only make problems worse.

Note that we have added two supplemental handouts that we believe can be useful for teens and families. These supplemental materials can be reviewed in the group if there is time, or during an individual therapy session if needed. These are Optional Handout 16a, "FOOD and Your MOOD," and Optional Handout 16b, "BEST Ways to Get REST: 12 Tips for Better Sleep." We developed these additional handouts to supplement the PLEASE skills, based on frequent struggles with food choices and sleep we have observed with teens. These latter two handouts have not yet been included in research.

Note to Leaders: Given the amount of content in this module, consider abbreviating the Orientation and Mindfulness module to 1 week instead of 2 to allow for an extra week of the Emotion Regulation Skills module. This would afford the possibility of spending 5 weeks covering emotion regulation content rather than 4.

SESSION 1

BRIEF MINDFULNESS EXERCISE
• • • •
HOMEWORK REVIEW
• • • •
BREAK
• • • •

EMOTION REGULATION SKILLS

Orientation of Clients to the Emotion Regulation Skills and Their Rationale

We want you to become the captain of your ship, the king or queen of your castle, the controller of your own emotions. So, today we are going to teach you how to stop your emotions from controlling you. No more being victimized by your emotions. Isn't that how it feels sometimes when you are depressed, or worried, or angry?

As clients in DBT, you have a biologically based emotional vulnerability. Emotion regulation skills will help you feel less emotionally vulnerable, feel more in command of your emotions, and learn how to experience emotions like a wave without drowning.

Why Bother Taking Charge of Emotions?

Refer participants to Emotion Regulation Handout 1, "Taking Charge of Your Emotions: Why Bother?"

Taking charge of your emotions is important because:

1. Emotionally dysregulated adolescents often have intense emotions, such as anger, frustration, depression, or anxiety. [*Ask group members if they agree with this statement.*]

2. Difficulties controlling these intense emotions often lead to impulsive or problem behaviors. [*Leader invites a few examples that are likely to include drinking, using drugs, risky sex, risky online behavior, anger explosions, missing school, avoiding people or responsibilities, suicidality, and disordered-eating behaviors.*] Do you agree with this statement?

3. Problematic behaviors, such as fighting, drugging, binge-eating, cutting, yelling, or walking away from someone when he or she is talking to you are often behavioral solutions to intensely painful emotions. This module will teach you more effective solutions. Here is how.

GOALS OF EMOTION REGULATION TRAINING

Refer participants to Emotion Regulation Handout 2, "Goals of Emotion Regulation Skills Training."

Understand the Emotions You Experience

You are going to learn why emotions are important. You are going to learn how to identify emotions by using your mindfulness (observe and describe) skills. You have to know what you are feeling in order to change it.

You are going to learn how to evaluate whether your emotional responses are effective. That means you will need to ask yourself whether your emotions are working for you or against you in this moment.

If the emotion is working for you, then let yourself experience it. For example, you are walking down a dark alley at night and you feel anxious. Use that emotion to be extra vigilant; walk carefully and quickly or turn around and go another way. Another example: You feel ashamed after being disrespectful toward a teacher whom you normally like. Use this emotion to apologize for your action and assure your teacher that you will not repeat that behavior. Then let it go and move on.

If the emotion is working against you, figure out which skill you need to use to change it. For example, you feel so worried about a test that you can't focus. Instead you get irritable, scream at your sibling, and watch TV instead of studying. Maybe you feel so angry that you hurt yourself, punch a wall, or curse at your parent. Maybe you feel so sad and depressed that instead of going to school, you lie in bed all day and get further behind and feel even worse.

Reduce Emotional Vulnerability

You are going to learn how to keep unwanted emotions from starting in the first place. And, if they do start, they hopefully won't get as intense, and they won't last as long as they do now. In other words, you are going to learn how to decrease your vulnerability to Emotion Mind. Wouldn't it be great if you didn't feel irritable as often?

You are going to learn how to increase positive emotions. Does anyone know how to increase positive emotions? If you want to feel happier, more engaged in life, and more in control, what do you do? Stay tuned; we're going to teach you those skills in this module.

Decrease the Frequency of Unwanted Emotions

By understanding what emotions do for you, learning to decrease emotional vulnerability and increase positive emotions, and practicing ways to reduce painful emotions when they occur, you will decrease the frequency of unwanted emotions.

Decrease Emotional Suffering

You are going to learn how to stop or reduce your suffering from unwanted emotions once they start. How can you reduce shame, reduce anxiety, reduce guilt, reduce anger, reduce sadness? First, you will learn how to nonjudgmentally observe and describe painful emotions, accept them, and even let go of them using mindfulness skills. Then you will learn how to change your emotions through opposite action skills—that is, taking an action that is opposite to the emotion you currently feel. We are going to teach that to you at the end of this module.

A Short List of Emotions

Refer participants to the Emotion Regulation Handout 3, "Short List of Emotions."

EXERCISE

Ask participants to take 2 minutes to look at the short list of emotions on this next handout and check off every emotion they have experienced in the past week. Then ask: "How many of you experienced more than one emotion? [*Wait for show of hands.*] How many checked off two to four emotions? [*Wait again.*] How many had five to seven? How many had eight to 12? How many had more than 12?" [*Most people tend to indicate high numbers of emotions. Ask for observations about the nature of group members' emotions.*] *Points to make include*:

- People have lots of different emotions.
- Emotions often change.
- No one has had the same emotion forever!

> **DISCUSSION POINT:** *Ask,* "Have people been paying attention to their positive emotions? What happens when you have positive emotions? When you have worry thoughts? When you focus on the negative?"

• *It is important to recognize and label emotions.* Being able to label (i.e., notice and put words on) emotions, in itself, helps to regulate them. What you cannot change from being mindful you can learn how to change through the use of other emotion regulation skills we will be teaching you.

THE FUNCTIONS OF EMOTIONS: WHAT GOOD ARE EMOTIONS?

Refer participants to Emotion Regulation Handout 4, "What Good Are Emotions?"

Emotions Give Us Information

Emotions give us information. They can signal that something is happening (e.g., feeling very nervous standing alone in a dark alley). Sometimes our emotions communicate by "gut feeling."

But emotions are not facts. It's a problem when we treat emotions as if they are facts about the world. For example: "I love him, so he must be good for me," or "I'm afraid, so there's a threat." My fear is not proof that a threat exists; it's only a signal that there may or may not be a threat. It is important to check the facts about a situation before making decisions. You want to make Wise Mind decisions that incorporate emotions in the decision making but avoid Emotion Mind decisions on their own.

Emotions Communicate to, and Influence, Others

Facial expressions and body posture say a lot about how you're feeling. Whether you realize it or not, your emotions, expressed by your words and/or your face and body language, influence how other people respond to you. They let people know when to move back, come closer, run, offer help, etc. For example, your sad face may cause someone to ask you if you are OK and to give you some support.

EXERCISE

The leader can demonstrate by looking sad and glum, putting head down on hands resting on table, and not speaking. Then ask: "What do you think I am feeling? What do you want to say or do in response to how I am behaving?"

> **DISCUSSION POINT:** *Discuss how group members communicate to, or are influenced by, others' emotional expressions.*

Emotions Motivate and Prepare Us for Action

Specific emotions have an action urge that is often biologically "hardwired." For example, when you hear a horn beep [*make an extremely loud horn sound, BEEEEEEEEEEEEEP!!!, many participants will jump out of their seats and become startled; point this out*], how you reacted to this sound is the point. If you are talking to your friend while crossing a busy intersection and you hear that horn blaring, you don't ask your friend, "Do you think we should hurry up?" You move forward or backward automatically. Your automatic, hardwired responses take over.

Emotions save time in getting us to act in important situations. We don't have to think everything through. For example, one teenage girl was hanging out on the playground with her 6-year-old sister. When she looked up she saw her sister hanging by her poncho, which had gotten caught on the playground equipment. She was now 8 feet up in the air with her feet dangling; she was having trouble breathing, and she was panic-stricken. The girl didn't think, "What should I do? Should I ask if you are OK? Should I call a friend?" No, without a second thought, she ran as quickly as she could, detached her sister from the equipment, and made sure she could breathe comfortably again. Then she took off her sister's poncho. They both sat down, calmed down, and then her sister got back on the slide again.

Are you ready to learn new skills to take charge of your emotions? Let's start by learning a model of emotions.

A MODEL OF EMOTIONS

Before asking the group to turn to Emotion Regulation Handout 5, "A Model of Emotions," one leader tells a compelling emotional story, while the co-leader draws the model's components on the board. (Looking at the handout first, out of context, can overwhelm members.) The co-leader should draw all the uni- and bidirectional arrows between the components, as shown in the handout. In telling the story, the leader shares his or her own experiences at each stage of the emotion, but also engages the group by eliciting what they might be thinking, feeling, having urges to do, doing, or saying, etc., in that situation. The following components of the emotion-inducing story could be explored:

- The prompting event
- Vulnerability factors preceding it that may make the emotional reaction stronger
- Thoughts about the event
- Internal body reactions
- Urges to act
- Facial expression, body language, words, and actions
- The emotion name(s)
- Aftereffects (including secondary emotions)
- A second prompting event

And so on, back through the components again. For example:

"When my daughter was younger, she wandered away from me in a sporting goods store. I figured she was just in the next aisle, so I walked around the immediate area; when I didn't see her, I began calling her name. So the *prompting event* was not immediately finding my daughter at Modell's. [*Co-leader writes in box, on left middle of board,* Losing daughter at Modell's.]

"Note that the event you experience could be located internally, such as a thought, memory, or body sensation, or in the environment, such as my not finding my daughter, something someone says, or getting a poor test grade. Also, paying *attention* to the prompting event is a central part of the chain of reactions it triggers. For example, if one successfully distracts from receiving a poor final exam grade by studying for the next final, the various emotion-related components and resulting negative emotions will be diminished.

"*Vulnerability factors* contributed to the intensity of my emotional reaction. They included being tired and hungry. [*Co-leader writes* tired, hungry *and puts a box around the words on far upper-left corner of the board, drawing an arrow from that box leading into the* Prompting Event *box*.]

"The first *thought*, or interpretation, I had when she didn't answer my call was, 'She's lost!' [*Co-leader writes* She's lost! *in a box below the prompting event of losing daughter.*] What other interpretations or thoughts do you folks think I might have been having?"

The leader takes a few suggestions from group members and the co-leader writes them in the same box below the prompting event. These might include, "She's missing!" "Someone took her!" "I'm a terrible parent!" *Now the co-leader draws a dotted line with an arrow pointing down from the* Prompting Event *leading to the* Thoughts *box, showing the link between the prompting events and the thoughts. Note that the line is dotted because sometimes an event leads to emotional reactions without being mediated by thoughts; leaders can point this out later.*

"Now, all this stuff started to go on *inside* of me, like brain changes, face and body changes, what I sensed or experienced, and urges. These were my *internal* reactions. So my adrenaline was making my heart pump, my face felt hot, I sensed a lump in my throat. I had the *urge* to run all over the store, shout her name, let out some profanities, and shake the security guard, yelling, have you seen my daughter?!?!"

The co-leader draws a much larger box to the right of the prompting event box. On top of the box, he or she writes the word Internal. *The co-leader draws an arrow from the* Prompting Event *box leading straight to this box, and also draws a dotted arrow from the* Thoughts *box to this box, indicating that the prompting event leads directly to these internal events, and that one's thoughts can also lead to these internal events. Inside the box, on top, the co-leader writes* Body Changes/What You Experience.

"These body changes can include neurochemical changes, muscle changes, sensations from nerve signals, blood vessels/pressure, heart, and temperature throughout the face and body."

Now fill in the upper portion: adrenaline pumping, face hot, lump in throat.
About two-thirds of the way down, write the words Action Urges. *Below those words write* run around, shout, curse, shake guard. *Now ask the group:*

"What might some of you be feeling, if you were in my shoes? Remember, an observer can't see this; it is only what you are experiencing internally."

Take a couple of descriptions and write them down in the proper place. They might offer experiences such as heart racing, muscles tensing, and sweating. Under action urges, they might offer urges to ask others for help, or urges to run outside and check the parking lot.

"In addition to everything going on inside me, there were *external* things happening, that if people were watching me, or I were being filmed, others could observe and describe. These include my face and body language, expression, posture, gestures, what I actually say and do."

The co-leader draws another big box, same size and shape as the Internal *box, to the right. On top of the box, he or she writes the word* External. *Inside the box, on top, he or she writes the words* Face and Body (expression, body language, posture). *About three-quarters of the way down, he or she writes the word* Actions (what I say and do). *Now fill in the upper portion, face and body:*

"You'd see my eyes wide and darting around, brow furrowed, jaw and fists clenched. What I actually *said and did* was this: I ran by all the aisles; I turned my head rapidly in different directions and repeatedly shouted my daughter's name, in an ever-louder volume."

Below the words what I say and do, *the co-leader writes* run around and shout her name. *Now ask the group:*

"For each of you, what might your face and body look like in this situation?"

Write down a couple of their contributions—these might include wide mouth, erect posture.

"What might some of you be saying and doing, that an observer could plainly see, in this situation?"

Take two or three more comments and write them in the proper place. Members might offer responses such as asking others for help, taking out phone and frantically dialing, etc. Now the co-leader draws an arrow leading from Internal *box to* External *box, and a second arrow leading from* External *box to* Internal *box. Also, the co-leader draws the arrowhead pointing back toward* Thoughts *from the* Internal *box, so that the arrow connecting these two boxes is bidirectional. Teaching points include:*

• *Urges and actions are not the same.* Notice that my action urges and my actions are not exactly the same. (*Leader gestures to bottom portion of both boxes and points out discrepancy between the urges in left,* Internal *box and actions in right,* External *box.*) Many of us have powerful emotions that create intense urges such as to scream, curse, throw things, run away, etc. Having the urge is not the problem; *acting* on the urge is often the problem. We want to cut this cord between *feeling* the urge and *acting* on the urge. (*Draw a line on the board between* Action Urge *and* Action; *then cut through it with another line.*) The key is to *observe* (via mindfulness) the urge without necessarily acting on it. Notice that although I did run around and shout, I did not curse or tackle the security guard at the front door!

• *Components of emotions can work in both directions.* Notice the bidirectional arrows. We often think that our internal sensations and our urges (*point to* Internal *box*) dictate what we say and do (*point to* External *box*). This *can* be true and, just as important but not as obvious, our face and body language and what we say and do can influence our internal bodily chemical reactions, our experience, and our urges! For example, have you noticed that if you are sitting down in a relaxed posture and speaking calmly and softly, it is hard to be as angry? We will talk more about that later in this module, particularly regarding the *acting opposite* skill.

Similarly, not only can thoughts affect how we feel and act, but how we feel and act can affect our thoughts. For example, if our heart is racing and we are running around shouting, we might have the thought "This is horrible—I can't stand this!"

- *Sometimes, the external, observable actions can come first!* For example, if a car speeds toward us (the event) and we dart out of the way, we're usually not aware of thoughts or internal experiences until *after* we've jumped to safety. *Then* we feel our heart pounding and think, "That could have killed me!" So, what emotion(s) do you think I might have been feeling at this point?

Co-leader writes members' responses in a new box right in the middle, labeled Emotion Name. *Emotions can include fear, panic, worry, regret, guilt, and others. Positioning the emotion(s) in the middle conveys that all of these internal and external events make up the emotion. The co-leader can also draw one big box, enclosing both the* Internal *and* External *boxes, indicating that both our internal experiences/urges and our external behaviors/actions make up the emotion.*

"So I'm tense, heart pounding, searching, running, shouting, panicking. What do you think the immediate aftereffects might be? And do you think I might have other, secondary emotions in response to the first emotion or set of emotions? Sometimes an emotional response sets off other emotions, such as shame about sadness or anger in response to feeling hurt."

Group responses might include still panicking, feeling ashamed about losing track of one's daughter and making a scene, being out of breath, sweaty, shaky. The co-leader writes two or three of these in new box labeled Aftereffects, *drawn on bottom center of the board. Note that other aftereffects might include engaging in an impulsive, harmful behavior. The co-leader draws arrows from the now enclosed* Internal *and* External *boxes leading to this new box, indicating that fired emotions, with their internal and external components, lead to aftereffects.*

"So I finally find my daughter across the store, oblivious, trying on and caressing the leather softball mitts. This is the next prompting event."

The co-leader draws new box labeled Prompting Event 2, *toward the lower left of the board, below the first* Prompting Event *and* Thoughts *boxes, and writes inside* find my daughter with softball mitts. *The co-leader draws an arrow going from the* Aftereffects *box toward the left, leading to* Prompting Event 2, *indicating that the emotional experience and its aftereffects can amplify our response to the next prompting event. The co-leader also draws an arrow from the* Prompting Event 2 *box going toward the right, into the* Internal *box, indicating that this new prompting event will lead to more internal reactions, external reactions, new emotions fired, and so on. The co-leader draws another dotted line and arrow going up to the* Thoughts *box, indicating that the second prompting event can also lead to more thoughts, which can affect the emotions experienced.*

"Now, my thoughts might be, 'Thank goodness, she's safe!!!' or 'How could she have walked away and then not heard me shouting?!' My internal reactions might be more shakiness, face feeling cool, blood pressure decrease, muscles relax, tears well up, and urges to hug *and* scold my daughter. My external behaviors might be sighing, shaking my head, hugging her, and asking 'How'd you get all the way over here? I was worried about you!' My emotions might be relief, perhaps tinged with happiness, frustration, and anger at myself for letting her out of my sight."

Teaching points:

- ***Aftereffects.*** Once we have been aroused by an emotion, other emotions are more easily triggered. We are more sensitive to prompting events and to having additional strong reactions. These can include secondary emotions, which are emotions triggered by prior emotions, such as experiencing anger or shame after feeling hurt or fear. This sensitivity to additional prompting events explains why intense emotions and impulsive behaviors can sometimes seem to continue and be self-perpetuating. My reactions to the next event might be more intense because my emotions were already running high from the first event. For emotionally sensitive and reactive folks who take a long time to return to baseline [*see biosocial theory in Chapter 5*], many day-to-day events can feel like this because we may already have vulnerability factors operating, and may still be experiencing a high level of emotions from a prior trigger.

- ***Emotions are complex.*** They have many components! When people tell us "just get over it already; what's the big deal?" they may not realize we have all these things going on—thoughts, body reactions, urges, face and body posture, what we say and do (*leader gestures to all parts of the model on a now filled-up whiteboard while speaking*). We can't simply "shut off" our emotions like a light switch.

After leading the group through the above exercise with an engaging story, refer members to Emotion Regulation Handout 5, which will now be easier to assimilate. If time allows, ask for another example from group members and run through the parts of the model again, even briefly. The following stories have elicited strong emotions and group participation while illustrating the model:

- Toddler twin daughters run in opposite directions.
- Fully dressed at a party, you accidentally drop your new phone into the swimming pool.
- Your friend cancels plans you were looking forward to at the last minute.
- You see kids talking and you're certain it's about you.
- While coaching a soccer game, you see two players collide at the end of the field. Parents on the sideline wave wildly for you to come over. When you do, you see your son with his arm clearly broken.
- You get stuck on a stalled train in a tunnel, with no cell phone reception, when a friend is waiting for you outside an arena with concert tickets for a show starting within half an hour.
- You drop your unzipped book bag running for the school bus and everything falls out all over the street. You crouch down in the middle of the street and begin picking it all up while the bus waits, and everyone on the bus seems to be looking and snickering.
- Your parent tells you that you cannot go to a concert or party to which you've been invited.

Many Places to Intervene

The good news is that the many parts of this model suggest ways we can start to intervene to change our emotional experience and our actions. This model is like an electrical circuit; if we break the circuit somewhere, we can change the emotion or its intensity. The DBT skills in this and other modules can help break the circuit.

Refer participants to Emotion Regulation Handout 6, "A Model of Emotions with Skills." This handout reinforces the aforementioned points that teens and parents can use a variety of DBT skills to help manage the various components of emotional dysregulation.

Emotion Regulation Handout 6 lists the skills within this module that will help you manage emotional sensitivity, reactivity, and difficulty returning to baseline. We can work on vulnerability factors using our ABC PLEASE skills. We can reduce at least *some* prompting events by using problem solving, and we can change our thoughts and emotions by checking the facts. We can notice our internal reactions and urges without acting on them (mindfuness to current emotion), and apply distress tolerance crisis survival strategies (Chapter 7) to avoid making the problem worse when our urges could turn into actions. We can use the opposite action strategy to reduce or change our emotion and its associated actions. For identifying the emotion name(s), we can use the "Short List of Emotions" (Emotion Regulation Handout 3) to describe the emotion(s). We can use our distress tolerance skills to reduce reactivity to prompting events (e.g., placing our attention on something else through distraction, and so on). Note that although not on the handout, we could also use interpersonal effectiveness skills (Chapter 10) or walking the middle path skills (Chapter 8) to reduce conflict and behavioral extremes and thereby help prevent prompting events.

ASSIGNMENT OF HOMEWORK

Assign Emotion Regulation Handout 7, "Practice Exercise: Observe and Describe an Emotion." Ask group members to fill out the model of emotions on the handout using a real-life example of their own from the week. They should fill in each component of the model with their event, thoughts, sensations, urges, actions, aftereffects, etc.

SESSION 2
BRIEF MINDFULNESS EXERCISE
· · · ·
HOMEWORK REVIEW
· · · ·

BREAK

> *Note to Leaders: Draw a scale on the board, with one side of the scale weighed down lower than the other. Write* Negatives *above the side of the scale that is weighed lower. Write* Positives *above the side of the scale that is higher. The point of this drawing and subsequent discussion is to highlight how there are fewer "positives" and greater "negatives" in each of their lives.*

ORIENTATION OF CLIENTS TO ABC PLEASE SKILLS AND THEIR RATIONALE

If each of you weighed your life right now, my guess is that the scale would look like this, with more negatives than positives. Starting with this session, we will learn how to actively increase the "positives" side of the scale by accumulating positive experiences and building mastery, while, at the same time, reducing the "negatives" side of the scale by reducing your vulnerabilities to Emotion Mind. You can remember the skills we will learn by the phrase: ABC PLEASE. [*Refer participants to Emotion Regulation Handout 8, "ABC PLEASE Overview."*]

> **DISCUSSION POINTS**: *Elicit examples from participants about the negatives in their lives, such as depression, financial problems, academic difficulties, peer difficulties, sleeping problems, etc. Then invite participants to list the current positives in their lives, such as a positive relationship with a sibling or spouse, satisfaction from their job, playing soccer or exercising regularly, enjoying piano lessons, enjoying a favorite TV show. Point out that there appears to be a greater number of negatives than positives and ask them if they'd like to readjust the scale so that there are more positives. Even if there is an even number of positives and negatives, the leader can point out that we still want our scale to have a clearly greater number of positives, if possible. Increasing positive experiences not only helps build a meaningful and rewarding life but also helps buffer the impact of the negative conditions or events.*

ACCUMULATING POSITIVE EXPERIENCES—SHORT TERM

How can we get more positives into our lives? [*Invite a participant to read the items in the first box on Emotion Regulation Handout 9, "Accumulating Positive Experiences—Short Term."*]

Why Bother?

Scheduling pleasant activities and getting active are treatments backed by research. They have been shown to reduce depression in some individuals regardless of whether they do anything else.

In addition, increasing pleasant activities can also reduce your emotional vulnerability. Think about a week when you've been having more pleasant, enjoyable things happening and a little thing goes wrong. Compare that to a week when you've been really down and stressed and one more little thing goes wrong. How do you react to it on a good week versus a tough week?

The Skill Is Doing the Activity

It seems so simple to increase pleasant activities; however, when you are depressed, angry, anxious, or emotionally dysregulated, it is in fact sometimes hard to get yourself to do presumably pleasant things. When you are depressed, your natural urge is to lie in bed and not do things. The skill is to get yourself up and do "pleasant" things when you're not in the mood to do pleasant things.

How to Do It

Schedule Appointments

I suggest you think of it as if it were a "doctor's appointment." For example, at 1:00 P.M. you have an appointment to play the piano. At 2:00 P.M. you are scheduled to call a friend. At 4:00 P.M. you have an appointment to walk on the treadmill. Put these appointments on your calendars or into your smartphone, add alerts, and let's get these activities going. *After* you accumulate some of these, they will increase your positive emotions.

Be Mindful of Positive Experiences; Be Unmindful of Worries

Going through the motions of a "pleasant" activity isn't enough. You have to be present and pay attention to it; you have to be mindful of it or you can actually miss it. [*Leaders can share one or more personal examples of not being mindful of positive experiences and allowing the mind to drift including drifting into worries.*] For example:

> "On some Sunday afternoons and early evenings, while sharing a pleasant family activity like playing cards, or ping-pong, or watching a sporting event, it is not uncommon for me to start thinking about what is going to be happening in the upcoming work week. Then I'll think about things that need to get done or stressful things that are going to happen, such as having to interview 15 internship applicants . . . and . . . [*dramatically demonstrating getting dysregulated emotionally, cognitively, physiologically*]. How mindful was I being of the card game I was playing with my family? I'd stopped being mindful of the current experience and now I was no longer enjoying myself. How do you think this lack of mindfulness of positive experiences was affecting my emotions? My relationships?" [*Invite participants to share similar experiences.*]

And here's another example:

> "While I was away on vacation on a beautiful beach, I heard that the weather back home was going to be bad, with a high wind advisory, on the day we were due to fly home. There were storms coming. So, even though flying was 2 days away and I was lying on a lovely beach, I found myself thinking about how my family was going to fare on a very turbulent flight. I started worrying about the flights being delayed or canceled, and whether we should spend an additional day. Was that even possible [*dramatically demonstrating nervousness, wringing of hands, etc.*]? For many hours, these worries interfered with my capacity to derive pleasure on the vacation."

DISCUSSION POINTS: *Invite participants to share and discuss how some of their positive experiences may have been destroyed by worries or by thinking about (1) when the activity would end, (2) whether they deserved this positive experience, or (3) how much more might be expected by them now.*

Pleasant Activities List

Refer participants to Emotion Regulation Handout 10, "Pleasant Activities List."

EXERCISE

Ask members to read this handout and check the activities they enjoy and may currently use. They should star activities they haven't done and might like to try. Point out the blank spaces at the end of the list. These are for writing in activities that might not be listed. This exercise can then continue with either a high-energy version or a low-energy version.

High-Energy Activity

Break the group into pairs, putting people with nonfamily members for "pleasant activity interviews" based on the handout. Write the following three interview questions on the board:

1. Which activities do you currently like to do?
2. Which activities have you done in the past that you'd like to do again?
3. What's one new activity you'd like to try?

The paired individuals are to interview each other and write down their partner's answers. They will have about 5 minutes for each interview. You will announce the half-way point when it is time to switch interviewer and interviewee. When time is up, go around and have each member of each pair report on one item for each of the three questions from his or her partner. Members can report what they found the most interesting, the most fun, inspiring, or just a great idea. Participants have a lot of fun with this exercise, getting to know each other better and getting motivated to engage in the activities. They seem to enjoy reporting on their partner's activities and feel less shy than when reporting on themselves. This is a great way to bring out quiet, socially anxious, or shame-ridden members.

Lower-Energy Activity

After writing the three questions on the board, ask clients to answer them by going through their lists silently and independently. Then ask for volunteers to report on one item for each question. If there is time and you want to encourage full-group participation and activation, go around and ask each group member to report on the three questions.

Parent–Teen Shared Pleasant Activities

Note to Leaders: Although Emotion Regulation Handout 11, "Parent–Teen Shared Pleasant Activities List," has not been included in research trials to date, we include it here as a variation of the standard DBT skill of engaging in pleasant activities, rather than as a new skill.

By the time families have sought DBT, there have usually been many stressors, conflicts, and difficult times within the family. Does this ring true for some of you? [*Allow for hands or head nods.*]

Often, our family interactions can get skewed toward the negative—rushing to doctor's appointments; cramming in sports and activities; nagging about schoolwork or cleaning up; conflicts about friends, electronic gadgets, and going out. The overall feeling can be down, stressed, anxious, angry, or burned out. Is this true for you?

Sometimes we stop making time for the positive interactions that family members can have with one another. What happens to family relationships if we focus only on the negative, the fighting, the struggles?

Emotion Regulation Handout 11, "Parent–Teen Shared Pleasant Activities List" is another way to accumulate short-term pleasant activities. These are activities that you can do together. They can help keep family members close, reduce emotional vulnerability, and be a buffer for negative family interactions. Of course, we still want to work on our interpersonal effectiveness skills with our parents and with our kids, but it is also helpful to spend time with your family member on positive activities. [*If time allows, or if shared activities is a priority for the particular group members present, do one of the exercises listed below. If time is short, leaders can let group members know they'll have a chance to practice this too, and assign it for homework.*]

Refer participants to Emotion Regulation Handout 11, "Parent–Teen Shared Pleasant Activities List."

EXERCISE

Break into groups by family. Have family members read the list of activities together, writing in some of their own activities as well. Ask them to discuss and check off the ones that they already do, star the ones they used to do and could maybe return to, and circle new ones they might like to try. Allow about 5 minutes.

High-Energy Activity

Then go around and ask members of each family (or a representative from each) to offer what they learned and what they will work on regarding shared activities.

Lower-Energy Activity

Ask for volunteers to share with group rather than proceeding around the whole group. This might be the exercise to choose if a person is there without a family member, or if families in the group tend to become dysregulated when interacting and derail the activity for themselves or the whole group.

ACCUMULATING POSITIVE EXPERIENCES—LONG TERM

Refer participants to Emotion Regulation Handout 12, "Accumulating Positive Experiences— Long Term."

What would happen if we focused *only* on short-term positive emotions and experiences? If we only spent our time going to the movies, hanging out with friends, listening to our favorite music, or playing board games with family members, we would not be working toward our long-term goals or building a future. If we want positive events and emotions to occur more often, we also need to build a life worth living where that will happen—and that's a long-term goal.

Before we start taking steps toward our long-term goals, we may realize we need help identifying what those goals are. How do you begin to build a life that's worth living? One way is to be clear on your values and priorities.

Wise Mind Values and Priorities

Working on long-term goals will not be particularly helpful if we do not pick them based on our values and priorities—on those things, principles, or ideas we find most important and meaningful to us in life.

Let's take a look at Emotion Regulation Handout 13, "'Wise Mind' Values and Priorities List." This handout lists some of the values and priorities that many people have. Take a few minutes to read this, check off the ones that are especially important to you, and write in your own if you want. Some of you might value close family relationships, some of you might value hard work, or integrity (e.g., honesty), or contributing to others (e.g., volunteering in your community). Listen to your Wise Mind as you review this list and see which ones truly resonate with *your* values—not your parents' or your friends' values.

> **DISCUSSION POINT:** *Ask,* "How many people checked at least one of the values? At least three values? At least five? Anyone with more than seven? For those who checked off only one or two or none, this is important information. You might want to work with your individual therapist on identifying what is most important to you in life. It's hard to choose meaningful goals if you aren't sure what you value the most. For those who checked several values, that's also important information. It means you already have a road map for selecting some important long-term goals—goals that can provide more positive emotions in your life and help create the life you want."

Taking Small Steps toward Long-Term Goals

Let's take a look at how values can help you set goals. [*Refer members back to Emotion Regulation Handout 12 and model a brief example, such as the following.*] A value of mine is to be healthy, and a goal to support that value would be to get in shape, to be more physically fit. That's a long-term goal. I can't make that happen right away. But I can begin to take some small steps that will get me moving toward my goal. Three small steps might be (1) to go online and look for gyms in my area, (2) to visit some local gyms and ask about costs, and (3) to buy sneakers. I might decide that the first step is to go online and search for gyms in my town. I feel I can go home and easily do it tonight in a few minutes.

Another example of a value is contributing to the community; a goal that expresses that value might be to start a recycling program in my school. Maybe you value having a good career that you love, and a goal might be getting into college; for a value of doing well in school, the goal might be passing math. But each of these goals consists of many, many small steps—the idea is to figure out what a first, manageable step would be, and then take it.

EXERCISE

Ask each person to take out pen and paper or distribute these. Then explain that group members are going to start identifying long-term goals and steps they can take toward those goals. As you walk them through the following steps, one at a time, each group member is to carry them out.

1. Identify and write down a value that is important to you.
2. Select and write down a couple of long-term goals based on the value.
3. Select one of the long-term goals.

4. Brainstorm some initial steps you could take toward that goal.
5. Identify and select a first step. If the step is too large or too hard, how can you break it down further?

Go around and ask, "What was the goal you chose to work on? And what was a first step? Did you have to break down your steps further to get to a doable, nonoverwhelming first step?"

> *Note to Leaders:* You may need to help members identify an easy first step if they are stuck. For example, if the value is to be educated, a long-term goal for a struggling 10th grader might be to graduate from high school and go on to college, but the student currently isn't even going to school. So, initial steps may be to get out of bed and go to just the first class in the morning. However, the actual *first* step may be smaller or more immediate: to buy an alarm clock or set a smartphone alarm and *not* hit the *snooze* feature.

The Effects of Moving toward Your Goals

Taking steps toward your long-term goals can have a direct and rapid impact on your mood, even if it isn't fun or immediately satisfying. (Of course, when you continue to work through the steps toward your goals, you begin to set up conditions for a life that will bring you more positive emotions in the long run.) For homework, we will ask you to identify a goal, steps toward the goal, and the very first step. Then, we'll ask you to take that first step this week! We will come back to this idea shortly with the notion of building mastery.

Pay Attention to Relationships

Our relationships affect the degree of contentment we have in our lives over the long term.

> DISCUSSION POINT: *Ask*, "How many of you notice that when your relationships are strained, distant, or broken, you feel less happy, if not downright unhappy or miserable?" *Acknowledge that when teenagers are depressed they often withdraw socially. And, the parents of teens who are struggling emotionally also tend to withdraw socially and focus primarily on their loved one. It is important for both teens and caregivers to attend not only to that relationship but also to building new relationships and repairing old relationships with their peers and other family members.*

EXERCISE

Ask group members to take 2 minutes to mindfully reflect on their various relationships. Have them rate the quality of their overall relationship portfolio on a scale of 1–10, with *1* being "not close to anyone," *5* being "generally OK but more work could be done to make them stronger," and *10* being "outstanding and not requiring any further work." Now ask them to identify a relationship that they would like to strengthen and then tell the group one thing they could do (or will do this week) to work on that relationship.

Avoid Avoiding and Avoid Giving Up

When we avoid and give up, we feel more emotionally vulnerable. When we feel more emotionally vulnerable and upset, we avoid or give up. It's a vicious cycle. For example, say I am feeling financially strapped and the electric bill comes. I don't want to deal with it right now, so I put it away in the desk drawer and I don't think about it. Then when the next bill comes, it shows that I owe for two months instead of one. Now I feel even *more* anxious and I am more inclined to want to bury this bill even deeper. What happens if I keep this avoidance going? My lights are turned off!

Here's another example. Imagine you were struggling emotionally, missed school, and got behind on your schoolwork. When you return to school, your teacher gives you a pile of "make-up" work. You get home and see this mountain of work and you feel like saying, "Screw it—I'm not doing this." Essentially you give up. In the short term, you feel some relief since the mountain of work is not staring you in the face and giving you that overwhelming sense of anxiety and dread. However, when you give up on something like your make-up work, you will inevitably feel worse about yourself and you will create bigger problems in due time. So, in the name of increasing positive emotions and reducing your vulnerability to Emotion Mind, we are suggesting that you do your best to mindfully *avoid avoiding* and *avoid giving up.*

EXERCISE

Ask each group member to think about something that he or she has been avoiding or giving up on recently. Invite them all to share and discuss what impact it has had emotionally. Ask participants if they can commit to *avoid avoiding* or avoid giving up on one of those issues this week, and, if not, at least be willing to discuss it with their primary therapist.

ASSIGNMENT OF HOMEWORK

Assign Emotion Regulation Handout 14, "Practice Exercise: ACCUMULATING Positive Experiences in the Short and Long Term.

1. In the short term. *Ask group members to commit to doing one pleasant activity each day and to then complete the homework sheet under "In the Short Term." Family members can select three activities from Emotion Regulation Handout 11, "Parent–Teen Shared Pleasant Activities List." If the family did not work on the shared activities list in the session or did not agree on activities at that time, they can select the shared activities at home. Referring to Emotion Regulation Handout 8, "ABC PLEASE Overview," remind group members to be mindful during these pleasant activities by focusing their attention on the activities as they are happening, refocusing attention when their minds wander, and participating fully in the experience.*

2. In the long term. *Ask group members to commit to taking one first step toward the long-term goal identified in the session, or to identifying one other value, goal, and first step and to taking that first step.*

CHALLENGES IN TEACHING ACCUMULATING POSITIVES

When assigning activity scheduling, members often say, "But I don't think I will enjoy them because I am too depressed [or upset or other emotion]." Leaders can respond that that is understandable. At the same time, they can ask whether it might be Emotion Mind talking, anticipating how it will feel. Once people fully participate in an activity, they will often find that they feel better and get some enjoyment out of it, even if not to the full extent possible. Remember the bidirectional arrow from the model of emotions: Not only does mood impact behavior, but behavior impacts mood! If people continue to participate in such activities, they will find themselves starting to accumulate more weight on the "positives" side of the scale.

Many people feel overwhelmed by their first steps toward long-term goals and thus may not take them. The key is for leaders to model and coach participants to break their goals down into baby steps and identify the very first one, no matter how small. If it still seems too hard, help them break down the goal into even smaller, more manageable steps.

SESSION 3
BRIEF MINDFULNESS EXERCISE
· · · ·
HOMEWORK REVIEW
· · · ·
BREAK
· · · ·

BUILD MASTERY, COPE AHEAD, AND PLEASE SKILLS
Orientation of Clients to the Build Mastery Skill and Its Rationale

We are now moving to the "B" portion of the ABC PLEASE skills. It stands for *building mastery*, which means increasing how effective and in control of your life you feel. Does anyone here have "to-do" lists that they can't keep up with? How does it feel when you accomplish something small, but maybe that's been nagging at you, and you get to cross it off your list? [*Allow responses.*] This is a way of building mastery. When you take the time to accomplish even little things, it can make you feel more in control. It can also help you avoid avoiding, as we discussed last time.

In addition to accomplishing the little things on your to-do list, building mastery can also involve honoring the truth about where you are in your life and where you want to go. It is saying, "I have not been going to school for the past several weeks while I have been depressed, *and* I know I want to pass my classes and move on to 11th grade. To do that, I will need to figure out a way to get myself back to school, gradually if need be, which will then result in my feeling effective and in control of my life." This is a form of *building mastery*—of feeling effective and more in control of your life. Going to work where I feel productive and am contributing to others is an example of building mastery. Learning how to drive, when you haven't driven before, is an example of building mastery. Getting better at a skill that is challenging, such as practicing a new song on the violin, is another example. Rebuilding relationships with someone with whom you had a falling out is another example of building mastery.

DISCUSSION POINT: *Ask*, "Should building mastery be fun and pleasant? If not, why bother? Why not focus only on pleasant events? Just as 'all work and no play makes Jack a dull boy,' it is also true that 'all fun and no work makes Jack a dull boy.' What we mean is that playing videogames *all* the time can lead one to feel empty, disconnected, and unfulfilled long-term. Although it may be fun to play videogames or be on Facebook for several days or a week, after a while you will feel bored, ineffective, and discontent with life (believe it or not). Thus, we recommend a healthy balance of pleasant activities *plus* mastery-building activities. Sometimes they may be the same thing—practicing the piano and learning a new song may involve both pleasure and mastery. Often, however, mastery is not 'fun,' yet it still increases your positive mood."

How to Build Mastery

Invite participant to read the Emotion Regulation Handout 15, "Building Mastery and Coping Ahead."

1. Plan to do at least one thing each day to feel competent and in control of your life.
2. Plan for success, not failure. Do something difficult *but* possible.
3. Gradually increase the difficulty over time. If the first task is too difficult, do something one rung lower on the ladder. [*Leader, draw ladder on board to highlight stepwise progression of building mastery.*]

DISCUSSION POINT: *Ask group members to think of some examples in which they are building mastery now. Then ask them to think of examples in which they would like to build mastery but have not felt able to do so. What is one small thing they could do today to cross off their to-do lists? Discuss.*

Orientation of Clients to Cope Ahead Skill and Its Rationale

The "C" portion of the ABC PLEASE" skills refers to coping ahead with potentially upsetting situations is an invaluable skill to learn. If you can visualize the situation in advance and decide which skills you will use, then you will be much more likely to cope effectively. Here are some examples of situations in which people might want to cope ahead:

- Upcoming social event where an ex-friend will be present; you're afraid it will ruin your night.
- Going to a party where there will be drugs and drinking and you don't want to use.
- Having to do a class presentation.
- You're going to your second driving lesson and last week the others in your group turned out to be mean kids.
- Going on a school field trip.
- Having to ask the teacher for an extension on a deadline.
- Having to go to a family event where a "difficult" relative will be present.
- Having to return to school after a 2-week absence due to a psychiatric hospitalization. You imagine everyone will ask where you've been, and rumors will get around.

How to Cope Ahead

Refer participants to the section on coping ahead in Emotion Regulation Handout 15, "Building Mastery and Coping Ahead" and briefly go through the four steps using an example such as one of the situations listed above or one suggested by a group member.

    1. *Describe an upcoming situation that is likely to create negative emotions.* Be specific in describing the situation. Name the emotions most likely to interfere with using your skills. For example, you are anxious about going on a school trip where you may be seated next to some kids with whom you don't feel comfortable.

    2. *Decide which skills you want to use in the situation.* Be specific and write out your plan. For example, "I will first take some deep breaths, notice how I am feeling, try to be non-judgmental, and get myself into Wise Mind. Next, I will use my distract skills from the Distress Tolerance Skills module.

    3. *Imagine the situation in your mind as vividly as possible.* Imagine yourself *in* the situation *now*, not watching the situation. Picture yourself seated near Jennifer, who has been mean to you in the past. Imagine feeling anxious, getting into Wise Mind, and then choosing a distract skill. For example: "I will take out my phone and text a friend of mine who isn't on the bus; then I will play with one of my apps; then, I will listen to some of my favorite music mindfully."

    4. *Rehearse coping effectively in your mind*. Rehearse in your mind exactly what you could do to cope effectively. Rehearse your actions, your thoughts, what you say, and how to say it. Practice this scene in your mind or practice with your therapist. You can even anticipate problems that might come up with your plan and troubleshoot them—that is, decide what you might do then!

EXERCISE

Ask group members to take a few mindful minutes to consider an upcoming situation that is likely to provoke negative emotions. Each participant should apply the instructions for coping ahead on Emotion Regulation Handout 15, "Building Mastery and Coping Ahead," to their personal examples. Then invite one member of the group to share the entire example. Invite the group to provide assistance in applying the coping ahead instructions and provide your assistance if needed.

Orientation of Clients to the PLEASE Skills and Their Rationale

The PLEASE skills are about taking care of the mind by taking care of the body. How we sleep, how we eat, whether we drink or use drugs, whether we exercise, whether we take care of our physical health—*all* affect how we feel emotionally, our overarching mental health, and our physical health. Lifestyle factors *are* powerful. These factors affect whether an anxious and depressed person feels more intensely anxious and depressed . . . whether an interpersonal conflict at school or work results in a person being mildly upset or having a full-blown angry outburst with further negative consequences . . . and even whether someone with bipolar disorder experiences another episode sooner.

    On the physical health front, we now know that cardiovascular disease, obesity, diabetes, and cancer can be strongly determined by lifestyle. Even small differences in lifestyle can make a major difference in health status (Walsh, 2011). But just as importantly for our purposes here, these lifestyle differences can affect your emotional health! So, we cannot emphasize enough how important it is to develop healthy behaviors for the sake not just of your health but of your *mood*. Take a hard look at each of five behaviors on Emotion Regulation Handout 16, "PLEASE Skills," and ask yourself what kinds of improvements you might need to make. Improvements help to reduce your vulnerability to Emotion Mind. They can be made gradually and in the long term, they will help your overall mental and physical well-being.

Note to Leaders: Invite participants to read each letter of the PLEASE acronym, on Emotion Regulation Handout 17. Then explain each item as described below. Ask participants to rate how they are doing on each of the behaviors; leaders can draw the anchor points on the board. We recommend using a (–5 to +5 scale) as shown in Figure 9.1.

Treat <u>P</u>hysica<u>L</u> Illness

Invite a participant to read from the handout: "Take care of your body. See a doctor when necessary. Take medications as prescribed." [Leaders can use a personal example, such as the following.]

> "I'm not sure about each of you, but when I'm sick, I am not a happy camper. I'm often irritable, I have trouble focusing and finding humor in things, I just want to get through the moment as quickly as possible with the hope that my sickness will pass with it.
>
> "When we do not take care of our physical health, whether by not keeping that doctor's appointment, not taking insulin for diabetes, or not taking medication as prescribed for depression, anxiety, etc., we are increasing our emotional vulnerability and keeping ourselves sick. Do you realize that by *not* treating your illness, you are keeping yourselves sicker for longer? Why do that? Why stay sick and, in turn, stay in a more negative emotional state longer?
>
> "In contrast, taking care of our physical health, promptly and thoroughly, can help us return more rapidly to emotional well-being as well as improved physical health."

Balance <u>E</u>ating

Invite a participant to read: "Don't eat too much or too little. Stay away from foods that make you overly emotional."

What we eat and drink can directly affect our moods. Caffeine, turkey, pasta, candy—each can affect mood in different ways. Have you ever noticed how certain foods either make you more energized, more wired, or more down and tired? Have you ever noticed that when you sit down in front of the TV with a bag of chips, the chips are gone by the time your show is over? You have to ask yourself, "Where did all of the chips go? How did they taste?" since you may not have noticed. That's called *mindless eating*. When we mindlessly eat certain types of food

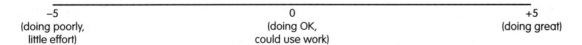

−5	0	+5
(doing poorly, little effort)	(doing OK, could use work)	(doing great)

FIGURE 9.1. Rating scale for PLEASE skills.

as well as certain portions of food (either too little or too much), we can feel bad physically and emotionally afterward. *Eating Mindfully* [Albers, 2003] or *Mindless Eating* [Wansink, 2006] are books about how to end mindless eating and enjoy a more balanced relationship with food.

DISCUSSION POINT: *Ask,* "How many meals do you eat per day? Do you skip breakfast and so start the day with no gas in your tank? It's the most important meal of the day. How is your mood and concentration by late morning? Do you end up bingeing when you haven't eaten for most of the day? What happens to your mood and energy level after that? Balanced eating means staying mindful of types of foods, frequency of meals and snacks, and portion control."

DISCUSSION POINT: *Many teens have little awareness of how drinking large amounts of caffeinated beverages (e.g., Coke/Pepsi, Mountain Dew) or having chocolate desserts before bed can not only hinder sleep but also adds tons of calories. Ask and discuss,* "Did you know how much your sleep and mood can be affected by what you eat and drink?"

DISCUSSION POINT: *Many teens do not eat enough fruits and vegetables on a daily basis and end up eating mostly fast food at odd times of the day and night. They overrely on fatty foods, salty packaged foods, and sugary snacks. As recent investigations have pointed out, these can wreak havoc on our food intake, energy, health, and mood (cf. Moss, 2013; Pollan, 2009), and tasty processed combinations of salt, sugar, and fat can even become addictive. Ask,* "How does eating this way affect your emotions?"

EXERCISE (OPTIONAL)

If time allows, go around the group and ask all members to identify one food that negatively affects their mood, for whatever reason. For families who need more education on the relationship between eating and emotional state, review the points on Emotion Regulation Optional Handout 16a, "FOOD and Your MOOD."

Avoid Mood-Altering Drugs

Invite a participant to read: "Stay off nonprescribed drugs such as marijuana, other street drugs, and alcohol."

Most people recognize that drugs and alcohol directly impact mood. Most people do *not* realize that alcohol is a depressant (not an antidepressant). Even though there is an initial disinhibition and possible lightening of one's mood, it never lasts. If someone is depressed, the worst thing he or she can do is drink alcohol in excess, since it further depresses the mind, body, and nervous system and, to top it off, it disrupts sleep. We're not claiming that all people should never drink because that would be a nondialectical statement. What we are saying is that if you are currently emotionally vulnerable and you want to reduce your vulnerability as much as *you* can, try to avoid nonprescribed drugs and alcohol until you are less emotionally vulnerable (not to mention, above the drinking age!). For the parents in the group, having *one* glass of wine or one beer with dinner is not likely to cause the adverse effects we're describing. That is moderate drinking and is not considered extreme or problematic.

Other drugs, including marijuana, also have negative effects on mood. Even though some states allow doctors to prescribe marijuana for helping patients cope with severe physical pain, research finds that marijuana can adversely affect attention, concentration, motivation, energy, memory, and actually worsen some people's anxiety and increase paranoia. Some people unwittingly use street drugs that are laced with other things, such as hallucinogens, and find themselves becoming psychotic. In research conducted with adolescents in an outpatient clinic, we found that those who were using marijuana were more likely to engage in nonsuicidal self-injurious behaviors [*Velting & Miller, 1999*]. So, if you are a teen or adult who is currently looking for methods to reduce your vulnerability to Emotion Mind, it is important to avoid nonprescription drugs and alcohol.

Balance <u>S</u>leep

Invite a participant to read: "Try to get the amount of sleep that helps you feel rested. Stay on a regular schedule in order to develop and maintain good sleep habits."

Many of us are sleep deprived, living our lives chronically fatigued because we're not sleeping enough. This includes many American teens. Many researchers have found the majority of teenagers get too little sleep (i.e., less than 8 hours) and as a result have a host of other health risk behaviors [McKnight-Eily et al., 2011]. "Raise your hands if you are getting less than 8 hours of sleep per night on average, not just on Sundays. [*Allow response.*] How many of you get 8 hours? 7 hours? 6 hours? Less than that, sometimes? What happens to your mood when you get such little sleep or erratic sleep? Your focus? Behavior?"

Undersleeping (and oversleeping) is a real problem for your mood, your functioning at school and work, and your health. Americans are also becoming more physically ill because they are not sleeping enough. Sleep problems potentially can reduce attention and concentration, and increase anxiety, depression, obesity, and accidents [cf. Thakkar, 2013].

Not getting enough sleep or significantly switching bedtimes can influence whether a teen diagnosed with bipolar disorder has another manic or depressive episode and whether that adolescent may be more prone to suicidal behavior. Sleep is *critical*!

Some of you are not sleeping because you may have insomnia, a discrete sleep disorder that is not related, necessarily, to your being depressed, anxious, etc. Are there other reasons you are not sleeping? [*Take a couple of responses.*] Some of these issues might require problem solving with your individual therapist.

[*Leaders can review Emotion Regulation Optional Handout 16b, "BEST Ways to Get REST: 12 Tips for Better Sleep," if time and interest indicate; family members can also take this handout to review at home or with their individual therapists.*] For sleep problems, you can review the sleep hygiene tips with your parents and make sure you are following them to the letter [*e.g., Epstein & Mardon, 2006; Morin, 1993*]. If good sleep hygiene is not established, it is important to get a consultation for either a short-term behavioral intervention for sleep disorder or a medication or both. The important point for you to understand today is *do not wait to balance your sleep.* Tonight's the night.

Get <u>E</u>xercise

Invite a participant to read: "Do some sort of exercise every day, including walking. Start small and build on it."

Exercise is one of the best antidepressants on the market. Research has found that for many people, exercise provides significant mood enhancement, anxiety and stress reduction, and sleep enhancement [e.g., Otto & Smits, 2011]. Usually, within 5 minutes of doing moderate exercise you will experience a mood enhancement effect. It's best to get your heart rate up, which can happen with fast walking. If you have not been exercising at all, try to build *gradually* up to 20 minutes daily.

What do some of you do for physical activity? Have you noticed a difference in your mood when you skip your routine physical exercise, or when you go through periods of inactivity?

DISCUSSION POINT: *Ask participants for their thoughts in reaction to each of the PLEASE behaviors.*

ASSIGNMENT OF HOMEWORK

Assign Emotion Regulation Handout 17, "Practice Exercise: Build Mastery, Cope Ahead, and PLEASE Skills." Ask group members to commit to the following over the next week:

1. Think of one way you can build mastery this week. Then do at least one thing each day to feel competent and in control of your life.
2. Describe a plan to cope ahead with a future emotional situation.
3. Practice two of the PLEASE skills this week.

SESSION 4
BRIEF MINDFULNESS EXERCISE
· · · ·

Refer participants to Emotion Regulation Handout 18, "The Wave Skill: Mindfulness of Current Emotions.

Often it can feel like emotions will never go away and we're stuck in them. That is part of why they can feel unbearable, and so we try to avoid them. But does avoiding painful emotions work? No, emotions just tend to flood back in. Today's mindfulness exercise is intended to help you recognize that emotions do come and go, that you are not your emotion, you do not have to act on your emotion, and by welcoming and radically accepting the emotion, we can bear the emotion skillfully.

The Wave Skill Instructions

Tell group members that this will be a guided mindfulness practice, and they should follow each instruction as the leader gives it. The leader should pace instructions so that there are 20–30 seconds or so between each of the following lines, with the whole exercise taking about 5 minutes. Begin by saying:

Experience your emotion as a wave, coming and going.
Step back and just notice.

Don't try to *get rid* of or *push away* the emotion.

Don't *hold on* to it.

Practice mindfulness of emotional body sensations; notice *where* in your body you are feeling emotional sensations.

Experience the sensations as fully as you can.

Observe how *long* it takes before the emotion goes down.

Remember: You are not your emotion; you don't need to *act* on the feeling.

Remember times when you felt differently.

Practice loving (or at least accepting) your emotion.

Don't *judge* your emotion.

Invite it home for dinner (that is, invite it *in* rather than pushing it *away*).

Practice *willingness*.

Radically *accept* your emotion.

Leaders can now ask for observations regarding the exercise.

HOMEWORK REVIEW
• • • •
BREAK
• • • •

CHECK THE FACTS AND PROBLEM SOLVING

Note to Leaders: Some clients might feel stuck and may need more help figuring out skills or generating solutions to cope effectively. These clients might benefit from Emotion Regulation Handout 19, "Check the Facts and Problem Solving." First, clients check the facts to determine whether the problem is as they view it. Sometimes emotions fuel our thoughts, and the problem turns out to be smaller or different than we thought it was. Assuming the problem remains, clients can go through the steps on the handout to brainstorm solutions, attempt a solution, evaluate it, and try a different solution if the first one does not work.

Clients can use the skills of checking the facts and problem solving and for a range of problems not limited to coping ahead. For example, a teen may face the problem of wanting to participate in the school play, but worries that she is not good enough and has the urge to avoid auditioning. Checking the facts may be a relevant skill to apply in this instance. Relatedly, problem solving may be relevant for this student if in fact she is selected for the school play. She recognizes that by participating in the school play as well as the yearbook and the track team, she will have major scheduling conflicts, and the time demands will likely be too high to do all three. Thus, some effective problem solving is necessary to consider what she may need to adjust to manage her various activities and responsibilities throughout the year.

Checking the facts and problem solving are also useful for changing or reducing painful emotions. For example, let's say a teen is distressed because she believes her friend is angry with her. She may talk to the friend and realize her belief was unfounded. Or, if indeed her friend is angry, she can use problem solving to help resolve the situation.

OPPOSITE ACTION

Orientation of Clients to the Skill of Opposite Action and Its Rationale

Today we're going to learn the skill called opposite action. When you decide that an emotion is not helping you, or is very painful, you can use this skill to change or reduce that emotion. How many of you feel that when you are experiencing strong, painful emotions, you don't know what to do to get them to go down? The skill of acting opposite the emotion can help you decrease the intensity of unwanted emotions. Remember the biosocial theory and the idea that people with emotional vulnerability experience high sensitivity, high reactivity, and slow return to baseline mood? Acting opposite to your current emotion can help you return to baseline.

Every emotion has an action urge, and those urges can serve important purposes. For example, fear urges us to run away and avoid what we fear. This response is extremely useful when a threat is real and we are in danger, like if a bear is chasing us in the forest. However, we can also be afraid when there is no threat or when a danger has passed. When this happens, fear and its urge to avoid aren't helpful. Instead, fear can unnecessarily limit your life as you avoid things that set off the fear.

What urges go with the emotion of anger? [*Answer: urges to yell, scream, attack, etc.*] What urges go with depression? [*Answer: to stay in bed, isolate oneself, be passive.*] What urges go with shame? [*Answer: to hide, avoid.*]

When to Use Opposite Action

Opposite action is most useful in either of the following two situations:

1. The emotion *does not fit the facts* of the actual situation, that is, it is not justified. For example, you feel terror when speaking in front of the class, but your classmates do not actually pose a danger to you. Plus you (and everyone else) have to do an oral presentation to pass the class.

2. Your emotion is too intense, it has lasted too long, or acting on the emotion *will not be effective* (or is no longer effective) in the situation, even if the emotion is justified. For example, your teacher wrongfully blames you for distracting the class; this makes you angry (with good reason), but acting on the urge to talk back to her will just make the situation worse. Or, your cat died 4 months ago, and you still are moping around, withdrawn from your friends, turning down their invitations because you don't feel like socializing. A mourning period is certainly understandable; yet, at a certain point, it feels excessive, and you believe it is time to try to change the emotion.

What Is Opposite Action?

The skill of opposite action consists of acting opposite to an emotion's action urge. Remember in the model of emotions how changing one component can change the emotion? We are talking now about changing behavior. So, to reduce or change fear, you approach rather than avoid what you fear. This is not easy, and once isn't enough. It takes repeated effort, but it can work. One of the most consistent research findings is that if you repeatedly face what you fear (e.g., dogs, airplanes, spiders) and nothing bad happens (e.g., the dog doesn't bite you), your fear will go down. Another amazing research finding is that if you are depressed, you can make yourself less depressed by becoming active (e.g., resuming exercise, going out to socialize even when you're not in the mood). The point is that *we can change our emotions by acting opposite to how we feel.*

Every emotion has an urge associated with it, as we said above. It is natural to want to act on the urge, and you may sense that that will relieve the emotion. It does seem to relieve it—but only in the immediate short term. The problem is that this doesn't really work; in fact, it just keeps the emotion around. For example, if you avoid speaking in class for half the year, do you suddenly become comfortable speaking in class one day? If you stay in bed and sleep all day when depressed and wake up at 5:00 P.M. as the sun is starting to go down, do you suddenly feel happy and upbeat? [*Group members tend to see the point that acting on the emotion urge just maintains the emotion.*]

Let's take a look at these ideas with regard to some specific emotions. [*Refer participants to Emotion Regulation Handout 20, "Opposite Action to Change Emotion."*]

Acting Opposite to Fear

The urge in fear is to *avoid.* The opposite is to *approach* and to do what you are afraid of doing . . . over and over: confront. When you do this, you will feel afraid. Don't try to suppress the feelings; allow them but don't hold on to them either. Let the opposite actions themselves do the work of changing the emotion. Do things to give yourself a sense of control and mastery.

For example, I used to be afraid of public speaking—which, by the way, is the number one phobia in the world. Now I can stand up in front of 300 or 400 people and not feel particularly anxious. How did that happen? I gave lectures, over and over again, participating fully in giving them. I get generally positive feedback and do not get any "boos" or tomatoes thrown at my head.

> **DISCUSSION POINT:** *Invite participants to give examples of things they are afraid to do or feel and ask whether they act on the urge or engage in the opposite action. Highlight how fear and anxiety go down when they act in an opposite manner. For example*:
>
> "Sometimes the fear goes down by staying in the situation (e.g., during a 10-minute conversation with a peer, a socially anxious teen might notice a decrease in anxiety after the first minute or two) or after repeated practice (e.g., after the fifth time within a week of approaching different people to ask a question, the same socially anxious teen might find this getting easier).
>
> "Do not act opposite when your fear is justified, however. When a car is suddenly barreling down on you as you cross the street, definitely run out of the way. If the dog is growling and snarling at you, do not approach and try to pet it."

Acting Opposite to Anger

The urge in anger is to attack. Its purpose is to protect us when we are threatened with the loss of important persons, things, goals, or rights. The opposite of the urge to attack is to *gently avoid*, which does not mean storming out or sulking, but rather quietly keeping our distance. It means taking some deep breaths or doing something calming until we have entered Wise

Mind. Then we can approach with kindness, rather than Emotion Mind, hostility, or blame. To help yourself be able to do this, put yourself in the other person's shoes. Rather than blaming, imagine sympathy or empathy for the other person.

For example, I came home one night and my spouse was preoccupied with work, barely acknowledging me. I started to feel angry because I'd looked forward to coming home and talking. I had the urge to attack and say angrily: (*highly accusatory tone*) "Hey, what's going on? Why are you ignoring me?" How was that likely to go over? [*Acknowledge group member feedback.*]

I'm likely to get an angry response, which would make me angrier, and still not get what I want. Thinking that attacking wouldn't go over so well, I left him alone for a few minutes while I took some breaths and thought about it. I then tried to put myself in his shoes and remembered that he was stressed and had a big work deadline coming up shortly. I was then able to approach him with kindness, gently asking: "Can I get you some coffee or something? You look like you're buried in work." He then looked up, smiled, and said, "Yeah, thanks. Sorry—it's just that this grant deadline is Friday, and I'm going crazy trying to get it all done!" I then responded supportively to that, engaged in some talk with him about his deadline, and felt my anger melting away. By acting opposite to the urge, I brought down my emotion.

> **DISCUSSION POINT**: *Ask participants for examples of anger and whether they acted on its urge or engaged in an opposite action. Highlight how anger dissipates when they act opposite to its urge. Note that when anger is justified, such as when you find out a peer has been spreading false rumors about you, you may not want to approach kindly or to gently avoid. However, it still may be the most effective thing to do to confront your friend and express your feelings in a controlled way, rather than, say, blowing up in public.*

Acting Opposite to Sadness

The urge in sadness is to withdraw, turn inward, and become passive. Its purpose is to help us figure out what is important and what to do when we have experienced a loss. The opposite of sadness is to approach, don't avoid, and get moving. Don't wait until you feel like it. Do things that make you feel effective and self-confident.

How many of you, when you feel sad or depressed, tend to lie in bed or on the couch, watching TV and just "vegging"? In some ways it feels soothing, cozy, and safe. Essentially, you are acting on your urge to withdraw and not move. But if you're depressed, it is the most unhelpful thing you can do. By staying inactive, you will stay depressed. It's hard for sad people to get themselves to act opposite—to act as if they're not sad and hope that they will feel better afterward. *Acting opposite* means going to school, scheduling pleasant activities and social plans, and trusting that if you do these things all the way—that is, throwing yourself into doing them—you may begin to feel less depressed *after* you keep this up for a while. It is hard to trust that this will work, but there is solid scientific evidence that it does. Teenagers actually feel better *after* they get behaviorally activated. Get up, get out, and move.

> **DISCUSSION POINT**: *For group members going through this module a second time, ask, "How many of you struggle with acting the opposite to how you're feeling? What have you tried and where do you get stuck? Do any of you give up too early on the Opposite Action to sadness skill?"*

Acting Opposite to Shame

Shame urges us to hide, to avoid, or to withdraw from people. We sometimes feel ashamed when we have violated our own sense of right and wrong and we know that others will be disappointed in us or even reject us. But we can also feel ashamed sometimes when we have not violated our values or harmed anyone, and there is nothing about us or our behavior that is objectively wrong. Shame may urge us to hide in this case because we believe that we will be rejected from a particular social setting—and sometimes this is true. For example, proudly showing all of your tattoos when on a job interview at a bank is unlikely to get you the job. Sometimes we are not likely to be rejected—for example, telling your open-minded best friend the truth about not having enough money to go away on vacation with the friend's family or that you are gay. When we have good reasons for feeling shame, we should come clean and repair the mistake. When we feel ashamed about who we are and will not be rejected for it, we should go public with the truth or the behavior.

• ***Feeling shame for good reasons.*** How many of you have difficulty apologizing for things that you know you did "wrong"? For example, you impulsively said or did mean things to someone you care about. You lied about your schoolwork and then got caught. You "borrowed" and kept things from a friend or sibling without asking. You forgot your friend's birthday and didn't say anything. You got so angry you screamed at a loved one in public, or got so behind you failed a class and let yourself and your parents down. Do any of these ring a bell?

A critical first step in helping to reduce shame, when it is justified, is by saying that you're sorry, *sincerely*. Saying "my bad" is not going to do it. Don't stop at the apology. Making up for what you did is called a *repair*. Your effort to repair is what lets people know that you are serious and not just giving lip service to the apology. What kinds of repairs do people make? They include helping prepare dinner, doing extra cleaning around the house, or whatever else is going to help the other person see that you really do care about him or her. You can help your little sister with her homework after you failed to pick her up at school earlier in the day. Accept the consequences for what you did and sincerely try to avoid making the same mistake in the future. After you follow the steps listed above, you then need to let it go.

• ***Feeling shame without good reasons.*** You may feel ashamed in the following situations but you had not done anything wrong or caused others to be disappointed in you. You turn down a friend's request for help when you have already overextended yourself helping him or her, or the requested help goes against your self-respect. You are ashamed about the way you look, that your uncle had schizophrenia, that your mom lost her job, that you live on the "wrong" side of town, that your clothes are not all designer labels like some of the popular kids at school are wearing.

If you feel ashamed but have done nothing wrong, and you will not be rejected in the situation, what do you do? You go public and hold your head up high. You do not apologize for things you did *not* do, and you do not hide. Clarify with your individual therapist why your unjustified feelings of shame remain and what other tools may be necessary to reduce the intensity of these emotions.

Acting Opposite to Guilt

When we are feeling guilty, we normally have urges to overpromise that we won't commit the offense again, or we go to the opposite extreme and disclaim all responsibility. Yet another possibility: We act in harmful ways (e.g., act with rage toward the one we wronged or punish ourselves excessively) to manage the feelings of guilt. We may hide, lower our head, or beg for forgiveness.

- *Feeling guilt with good reason.* When the guilt is justified because your behavior violates your own moral code or has hurt the feelings of significant others, the opposite action is to *face the music.* This means accepting responsibility for your actions and allowing yourself to experience the guilt. You can apologize and ask (but don't beg) for forgiveness and accept the consequences. Importantly, you can repair the transgression and work diligently to prevent it from happening again. Doing something to repair the hurt helps not only your guilt but also the relationship.

- *Feeling guilt without good reason.* If we did not do something that violates our moral code or to hurt another, we may still feel guilty. For example, you may feel guilty about your parents' divorce, guilty that you didn't let your friend cheat and then she failed the test, guilty that you broke up with a partner who treated you terribly, guilty that you made team captain and your buddies did not. In cases in which guilt is not justified or is excessive, don't apologize or try to make up for it. If the guilt is without good reason, then change your body posture, stand up tall to look innocent and proud, pick your head up, puff up your chest, maintain eye contact, and keep your voice steady and clear.

Acting Opposite to Jealousy

When we are jealous, we believe a valued relationship is being threatened, may have to be shared, or may be lost. Jealousy may urge us to make verbal accusations, attempt to control the other person, act suspiciously, snoop as to his or her whereabouts and activities, and push away the threatening person.

Jealousy is often not justified or not effective. Even if the relationship is in danger, holding on and controlling behavior tends to backfire and drive the person away. The opposite actions for jealousy include letting go of controlling others' actions, stopping spying or snooping, and relaxing your face, body, and voice tone.

Opposite Actions for Love

Love can be a highly positive emotion. However, there are times when love is not justified or effective. If a relationship is clearly over or is clearly unattainable (e.g., your college-age neighbor who is engaged, your math teacher), or the object of your love is abusive to you, it is helpful to reduce loving feelings by taking the opposite action.

Urges for the emotion of love include saying "I love you," making an effort to spend time with the person or know what he or she is doing, doing what the other person wants and needs, and showing affection.

You can act opposite to that feeling of love by *stopping* the expression of love (when not justified or effective), by avoiding the person and distracting yourself from thoughts of the person, by reminding yourself of why love is not justified and rehearsing the "cons" of loving this person. You can also avoid contact with things that remind you of the person (e.g., stop looking at pictures, "unfriend" them on Facebook, remove contact from your phone).

How to Do Opposite Action

Taking opposite action as an emotion regulation strategy requires the following eight steps:

1. Figure out the emotion you are feeling (use mindfulness, observe, and describe skills).
2. What is the action urge that goes with the emotion?
3. Ask yourself: Does the emotion fit the facts of the situation?
4. *If yes*, ask: Will acting on the urge of the emotion be effective?
5. Ask yourself: Do I want to change the emotion?
6. *If yes*, figure out the opposite action.
7. Do the opposite action—all the way!
8. Continue doing the opposite action until the emotion goes down enough for you to notice.

Doing Opposite Action "All the Way"

Doing this skill "all the way" means adopting not only actions but also words and thinking that are opposite to the emotion you want to change. Pay attention to your facial expression, voice tone, and posture and make those opposite to the emotion you want to change.

It is very easy to think you are using opposite action when you are not. When you are feeling depressed and you get yourself out of bed to then lie on the couch to watch TV, you are not using opposite action. Why? It's because it is not done *all the way*. How could it be done *all the way* in this example?

> **DISCUSSION POINTS:** *Say,* "If you are experiencing social anxiety about going to a party with many new people attending, which of the following examples is using the opposite action skill:
>
> "1. Go to party, say hello to the host, and then find a chair in the corner of the room and wait for people to introduce themselves to you.
> "2. Go to party, say hello to the host, find the food and drink, and sit down in the kitchen and eat it quietly.
> "3. Go to party, say hello to the host, and then skillfully (with a smile and a firm handshake) introduce yourself to people who look toward you as you're walking by. If you are not abruptly interrupting their conversation, ask them their names and a follow-up question (e.g., how do they know the party host?)."

> **DISCUSSION POINT:** *Ask participants to observe and describe their typical responses to certain problematic emotions and what would be different in their voice, posture, eye contact, attitude, and behavior if they used opposite action all the way.*

Keep Repeating the Opposite Actions

One misunderstanding people have about the opposite action skill is that it should work quickly. Although it can work quickly, it often takes an extended period of time of repeated opposite actions before the emotion starts to go down. If you are anxious at a party, it may take several introductions and your tolerating the anxiety for 30 minutes or so before you find yourself engaged in conversation with your new acquaintance and then less anxious.

Role-Play Activity for Group Members

Break group members into four small groups of two or three. Give each group a scenario describing a brief scene that relates to a particular emotion. Leaders can write these scenarios on index cards ahead of time. We provide sample scenarios of anger, fear, sadness, and shame in the following sections; additional emotion scenarios (i.e., for guilt, jealousy, love) could be created if you have more than four groups.

Tell groups they will have 5 minutes to plan how they will (1) act out the urge that goes with the emotion and (2) act opposite to the urge. Each group will have 2 or 3 minutes total to present their two-part role plays. After each, the other group members will be asked to guess the emotion and the opposite action and to comment on how the situation worked out when participants acted on the emotion urge, and how it worked out when they acted opposite to it. Did taking the opposite action work to reduce the intensity of the emotion? Were there any other benefits?

During planning time for this activity, leaders should walk around, check in with each group, and offer coaching for coming up with emotion urges, opposite actions, and role-play tips. Examples of acting on urges might include:

- *Yelling or storming away for anger*
- *Freezing or shaking and avoiding for fear*
- *Displaying lethargy, flat voice tone, and unhappy facial expression for sadness*
- *Looking down, slumping shoulders, and avoiding eye contact for shame*

Groups can look at their handouts if they need help recalling actions opposite to the emotion urges. In our experience, members quickly pick up the concepts, have fun, and fully participate in this activity. Typically the second role play, displaying opposite action, will appear more effective.

Scenarios for Role Plays

Sample scenarios for role plays follow. Under each are notes to group leaders to ensure that opposite action is appropriately understood and demonstrated by group members.

1. You come home and your parents are busy and ignoring you, even though you really want to tell them about your day. You feel <u>angry</u>. [*The opposite action could include either gently avoiding the parents or approaching them with empathy and kindness.*]

2. Two of your friends are showing off their new cars. They want to know when you will be getting one of your own. It seems like everyone is getting a new car lately. But your family cannot afford to buy you one, so you feel <u>ashamed</u>. [*You can change the content in the above exercise to be appropriate to age, culture, and setting. For example, the friends are taking trips and they want to know where you will be going over vacation, or the friends have new iPads, bicycles, sneakers, and so on. Once group members guess the emotion, leaders can ask if the shame is justified. It is not, in this case. The acting opposite role play would include holding oneself upright, speaking confidently, not lying or avoiding, and saying something like, "Well, the money just isn't there right now for that, but I hope maybe one day . . . so, when can I go for a ride in your beautiful new car?" or "Those are awesome sneakers!"*]

3. Your friend takes you to a carnival, but you are feeling <u>depressed</u>. [*The opposite action in this case might look like the person acting energetic, smiling, talking, and saying positive things about the carnival.*]

4. You often think you know an answer in biology class, but you feel <u>afraid</u> to raise your hand and speak in front of everyone when the teacher asks a question. [*The opposite action in this case would involve raising one's hand confidently rather then sheepishly, looking at the teacher, and answering in a clear and appropriately loud voice.*]

Additional Scenarios

- You are feeling bad because your friend, who didn't study, asked you if she could cheat off your test. You said no. She got a D, and you are feeling <u>guilty</u>.
- Your girlfriend has a cute lab partner in science and you are feeling <u>jealous</u>. You keep peering into the classroom and demand to know what they were talking about when your girlfriend walks out.
- Your 25-year-old engaged Spanish teacher is attractive and friendly to you and you think you are in <u>love</u>. You begin waiting for him after school, stalking him online, and finding out everything you can about him. It interferes with your learning and your friends start to comment and get concerned that it is more than just an innocent crush.

ASSIGNMENT OF HOMEWORK

Assign Emotion Regulation Handout 21, "Practice Exercise: Opposite Action." Ask group members to commit to practicing opposite actions during the week. Explain that they should choose an emotion they experience during the week that they would like to decrease, either because it is not justified (does not fit the facts) or it is ineffective (excessive, too long-lasting, or interfering with their goals). They should identify the emotion, the action urge, and the opposite action. They should then act opposite to the emotion urge, all the way (including facial expression, body posture, and voice tone). Lastly, they should report how they feel after acting opposite to their urge. Did acting opposite lower the intensity of the emotion? Members write their experiences on the handout.

CHAPTER 10

Interpersonal Effectiveness Skills

SESSION OUTLINES

Session 1

▶ Brief Mindfulness Exercise

▶ Homework Review

▶ Break

▶ Orientation of Clients to Skills and Their Rationale

▶ Goals of Interpersonal Effectiveness

▶ Factors That Interfere with Interpersonal Effectiveness

▶ Maintaining Positive Relationships: GIVE skills

▶ Assignment of Homework: Interpersonal Effectiveness Handout 4, "Practice Exercise: GIVE Skills"

▶ Session Wind-Down

Handouts and Other Materials

▶ Interpersonal Effectiveness Handout 1, "What Is Your Goal and Priority?"

▶ Interpersonal Effectiveness Handout 2, "What Stops You from Achieving Your Goals?"

▶ Interpersonal Effectiveness Handout 3, "Building and Maintaining Positive Relationships: GIVE Skills"

▶ Interpersonal Effectiveness Handout 4, "Practice Exercise: GIVE Skills"

▶ Whiteboard or other writing surface

▶ Mindfulness bell

Session 2

▶ Brief Mindfulness Exercise

▶ Homework Review

▷ Break

▷ Getting Someone to Do What You Want: DEAR MAN Skills

▷ Assignment of Homework

▷ Session Wind-Down

Handouts and Other Materials

▷ Interpersonal Effectiveness Handout 5, "Getting Someone to Do What You Want: DEAR MAN Skills"

▷ Interpersonal Effectiveness Handout 6, "Practice Exercise: DEAR MAN Skills"

▷ Whiteboard or other writing surface

▷ Mindfulness bell

Session 3

▷ Brief Mindfulness Exercise

▷ Homework Review

▷ Break

▷ Maintaining Your Self-Respect: FAST Skills

▷ Challenging Worry Thoughts that Interfere with Interpersonal Effectiveness

▷ Assignment of Homework

▷ Session Wind-Down

Handouts and Other Materials

▷ Interpersonal Effectiveness Handout 7, "Maintaining Your Self-Respect: FAST Skills"

▷ Interpersonal Effectiveness Handout 8, "Worry Thoughts and Wise Mind Self-Statements"

▷ Interpersonal Effectiveness Handout 9, "Practice Exercise: FAST Skills"

▷ Whiteboard or other writing surface

▷ Mindfulness bell

Session 4

▷ Brief Mindfulness Exercise

▷ Homework Review

▷ Break

▷ Factors to Consider When Deciding How Intensely to Ask or Say "No"

▷ THINK Skills (Optional)

▷ Using Multiple Interpersonal Effectiveness Skills at the Same Time

▷ Assignment of Homework

▶ Assignment of Homework

▶ Assignment of Homework (Optional)

▶ Session Wind-Down

Handouts and Other Materials

▶ Interpersonal Effectiveness Handout 10, "Factors to Consider in Asking for What You Want"

▶ Interpersonal Effectiveness Handout 11, "Practice Exercise: Factors to Consider in Asking or Saying 'No'"

▶ Interpersonal Effectiveness Handout 12, "Practice Exercise: Using Skills at the Same Time"

▶ Interpersonal Effectiveness Optional Handout 13, "THINK Skills"

▶ Interpersonal Effectiveness Optional Handout 14, "Practice Exercise: THINK Skills"

▶ Whiteboard or other writing surface

▶ Mindfulness bell

TEACHING NOTES

> Love is like a precious plant. You can't just . . . think it's going to get on by itself.
> You've got to keep watering it. You've got to really look after it and nurture it.
> —JOHN LENNON

> When people talk, listen completely.
> —ERNEST HEMINGWAY

ABOUT THIS MODULE

This module focuses on skills for building and maintaining positive relationships. While other DBT skill areas of increasing awareness and focus, tolerating distress, reducing extreme thinking and behavior patterns, and regulating emotions no doubt will improve relationships, this module does so directly by teaching specific relationship skills. In turn, improving the quality of one's relationships will positively affect one's other skill capacities. For example, a solid social support network helps one tolerate distress, and fulfilling, low-conflict relationships help build positive emotions and buffer against negative ones. The skills set highlights obtaining three important interpersonal goals: (1) building positive relationships and reducing conflict escalation (the GIVE skills), (2) effectively asking for what one wants or saying "no" to another's request (the DEAR MAN skills), and (3) maintaining self-respect (the FAST skills). Note that we provide numerous scenarios for role playing the GIVE, DEAR MAN, and FAST skills because in-session practice with feedback until mastery is obtained is critical for generalization.

The module also covers how to use the three skill sets at the same time, how to challenge worry thoughts that can interfere with interpersonal effectiveness, factors to consider when asking for something or saying "no," and taking another's perspective (the THINK skills). Note that the THINK skills were not part of standard DBT and have not as yet been used in clinical trials; thus they are optional handouts. Noticing that teens and families often assumed the worst about others' intentions (which intensifies negative emotions), we developed the THINK skills based on Crick and Dodge's (1994) social information-processing model. This model points to the interpretations we make of another's behavior that bias our response choices toward the negative; thus, the skill aims to correct faulty negative assumptions. This module is designed to be covered in four sessions but could be extended to five if time allows.

SESSION 1
BRIEF MINDFULNESS EXERCISE
· · · ·
HOMEWORK REVIEW
· · · ·
BREAK
· · · ·

INTERPERSONAL EFFECTIVENESS SKILLS

Orientation of Clients to Interpersonal Effectiveness Skills and Their Rationale

Do certain relationships sometimes get stressful? Maybe problems get out of hand, and you don't know how to resolve them. Do you ever feel that you could use some help with them? [*Allow for responses from group members.*]

Maybe at times your friends have turned on you, or you feel like you don't have any friends at all. Or you're being bullied or you watch kids bully other kids, and you don't know what to do. When your relationships aren't going the way you want them to, do you find that you feel bad, and your emotions get more intense? [*Allow for responses.*] Maybe you want something and don't know how to ask for it. Or maybe someone asks you for something and you don't know how to say "no" and make it stick.

Skills for Maintaining Relationships and Reducing Conflict

In this module we will learn skills for maintaining relationships and reducing conflict, while also getting what we want and need for our own self-respect in those relationships. We'll also try to understand the many things that can interfere with obtaining these things. If these were not enough reasons, it is important to note that people who have really well-honed interpersonal skills tend to get hired more easily for jobs, and promoted more readily, and thereby can even end up more successful in the workplace because of good relationship skills.

In order for these skills to work, you will all need to practice them often, not only in here but also outside of group.

GOALS OF INTERPERSONAL EFFECTIVENESS

Refer participants to Interpersonal Effectiveness Handout 1, "What Is Your Goal and Priority?"

This module has three main goals and a set of skills for accomplishing each goal:

1. Keeping and maintaining healthy relationships: GIVE skills.
2. Getting someone to do what you want or saying "no" to another's request: DEAR MAN skills.
3. Keeping your self-respect: FAST skills.

Ideally, we want to have all three goals met in any interaction—to get what we want from others, while we keep a good relationship with them and keep our self-respect. We can think of these goals as three balls we are juggling. Trying to keep them all in the air without dropping any is the challenge.

Keeping Healthy Relationships

DISCUSSION POINT: *Ask*, "Have you ever known people who worked so hard on keeping a relationship that they sacrificed their needs and their self-respect?" [*Allow for nods of recognition.*]

• *Sacrificing your wants to keep a relationship doesn't work.* Many people believe the myth that if they sacrifice their own needs and wants, the relationship will go more smoothly, approval will come, and no problems will arise. This does not work. What happens if you push away your own feelings and needs for too long? One of three possibilities:

1. You blow up and risk the other walking out, or . . .
2. You get frustrated and leave the relationship yourself, or . . .
3. You stay in the relationship and feel miserable.

Either way, the relationship comes to an end or is put in serious jeopardy.

DISCUSSION POINT: *Ask*, "On the other hand, have you ever known someone who could forcefully assert what they wanted, and they got it but it hurt the relationship? Or have you ever said 'no' to someone's request and that also hurt the relationship?" [*Allow for responses.*]

• *Getting what you want while keeping the relationship.* It is possible to ask for what you want in a way that makes the other person actually *want* to give it to you. You can also learn to refuse others' requests in a way that leaves them feeling good about you. Using DEAR MAN skills helps you get what you want from others; they can also help make your "no" stick. When you use DEAR MAN skills together with the GIVE skills, you can keep, and even improve, your relationship with the other person.

• *Keeping your self-respect.* Some people may feel that the only effective way to get what they need is to fight dirty, give in, or act in other ways that violate their own values. They may get what they want, but there is a price—it leaves them feeling bad about themselves. Keeping your self-respect in an interaction can be just as important, or more important, than getting what you want and keeping a good relationship. Keeping self-respect means:

○ Acting in ways that fit your own sense of values and morality and
○ Acting in ways that make you feel competent.

For example, sacrificing your own needs to keep a relationship usually does great damage to your self-respect. The FAST skills are about keeping or improving good feelings about yourself while you try to get what you want from others.

> **DISCUSSION POINT:** *Ask,* "When have you done things that reduce your sense of self-respect? Like lying to get out of doing something, or going along with friends when you didn't like what they were doing?"

Clarifying Your Priorities

Before you go into a specific interaction, it helps to know which of the three goals we've been discussing is most important to you. If you can't get what you want, *and* keep a good relationship, *and* keep your self-respect, then which one is the most important to you? Which is least important? Sometimes, we have only one goal in an interaction and the task becomes identifying that goal. Maybe your boss or your teacher has called you in for a meeting and that doesn't sound good. Maybe the only thing you want out of the meeting is not to get fired or flunked. In other words, you want the other person to think well of you at the end of the meeting. Knowing that goal tells you to focus on using the GIVE skills for maintaining a healthy relationship.

The questions under each goal on Interpersonal Effectiveness Handout 1, "What Is Your Goal and Priority?" can help you think about the three goals and their relative importance to you in a particular situation:

1. How do I want the other person to feel about me when we finish talking?
2. What is it I want from this person? Or how do I effectively say "no"?
3. How do I want to feel about myself after the interaction?

Identifying your goals and priorities might take some mindfulness. Stop and ask your Wise Mind: What is my goal here? What am I trying to accomplish? Do I focus on maintaining the relationship, getting what I want (or saying "no"), or keeping my self-respect? Do I want some combination of these?

Let's consider this example. A college student is moving out of a rental apartment at the end of the lease. She's kept the place in good shape, but the landlord is unfairly keeping the security deposit. The student might rank her priorities this way:

1. Objective: Get the deposit back.
2. Self-respect: Not losing self-respect by getting too emotional, fighting dirty, or giving in.
3. Relationship: Since she's moving out, keeping the landlord's good will and liking is not a high priority. Yet, alienating or angering him would make it less likely he'd return the deposit.

FACTORS THAT INTERFERE WITH INTERPERSONAL EFFECTIVENESS

Refer participants to Interpersonal Effectiveness Handout 2, "What Stops You from Achieving Your Goals?"

What stops you from achieving your goals? There could be several reasons.

- Lack of skill
- Worry thoughts
- Emotions
- Can't decide
- Environment

> **Note to Leaders:** For the example that follows, present the situation, read each interfering factor, and indicate into which category it falls. You can move through Interpersonal Effectiveness Handout 2 quickly; the main point is to acknowledge that it can be hard to get our wants and needs met in relationships, and that throughout the DBT skills modules, we teach skills that can help you do it.

Imagine that you are in danger of failing math class this quarter because of your test grades. You want to approach the teacher and try to solve the problem, perhaps by doing some extra credit work or retaking a test. What might interfere with your being interpersonally effective in this situation? Perhaps it is that:

- You don't know what to say or do [*lack of skill*].
- You believe the teacher will get angry with you [*worry thoughts*].
- You feel panicky when you start to approach her, so you back away [*emotions*].
- You don't know whether it is better to bring attention to yourself by asking for a special arrangement, or keeping a "low profile" and promising yourself you will study hard and do better next quarter [*can't decide*].
- You do ask, and she simply refuses to negotiate and says to try to do better next time [*environment*].

Getting Unstopped

So in these situations, what can we do? For each factor that interferes, there are skills that can be applied.

- For lack of skill, we will teach you specific interpersonal skills to handle such situations skillfully, based on your goals in the situation.
- For worry thoughts, we will teach you Wise Mind statements you can say to challenge worries that get in your way of being interpersonally effective.
- For emotions, you can use mindfulness skills to observe and describe your emotions and urges and to help you stay focused and do what works; in other modules we will teach you distress tolerance skills and emotion regulation skills for managing emotions and asking effectively even in the presence of the emotion.
- For can't decide, you can use mindfulness to make a Wise Mind decision about what feels right. You can also consider your values (emotion regulation values skill) in helping you decide whether you want to ask, have the right to ask, and what you are asking for.
- When it is the environment that interferes, you may have to use the skill of radical acceptance to accept that you will not get what you want (e.g., in the example with the math teacher). Distress tolerance skills can also help you to tolerate not getting what you want.

When using interpersonal effectiveness skills, it is important not only to identify what your goals are, but also to figure out what might be interfering with your using interpersonal effectiveness skills. In the remainder of this module, we teach you what to do when it is a lack of skill or worry thoughts that interfere; the other modules teach skills that help when emotions, not being able to decide, or the environment interferes.

MAINTAINING POSITIVE RELATIONSHIPS: GIVE SKILLS

Refer participants to Interpersonal Effectiveness Handout 3, "Building and Maintaining Positive Relationships: GIVE Skills."

When you want to maintain relationships and reduce conflict, remember the word *GIVE*.

> **Note to Leaders:** The leaders can introduce the handout and read through it with the group. We find it especially engaging to use one of the following three exercises: (1) a group member reads the GIVE descriptions from the handout while a leader acts the opposite; (2) a co-leaders role-play; or (3) a mindfulness exercise is used. Each is described in more detail below.

Orientation of Clients to the GIVE Skills and Their Rationale

EXERCISE 1: LEADER ROLE-PLAYS THE OPPOSITE

One playful way we teach this skill is to pick someone in the group to read Interpersonal Effectiveness Handout 3 aloud. As the member reads the description of each letter in the acronym, GIVE, a leader does the opposite of what the item instructs, as described more below. This should be done in a good-humored, outlandish way that is clearly exaggerated to get the group laughing and seeing how it looks to not use one's GIVE skills.

- **Be gentle.** Ask a participant to read the description of each GIVE skill on Interpersonal Effectiveness Handout 3. While the person is reading everything under "Be gentle" on the handout—("Be nice and respectful. Don't attack, use threats or judgments. Be aware of your tone of voice.")—the leader might attack and threaten, "Come on, slow poke! Hurry up already," or "This is awful! I ought to pick someone else to read!"

- **Act interested.** As the participant reads, the leader says, "Yeah . . . whatever," rolls his eyes and sighs loudly, or interrupts and brings up something off topic addressed to the group: "Hey, did you catch that football game last night?"

- **Validate.** While the participant is reading (probably more cautiously now after the interruptions), the leader invalidates the speaker with more ribbing: "You shouldn't be hesitating. There's no reason to be slowing down or feeling nervous. Come on, just get through this handout already!"

- **Use an easy manner.** While the participant is speaking, the leader can say, very seriously, firmly, and stiffly standing over the participant with arms crossed over chest, "I would like to talk to you now. I need to teach the group these skills and I would like you to finish up already!"

Then, the leader asks what it was like for the reader and how it made him or her feel about the reading and the relationship (e.g., the leader might add, "I'm guessing I wasn't your favorite person in the world at the moment!"). Usually, readers will report that they did not feel like continuing to talk. Leaders ask the group for comments and observations as well. *Ask:* What is it like to try to keep on talking when someone is not using these skills? What does it do to the relationship interaction?

EXERCISE 2: LEADERS ROLE-PLAY BOTH SCENARIOS

An alternative way of introducing the GIVE skill is with a role play between group leaders. Group leaders first role-play a scenario without using any GIVE skills, then role-play the same scenario using all of the GIVE skills. For example, one leader can ask the other to buy different kinds of snacks for the session break, explaining that he or she thinks the other is not doing a good job selecting them. The leader requesting the change can attack, be judgmental, have an attitude, and show no interest in what the co-leader has to say. In response to this attacking approach, the co-leader can then snap back with more attacks, show no interest in or validation of the first leader, finally ending in an angry, "WHY DON'T YOU JUST BUY THE #@$&% SNACKS YOURSELF!"

After observing, group members are asked how they think this interaction went. What went wrong? Where did the communication between the two break down? How is each leader feeling now about the relationship, about continuing to work with the other? How could it have gone better? Group members are usually astute observers and generate many elements of the GIVE skills intuitively. When the leaders role-play the same scenario using the GIVE skills, it should demonstrate a much better outcome in terms of the relationship.

Another scenario leaders could role-play is a parent–teen conflict, such as the teen's wanting to quit the soccer team when the parent has just bought all the equipment and paid the team fee. For the first scenario, each leader could just "let it fly," and then repeat the scene using their GIVE skills. A point to illustrate and highlight is that even if the role players during the GIVE scenario don't necessarily solve the problem, they are not angry and they remain in the conversation without escalation. For example, in the soccer scenario, the parent might end up saying that he or she would really like the teen to stick with the commitment made and carry on, at least through this year's season. Because each is gentle, interested, validating, and uses an easy manner (i.e., the GIVE skills), the issue does not blow up into a fight, even though the teen does not get the desired outcome. And, they still feel good about each other after the interaction—hence, the goal of keeping the relationship is achieved.

EXERCISE 3: MINDFULNESS EXERCISE

A third way to introduce these skills is with a mindfulness exercise. Have each group member turn to the person next to him or her to form pairs. Select one person in the pair to be the speaker and the other to listen. When the mindfulness bell rings, the speakers are to begin speaking about anything they are willing to share, such as their day, their commute to the DBT skills group, or a movie they recently watched. Meanwhile the listeners are instructed not to listen or pay attention, to act completely uninterested and distracted. After about 2 minutes, ring the mindfulness bell again, and instruct the listeners to switch to being fully present, showing interest, and fully focusing on what the speaker is saying. Then, leaders ring the mindfulness bell again, and participants stop and report observations, particularly the contrast between the two conditions.

Speakers inevitably report that they got angry, hurt, or distracted, and that it was very hard to stay focused on what they were saying or to be motivated to continue speaking. Those in the listener role often say how hard it was for them as well to ignore the other fully, and how they felt it was cruel and insensitive, and they could see the ill effects of not listening. If members have not already mentioned it, group leaders also make the point of how listening with focused attention is a form of validation because it conveys that you are taking the other person seriously. This exercise allows participants to experience the effects of central components of GIVE before leaders have formally taught it.

Leaders then turn back to the handout, define each skill, and discuss the benefits of practicing and using each. Leaders invite group members to conduct a self-assessment as each skill is reviewed, as indicated in the following material. As each skill is defined, leaders can also tie it back to what group members observed or experienced in the opening exercise. Examples follow.

- *Be gentle.* Can you think of some examples of attacks? How about: "You never do anything around here; you are lazy!" For threats, let's try this: "If you don't let me go to the party, I'll . . ." What about a gentle voice tone? What is the difference between speaking in a gentle or harsh tone of voice? How do people feel when we speak to them in a brusque or curt or gruff manner? How many of you need to improve your ability to communicate in a gentler way?

- *Act interested.* Do any of you multitask when speaking with others? Do you look at your iPhone, search the Internet, stare at the TV, read, cook, clean up, shoot hoops, and so on, when listening to others? How do you feel when people do that when you are trying to talk to them? How can we show we are listening and truly interested in what the other person is saying? [*Take answers from the group; these should include things like eye contact, nodding, making utterances such as"mmm-hmm," asking relevant questions, and a body posture that is open with arms uncrossed and turned fully toward the speaker.*] How many of you need to improve your skills in acting interested [*wait for show of hands*]?

- *Validate.* Validation is conveying that you understand where the other person is coming from, even if you do not agree. [*Group members have learned about validation from the biosocial theory taught during Orientation, and also from the Walking the Middle Path module if they have gone through it already.*] With validation, we communicate that the other person's feelings make sense. How many of you need to work on explictly, verbally validating others? Some of you may be acting in a validating way; however, we would like you to validate with words too.

> *Note to Leaders:* We find that some parents have a great deal of difficulty validating others' emotions instead of behaviors. For example, one father felt comfortable telling his daughter that he recognized her effort, but he had great difficulty validating her emotions (disappointment, sadness) about getting a poor grade on a project. Remind parents that it behooves them to practice validating emotions more since those near and dear to them will feel better understood, will likely deescalate their emotions, and will feel closer to them.

- *Easy manner.* Often when discussing something with others, especially if the content is serious, we display a very serious, grave, or harsh stance. Some talks can be lightened and relationships enhanced by using a lighter tone. You can do this through word choice, smiling, having a relaxed body posture, or using a little humor. This may involve sitting down next to someone who is already seated before speaking instead of standing or leaning over them.

Practice Exercises for GIVE Skills

> *Note to Leaders:* It is important to devote time to allow group members to learn, practice, and master this skill. Not only is the GIVE skill helpful for all relationships, it is critical for

family functioning. The lack of GIVE skills often precludes effective family communication and problem solving, and can cause family sessions to escalate in an unproductive way.
GIVE skills can be practiced in session by dividing all group members into pairs or selecting one pair to role-play the skills for the whole group.

Practice in Dyads

In the dyads, we ask members to select a topic and choose who will be the speaker and who the
listener. Be sure to explain that GIVE skills can be used either while listening to someone else
speak or for the primary speaker to use while discussing something or making a request. The
speaker is then to talk about something moderately, but not extremely, emotional. It is important that the topic not be too personal or too dysregulating. Leaders can give examples to help
members select topics. This could be something they enjoy, such as their pet, their little cousin,
a gift they loved, or a favorite movie or actor or musical band. It could also be something negative, such as a recent scary or sad movie, a frustrating situation such as arriving at the movies
and finding the tickets sold out, or a frightening situation such as being caught in a huge thun-
derstorm. Each dyad can work with the same topic or pick topics written on paper slips from
a bowl. As the speaker talks about their topic, the listener uses all of the GIVE skills. Leaders
need to go around and listen to each dyad briefly. At the end of a few minutes, each dyad can
share with the group how it went and what was learned.

Role Plays for Dyads or the Whole Group

*Demonstrations involving the whole group are important to ensure that each group member
views and practices correct application of the GIVE skills with coaching and feedback. For
these, we either ask for topics from group members or we have prepared topics ready to use for
role-play demonstrations. Leaders can ask members to first discuss without GIVE skills, and
then try again, using GIVE skills. Demonstrations can illustrate using GIVE as a speaker and
as a listener.*

*The following role-play topics can be used for practicing GIVE skills in dyads or in the full
group and can emphasize one or both parties' use of GIVE skills:*

- Parent asks the teen to clear all his or her stuff off the dining room table *now* because
  tomorrow is a holiday and the parent has to clean the room and set the table. The teen is
  on the way out the door to meet a very upset friend who called, crying, and said "I really
  need to talk," and so the teen says "no" to the parent.
- You are concerned that your good friend always hangs out with another friend who is
  mean to you. You want to ask your friend to at least be willing to not talk about you with
  the friend and to stand up for you.
- A mom promised her teen that she would take her shopping for her birthday. The mom's
  first free day arrives and the teen asks her mom to go shopping today. The mom explains
  that she is too tired.

DISCUSSION POINT: *Ask,* "What is the difference between how these conversations go when people use their GIVE skills and when they don't?"

EXERCISE: ROLE PLAY ON VALIDATION

Another role-play exercise involves elaborating on the skill of validation. The leader goes around the group and tells each member, one at a time, one of the statements in the list below. The group member's job is to respond using GIVE skills with an emphasis on validating the other person, even if it is difficult, and even if he or she does not agree.

Statements for validation practice:

- "My teacher is being so mean to me lately! I want to drop advanced math so I don't have to have her anymore."
- "Everyone's telling me I'm too emotional and too negative—so I don't know who I'm supposed to talk to or go to for help anymore . . . I feel so alone."
- "My father's going to kill me when he finds out I'm getting a C in biology!"
- "You need to eat dinner with the family even though you have a test to study for. It's the only time we all sit together without distractions, and it is important to us."
- "I love Gus! He's the best! I want to hang out with him all the time!"
- "Nobody likes me—I feel like I don't have any friends."
- "I'm obsessed with the TV show _____! I'm just dying that the season is over and I won't get to see it for months. I cried when the season was over!"
- "I'm furious that she came into my room and took my hairbrush!"
- "I love the theatre club! It's my favorite afternoon of the week! So you need to cancel that doctor's appointment you made because I absolutely can't miss it!"
- "I went to the audition and the kids were really unfriendly and clique-y—now I don't know if I want to be in the show."
- "I feel like my teacher was singling me out today and being really harsh—and I was trying my best!"
- "I was *so* excited to get tickets to the concert, and when I logged onto the site, they were sold out!"
- "I'm so upset with you! I feel like you were mean to me half the time at the party and ignoring me the other half of the time!"
- "I'm sure I failed the test—it was ridiculously hard!"
- "I'm so depressed—I went to sign up for my favorite dance class and it was closed out!"
- "I'm really devastated that you're going away for a week—I have so much going on and you won't be here! You can't go!"
- "I can't stand how my boss treats me—it makes me so angry—I think I'm going to quit my job!"
- "I missed the train, and then had to wait another half hour on the platform in the pouring rain!"

> ***Note to Leaders:*** Alert the group that it is your expectation that the acronym GIVE will become overlearned and overused.

- *Practice even when it's hard.* Sadly, many people working hard at school and at work come home and need to "stop working so hard," which sometimes looks like anti-GIVE behavior. It is critical for all group members to be extra mindful of this natural tendency. This focus will hopefully lead to more effortful and skillful GIVE-based interactions with the people whom you love and care about. In the future, if you forget to use GIVE with your family, peers, or co-leaders in this group, we will remind you, gently, using an *easy manner* about applying your "GIVE" skills in the moment.

Challenges Teaching GIVE skills

• **Validating versus complimenting.** Many people confuse validating with complimenting, praising, reassuring, or otherwise offering support. For example:

"Oh, come on, I'm sure your father will understand."
"I'm sure you did fine on the test—you always do!"
"Come on, you have lots of friends and you are well liked!"

Leaders may have to point out the difference and explain how well-meaning praise or reassurance can be perceived as invalidating and intensify emotions. For example: "No, you don't get it! My father really *is going to kill me!*"

• **Validating a perceived overreaction.** *Members also get caught up with whether they should validate when they think that someone is making* way too big a deal *out of something. In other words, they don't believe the emotion fits the facts. For example:*

"You are really getting this angry over a hairbrush? Don't you think you are making too big a deal out of it?"
"You're thinking of dropping out of advanced math—are you *crazy?*"

Leaders can also point out how this kind of response backfires and demonstrate in a role play; the minimizing or dismissing stance will nearly always result in an intensification of the emotion.

Sometimes the emotion is not stated, and validation involves educated guessing on the part of the listener. For example, you missed the train and had to wait for the next one while standing in the rain. A validating response might be, "That must have been awful! And so frustrating!" This is opposed to the invalidating response, "Next time, just leave earlier!"

• **Validating versus teaching responsibility.** *Another question that comes up often for parents is, "If I validate, am I somehow condoning the behavior?" Regarding the example directly above, a parent might ask, "Shouldn't I teach the responsibility of leaving on time, rather than feel sorry for them that they were stuck waiting in the rain?" A helpful response is to discuss which response is more effective, and to help the parent identify goals in the interaction. A validating response might convey understanding and highlight the natural consequence of leaving late for the train. An invalidating response will likely just annoy the teen and make him or her feel more distant from the parent.*

ASSIGNMENT OF HOMEWORK

Assign Interpersonal Effectiveness Handout 4, "Practice Exercise: GIVE Skills." Ask participants to commit to using the GIVE skills in two situations over the next week. They are to record the situations and the outcomes on this handout.

SESSION 2
BRIEF MINDFULNESS EXERCISE
. . . .
HOMEWORK REVIEW
. . . .
BREAK
. . . .

GETTING SOMEONE TO DO WHAT YOU WANT: DEAR MAN SKILLS
Orientation of Clients to DEAR MAN Skills and Their Rationale

DEAR MAN skills are often introduced either with a personal story told by the group leader or with a series of three role plays conducted by two group leaders.

The personal story method should involve the group leader's briefly giving some background to a challenging real-life interpersonal situation. Then, without identifying the specific skills, the group leader describes how he or she got what he or she wanted. DEAR MAN and GIVE skills should be embedded in the example.

Example of Personal Story Method

Two weeks after my son was born, he was throwing up more than your average baby and appeared to have severe reflux. By week 3, he began losing weight, which is very dangerous for a newborn. He was brought to the emergency room and it was determined that he had a condition called *pyloric stenosis*. This means that the muscle at the base of your stomach gets too tight and doesn't allow food to pass through. So, if food stops going down, there's only one direction for it to go—that is up! We were told he needed surgery.

So, in the face of tremendous anxiety, we agreed and went to an expert surgeon (Dr. W) who was well known for his excellent work with newborns who had pyloric stenosis. Our son was on an inpatient medical unit for days, waiting for his surgery because other surgeries were more urgent, we were told, and were given priority for the operating rooms. He was hooked to IVs and monitors and we were emotionally depleted. Finally, the morning of his surgery arrived. A woman swept into the room and announced, "I'm Doctor B, and I'll be doing the surgery." I remarked that we were told that Dr. W was doing the surgery. She said defensively, "I'm the chief resident and I will do the surgery. Dr. W will be in the OR with me." I quickly retorted, "Dr. B, we came here for Dr. W. He's the expert. I'd like to speak with Dr. W before anyone does this surgery." Dr. B got angry and stormed out of the room. My wife and I were taken aback by the entire interaction. One thing we knew was that we wanted the attending surgeon and not the resident operating on our 3-week-old son. An hour later, Dr. W calmly and confidently entered the room.

I said, "Dr. W, thank you so much for coming into the room and speaking with us. [*Describe:*] As you may have heard, Dr. B, your chief resident, introduced herself to us earlier and informed us that she was going to do the surgery. We came here specifically for you and your reputation. [*Express:*] I was surprised and irritated at Dr. B's gruff response, and now I am anxious that there is possibility that you won't be the surgeon after all. [*Assert with validation:*] Although I am a psychologist at another local teaching hospital and I strongly believe in training residents, I was expecting that you would be the surgeon, and I would like to request that you conduct this surgery. [*Reinforce:*] Given that this is my 3-week-old son, I only wanted you, who by all accounts is *the* man when it comes to pyloric stenosis, to do the surgery. As a parent, you only want the best, and I would feel eternally grateful if you could assure me it will be you.

[*Be mindful:*] Dr. W validated my concerns and said, however, that because this is a teaching hospital, his chief resident does the surgery under his supervision now. [*Broken record:*] I stayed focused on my goal and repeated myself, expressing again my concern that he would not be the surgeon, asserting that we came here specifically so he could do the surgery, and repeating how grateful we would be. [*Appear confident:*] I was gentle *and* confident as I said these things, with good eye contact and a firm handshake. [*Negotiate:*] I said we'd be willing to wait until any point in the day that was best for him to do the surgery. Dr. W stated that he heard my concerns and although he was confident in Dr. B's skills, he gave me his word that he would do the surgery and that Dr. B would assist, instead of the other way around. I said I was very satisfied with that and expressed my deep gratitude and appreciation for his time and his word.

> **DISCUSSION POINT:** *Ask the participants what elements of the interpersonal interaction were effective in this above example. The elements can then be labeled and tied in with the teaching of DEAR MAN.*

Leader Role-Play Method

Another effective method of introducing DEAR MAN is for leaders to role-play a situation. We start by stating what the person's goal is (e.g., a teen asking her parent to buy her a guitar and pay for guitar lessons).

First, we role-play an aggressive approach. The requesting leader angrily yells and makes demands of the other leader, who slinks away and looks horrified, or alternatively, starts yelling right back. Second, we role-play a passive approach. The requesting group leader beats around the bush, hints a bit, maybe uses some guilt, and then, when the other group leader is unresponsive, ultimately backs off from the request.

After each role play, we ask group members for observations about whether the actions taken to make the request were effective, and why or why not. We ask them what would have made the request more effective, and in doing this, the wisdom of group members typically comes through as they identify components of the DEAR MAN skills without having yet learned them.

Review DEAR MAN Skills

Refer participants to Interpersonal Effectiveness Handout 5, "Getting Someone to Do What You Want: DEAR MAN Skills." Introduce this handout and link it to the goals of asking for what you want or saying "no." Read (or have members read) and define each letter in the acronym.

Describe the situation. No judgments, no opinions.

Express feelings and opinions. "I feel" or "I prefer" but not "you should."

Assert by asking for what you want or need or by saying "no" directly.

Reinforce or reward the person ahead of time by expressing appreciation, letting the person know how granting your request will help him or her, help you, or help a situation. Explain the benefits of granting your request or accepting "no."

(Be) **Mindful**. Stay focused on your goals. Do not get distracted or allow yourself to get sidetracked. Return to your goals and your request again and again, like a broken record.

Appear confident. Appearing confident can include voice tone and strength, eye contact, posture (shoulders and back straight and tall, head held high), physical appearance (being well dressed and groomed projects confidence). All of this will help you to be taken seriously. [*Leaders can do a quick role play or request volunteers from the group to model the difference between a nonconfident request or decline and a confident one. Have group members observe the differences.*]

Negotiate. Offer to give to get. Say what you are willing to do to help the other person meet your request or accept your "no." If you cannot think of what to offer (e.g., "I can't do this, but I *am* willing to do this"), turn the tables: Ask the other person whether he or she has any ideas: What would help that person to be able to grant your request or accept "no"? For example, ask, "How do you think we can solve this problem?" [*Leaders can emphasize that in negotiating, the goal is not to defeat the other party, but to convey joint responsibility, effort, or openness in solving the problem. This approach can leave both parties feeling more accepting of the request or the "no."*]

Practicing the Skills

It is important to conduct role plays to give group members the chance to practice their DEAR MAN skills. These can be done in dyads, triads (where two people have the conversation and one observes, coaches, and gives feedback), or in a full-group format where volunteers role-play the skills and leaders and other group members coach and give feedback. Here are some examples for DEAR MAN role plays/discussions:

- Family member or friend asks for a ride at a time that is inconvenient. [*Role play can involve making the request or saying "no."*]
- Borrowing a large sum of money. [*Role play can involve making the request or saying "no."*]
- You want to ask for time off your job to take a trip.
- You want to ask a family member to spend more time with you.
- Parent wants teen to come home earlier from a planned night out; teen wants to stay out later.
- You want to ask your coach for more playing time.
- Turning down a request to hang out with a friend.
- Turning down your boyfriend or girlfriend who wants to do more with you sexually than you feel ready for.
- Parent wants to say "no" to teen who is asking to sleep over at a friend's house when there will not be a parent in the home.
- Someone puts you on the spot with a request, and worry thoughts, emotions, and indecision interfere. You really don't know whether you should say yes or no. [*The idea here is to use DEAR MAN to ask for time to think it over—and not impulsively say "yes" on the spot. Many clients have found it extremely helpful to learn that they do not have to make an in-the-moment, impulsive decision. The practice here is using the skills to assert "I need to think about it."*]

Challenges Teaching DEAR MAN Skills

Common questions raised by group members and suggested responses include the following:

• *What do you do when the* other *person isn't being interpersonally effective?* This can be tough and frustrating! Lots of times other people drag us down by not granting our request or by invalidating us, stonewalling us, picking on us, yelling at us, criticizing us, or otherwise hurting or frustrating us. Ultimately, you will be more likely to get what you want if you use your best DEAR MAN skills, emphasizing the broken record in staying mindful of your goals. We cannot control another person's skillfulness; we can only maximize our own use of skills. We also may want to add in GIVE skills or the upcoming FAST skills, which we will teach you; these might enhance the outcome.

At times, even using our best interpersonal skills with the person will not be enough. In such cases, we may want to enlist a number of other skills. We may want to use interpersonal effectiveness skills with someone else to get help with the situation, such as a school authority if a peer is harming you, or a friend or parent as a "sounding board." We will need mindfulness to notice our reactions and urges and either do what works (be effective according to your goals), or possibly focus one-mindfully on a distress tolerance skill such as distraction, self-soothing, improving the moment skill, pros and cons of a particular response, TIPP, or radical acceptance. We might want to use an emotion regulation skill such as engaging in a pleasant activity, working toward a long-term goal based on our values, ending the relationship (if possible) or working on current or new ones, or building mastery. The point is, when we don't get what we want in an interpersonal situation, there are many ways we can respond to reduce our misery.

• *What do you do when the other person is "DEAR MANing" you back?* Maybe you are using DEAR MAN to make a request, and the other person uses it to say "no." How does it work out? You will increase your chances of getting what you want if you stay mindful of your goals and emphasize the reinforcement (telling the person the benefits of giving you what you want) and the negotiation (be willing to give to get, or ask how the other person thinks you two can solve this problem, so he or she has some input). Nevertheless, you may not always get what you want, and you may have to accept this. It is still better in the long run to practice asking and negotiating skillfully.

• *Isn't it "groveling" to use DEAR MAN with kids to make a basic request?* Some parents have expressed concerns that using DEAR MAN to make basic requests (e.g., to help prepare for a holiday meal, or to babysit little sister when a grandmother is in the hospital) is somehow "groveling." They might say, "When I was a kid, my parents just told me to do it, and I wouldn't have even thought to question it!" They ask: Doesn't it send the message that this is a lot to ask or that it is somehow negotiable and thereby reinforce a culture of entitlement and of kids not taking responsibility? We always ask those parents how it is working now for them when they just try to "lay down the law" with their teens. If it is not working and ending up with conflict or rebellion, then using these skills might be a more effective strategy. Additionally, our teens will feel more respected when spoken to using DEAR MAN skills than given orders. Parents are also modeling effective interpersonal skills for their teens to use toward them and in other relationships.

ASSIGNMENT OF HOMEWORK

Assign Interpersonal Effectiveness Handout 6, "Practice Exercise: DEAR MAN Skills." Ask group members to commit to practicing the DEAR MAN skills in one situation during the next week and record on this handout. Members should write down the situation, their specific goal for the DEAR MAN skills (e.g., "I wanted to tell Maria I couldn't lend her the money"), how they used each component of the skill, and the outcome.

SESSION 3

BRIEF MINDFULNESS EXERCISE
· · · ·
HOMEWORK REVIEW
· · · ·
BREAK
· · · ·

MAINTAINING YOUR SELF-RESPECT: FAST SKILLS

Orientation of Clients to FAST Skills and Their Rationale

Sometimes being true to ourselves and feeling good about ourselves are the central goals. The skills we will learn today are about:

- Not being exploited
- Feeling good about yourself
- Not selling out
- Feeling good about how you are treating others

Refer participants to Interpersonal Effectiveness Handout 7, "Maintaining Your Self-Respect: FAST Skills."

A way to remember these skills is through the acronym FAST:

(be) **Fair** to yourself and the other person.

(no) **Apologies:** Don't over (*or* under) apologize. You don't have to apologize for sticking to your principles, for being you or being alive.

Stick to your values: Do what is right for you according to your Wise Mind values.

(be) **Truthful:** Do not lie, exaggerate, or act helpless.

EXERCISE: GROUP LEADERS ROLE PLAY

Leaders can role-play not using and then using FAST skills in the following situation:
Your uncle asks you to come work with him in the family business. Your parents are thrilled! Your heart isn't in it. You have other plans for yourself, but you feel really bad letting your uncle down. FAST skills might come in handy here.

Afterward, leaders can walk group members through each letter and ask: Was she fair to herself? Fair to her uncle? Did she apologize too much? Did she stick to her values? Was she truthful? Leaders can ask group members to comment on why each of these steps is important.

Group Practice of the Skills

Have group members practice their FAST skills. They can generate their own examples or leaders can select from the following.

- Your friend wants the two of you to take another friend out for his birthday at a really expensive place. You need to respond, and you are feeling you can't spend the money.
- You just got your license and lately you're always the one to drive everyone home late at night. This is making you get home past your curfew. You have worry thoughts, guilt, and so on. [*This situation can also be used for factors that interfere with interpersonal effectiveness.*]
- Your friend asks if you can raid your parents' liquor cabinet.
- You see your buddies at school leaving out another kid, not inviting her to hang out and ignoring her in the cafeteria, and you'd like to ask them to include her.
- You are going to a party where everyone is drinking and drugging and you don't want to.
- Your teacher embarrasses you by revealing personal and private information in front of the class.
- This guy says that if you don't send him naked pictures of you, he's not interested in hanging out with you.
- Your family member asks you to go somewhere with him or her and you have other priorities today.
- Your friend asks you for a lot of help with her paper when you are busy this week and trying to keep up your own grades.
- Someone close to you is invalidating your emotions and putting you down.
- A friend who's had too much to drink says, "Come on, I'll drive you home!"
- Your friend has play-off tickets and invites you to the big game, but it involves cutting out of work or school and lying about it, since you believe your parents would never let you. [*This role play could involve using FAST skills with the friend or with parents.*]
- At a holiday dinner, a relative makes derogatory comments stereotyping a group (by ethnicity, sexual orientation, age, ability, socioeconomic status, etc.). You are offended, but you don't want to start an argument.
- At a sleepover, friends pressure you to do a dare that makes you feel embarrassed or uncomfortable (e.g., dance for them, post something mean online about someone at school, reveal something private about yourself).

CHALLENGING WORRY THOUGHTS THAT INTERFERE WITH INTERPERSONAL EFFECTIVENESS

Refer participants to Interpersonal Effectiveness Handout 8, "Worry Thoughts and Wise Mind Self-Statements."

Orientation of Clients to the Topic

Worries sometimes get in the way of our using our skills. Some worries may also be myths we hold about getting along with others. We can counter these worries by challenging them with our Wise Mind or by trying out interpersonal skills with other people to see whether or not our worry thoughts are true: for example, by standing up for our values, even when we are worried that it might make a person not like us anymore.

> *Note to Leaders:* One way to introduce these ideas is with a personal story from a leader about a time when worry thoughts got in his or her way. An example follows.
>
> "My daughter was having a problem with a teacher in middle school. When my daughter could not handle it herself, I wanted to speak to the teacher to resolve it. However, worry thoughts stopped me at first. What if it does not work? What if she thinks I am making unfair demands? What if this ends up hurting my child more than it helps? The result was that it slowed me down from skillfully communicating to the teacher and trying to resolve the problems."

Not All Worry Thoughts Are Harmful

Sometimes worry thoughts can come in handy as a way to *stop* the action, slow you down, and think about whether you are saying something impulsively. It is important to check the facts, your emotions, and Wise Mind: Is it effective to ask or say this right now? Is it mainly worry thoughts that are stopping you?

Ways to engage group members with the above material include:

- *Have group members challenge each worry thought listed on Interpersonal Effectiveness Handout 8.*
- *Use a devil's advocate strategy: Argue each worry thought strongly, getting group members to argue strongly against them.*
- *Discuss the differences between rational and emotional agreement with the worry thought and with Wise Mind agreement.*

Exercises for Creating Wise Mind Statements

From the bulleted list of scenarios for worry thoughts and challenges below, try one or more of the following exercises.

- *Practice in your mind. Tell group members they should imagine themselves in an interpersonal conflict that you then describe (see the following scenarios for examples). Check that group members are really getting into the scene. Instruct them to say a Wise Mind statement to themselves, as if they mean it. Now go around and share statements used.*

- *Think-aloud practice. Describe another conflict situation. Go around the room and ask each member to say a Wise Mind statement out loud. More than one person can use the same one.*

- *Drawing thoughts. Draw a cartoon character head with two empty thought bubbles coming out. Then use one of the scenarios below and ask members for a worry thought to fill one bubble and a Wise Mind self-statement to challenge the worry thought for the other bubble.*

Scenarios for Worry Thoughts and Challenges

- You want to ask your parent to treat your boyfriend or girlfriend a little more nicely, but are afraid the parent will just get angry and tell you he or she doesn't like your boyfriend or girlfriend.
- You want to ask your teen to miss hanging out with friends this weekend to join you in spending time with the family, but you are afraid of a big blow-up.
- You want to share your opinion in class, but you are afraid you will look stupid.
- You want to ask for some help with your work, but you are afraid the (teacher, boss, friend, relative) will think you are incompetent.

Sample Wise Mind Self-Statements to Challenge Your Worry Thoughts

The following might be something you would say to your friend or loved one, but are not as likely to say to yourself. Practice saying these to yourself!

- "Just because I didn't get what I wanted last time doesn't mean that if I ask skillfully this time, I won't get it."
- "I can stand it if I don't get what I want or need."
- "It takes a strong person to admit that he or she needs help from someone else and then ask for it."
- "I can understand and validate another person and still ask for what I want."
- "If I say 'no' to people and they get angry, it doesn't mean I should have said 'yes.'"
- "I can still feel good about myself even though someone else is annoyed with me."

ASSIGNMENT OF HOMEWORK

Assign Interpersonal Effectiveness Handout 9, "Practice Exercise: FAST Skills." Ask group members to commit to practicing the FAST skills in two situations during the week. They are to use this handout to describe the situations and the outcomes.

SESSION 4
BRIEF MINDFULNESS EXERCISE
· · · ·
HOMEWORK REVIEW
· · · ·
BREAK
· · · ·

FACTORS TO CONSIDER WHEN DECIDING HOW INTENSELY TO ASK OR SAY "NO"

Refer participants to Interpersonal Effectiveness Handout 10, "Factors to Consider in Asking for What You Want." Leaders can have clients read through the items on the handout and then discuss each one. Then leaders can present some situations (see examples below) or ask for examples from the group to practice considering these factors and deciding how intensely to pursue the matter or how firmly to decline.

Sometimes we may have the skills, but we are not sure how intensely to ask for something (or whether to ask) or how firmly to say "no." In such cases, we have to attend to the social nuances and context of the situation to get more information. Considering the following factors and asking ourselves these questions can help us decide:

- *Priorities*: What are my priorities in asking? Keeping the relationship? Getting what I want or saying "no"? Maintaining self-respect? This skill orients us to first consider our interpersonal goals and priorities, which then helps us determine whether to emphasize GIVE, DEAR MAN, FAST, or some combination.
- *Capability*: Does the person have the ability to give me what I want? Do I have the ability to give him or her what is asked of me? We've got to consider capability; for example, if I'm thinking of asking my cousin with a broken leg to play Frisbee, I should probably find someone else to play. If a friend asks me to borrow money but I'm broke that week, I feel clearer about saying no.
- *Timeliness*: Is now a good time to ask? Is it a good time for me to agree to a request? Have you asked to discuss something important just as the other person was starting a movie or going to sleep? Have you approached someone to settle a problem while feeling emotional? While in public? Has someone ever asked you to clean up your stuff just as you were running out the door? Tried to talk to you when you were focusing on school or work? These are factors we've got to consider when asking for something or deciding about agreeing to a request.
- *Preparation*: Have I checked out the facts, done my homework, or prepared myself before asking? Has the other person? For example, it may be better to know details about cost and content before asking a parent for money for a class you want to take, or to have the information regarding the supervision and location of a party before asking your parent if you can go. Have you practiced your instrument diligently before asking your music teacher for a solo in the school concert?
- *Relationship*: Is what I am asking (or what the other person is asking of me) appropriate to our relationship? How well do I know this person? What is the nature of our relationship? What can I (or the other person) reasonably expect? Consider the nature of your relationship before asking or granting a request. Examples: Are we close enough that I can trust this person if I reveal something private about myself? I might ask an older and trusted friend for a ride, but not a teacher. I might ask a teacher if I can come for extra help in Spanish, but I might not ask a kid at school I hardly know for Spanish help.
- *Give and take*: Has the person been asking a lot of me lately, and have I granted it or said "no"? Have I been asking a lot of the other person lately? Have we been treating each other in a balanced, fair way? We need to consider whether we are on fairly equal footing or not when considering asking for something or saying no to a request. For example, have you asked the same kid to borrow lunch money again and again? Is someone always asking you to spend time at his or her place but never willing to come to yours?

Sample Practice Scenarios

Leaders can present a couple of scenarios and ask group members what factors would be relevant to consider in each case in making a decision about whether to ask for what is wanted or say "no" to a request.

- A relative is staying at your house and smoking. You would like to ask him or her to stop smoking in the house, but are not sure whether you have the right to do this.
- An acquaintance you recently met asks if you will come over this weekend and help her paint her room. You are thinking of saying "no" but are not sure if that is the right thing to do.
- Your sister is spending a lot of time hanging out with your ex-boyfriend, which you believe is disloyal to you. You are upset, and you're considering whether you have the right to ask your sister to decrease or end her contact with him.
- Your friend is throwing a party and invites you. You have something else you'd like to do earlier that evening and are considering telling her that you will be an hour late to her party.
- A family member has been doing some things that feel invalidating to you. You would like to make a time to talk about it with him or her, but are not sure whether to ask.
- You would like to ask a neighbor to drive you to a doctor's appointment because you don't have a ride. You know the general area but don't yet have the address or know how long it will take.
- You got your hair dyed and the hairstylist messed up the color. You want to return to the shop and ask her to fix her mistake.

THINK SKILLS (OPTIONAL)

> *Note to Leaders:* This skill (see the Interpersonal Effectiveness Optional Handout 13, "THINK Skills") derives from the social information-processing model by Crick and Dodge (1994). It helps members practice taking another's perspective and considering multiple and benign interpretations for another's behaviors. Because the THINK skill was not part of standard DBT (Linehan, 1993b) and has not yet been used in research, it is optional. Skills trainers can teach this material if time allows and if members demonstrate a need for this skill. Or individual therapists can teach the skill, if needed, with an individual client or family.

We developed the THINK skills after noticing that clients in DBT often jump to conclusions, assume the worst about others' intentions, and sometimes have trouble considering others' viewpoints. The social information–processing model highlights how negative interpretations of another's behavior (e.g., "He's being mean"; "She's trying to manipulate me!") bias our response choices toward the negative (e.g., "I won't tolerate this!"). The THINK skills thus aim to minimize negative attributions and prompt clients to consider other, more benign interpretations (e.g., "He's frustrated and worried about me because I keep breaking curfew"; "She's expressing her distress"), and then consider and select responses in accordance with those more benign interpretations (e.g., "I'm going to pay attention to what's being expressed!"). The skills also prompt clients to consider ways that others in an interaction may be feeling, may have been trying to improve the relationship recently, or may themselves be struggling with painful emotions or circumstances. Applying the THINK skills is thus likely to lower negative emotions that might be unjustified, and reduce hostile or otherwise ineffective interpersonal behaviors.

Orientation of Clients to the Skills and Their Rationale

Sometimes we feel upset in our relationships and we assume the worst about others' behavior or intentions. Maybe we think they don't care about us, hate us, are ignoring us, are selfish, deliberately trying to hurt us, or are otherwise doing something heartless, inconsiderate, or rejecting.

> **DISCUSSION POINT:** *Ask,* "Can you think of times when this has happened to you—when you assumed the worst? How did you feel?" *Most will identify increased negative, painful emotions.* "When you feel that way, how do you usually handle it with the other person?" *Most people will say they either attack or avoid the other person—neither of which is effective in maintaining or enhancing the relationship.*

Sometimes we don't know the facts and assume the worst, when the truth may be something completely different from what we are thinking. THINK skills help us consider other motivations for people's behaviors.

Why THINK about Other Motivations?

When we interpret situations as negative, our responses tend to be more negative or hostile in return. Even if we are partly or fully right in assuming negative intentions, it is usually not effective to approach the other person believing the worst to be true. For example, if a teacher is not providing you with extra help because he truly does not like you and does not believe in you, will it be effective to go on the attack and accuse him of this? Will this get the teacher to like you more or want to spend the time helping you? It is usually more effective to give people the benefit of the doubt, to consider their perspective, and then act on that basis. When you want to reduce conflict and negative emotions such as anger and hurt, THINK about it differently.

How to THINK

Refer participants to Interpersonal Effectiveness Optional Handout 13, "THINK Skills."

Think about it from the other person's perspective.

Have empathy. Try to think of what the other person might be feeling. Might they feel sad? Worried? Frustrated? Hopeless? Confused?

Interpretations. Come up with several possible reasons for the person's behavior. Make sure to come up with at least one good, positive, not ill-intended interpretation. Examples: Might the person be worried about what you are doing because she cares? Might he be not helping you right now because he is overwhelmed or doesn't know how? Might she be increasing her intensity because it is important and she doesn't know how else to be taken seriously?

Notice. In what ways has the person been trying to show caring or improve the relationship? Maybe the person is not cooperating or being supportive in this case, but perhaps he has made a real effort at other times or shown caring in other ways. Notice how the person may be struggling, perhaps going through hard times that make it hard to be there for you in the way you want right now.

Kindness. Can you assume there are more benign (i.e., not mean, evil, or hostile) reasons for the other person's behavior? Can you consider the ways she has expressed caring or ways she may be struggling herself? Keeping these possibilities in mind, use kindness and gentleness in your response to the person. How can this help the situation?

Sample Scenarios for Talking about THINK Skills

The leaders can present one or more of the following examples and then go through the steps on the handout, asking the discussion questions that follow the examples.

- A girl whose mom is traveling a great distance at great expense to bring her to therapy assumes her mom does not care about her because she does not run to her or react strongly every time the girl expresses distress.
- A teen who's been hospitalized is angry with his friends for not being there for him at a time like this; he assumes they are all selfish.
- A mother is upset when she comes home from work and finds her partner with eyes fixed to the computer screen, not paying any attention to her. She assumes her partner is angry at her and ignoring her.

Discussion Questions

- What might the other person's perspective be on the situation?
- What might the other person be feeling right now? What pressures or other demands might be on him or her?
- What are several possible interpretations or explanations for the person's behavior, beyond the first interpretation?
- Can you notice or look for ways that the other person has been trying to attend to the relationship? Notice ways the other person might be struggling with his or her own stress, problems, difficulties at home, school, or work.
- Can you think of a kind way to approach the other person? What would you say or do? How would that be helpful?

USING MULTIPLE INTERPERSONAL EFFECTIVENESS SKILLS AT THE SAME TIME

At this point in the module, it can be useful to "test" the members by having them practice a situation that requires use of multiple skills. This can be done in a couple of ways. For the first option, leaders can have group members role-play a scenario, orienting the group as to which skills they will want to access, and coaching them through the role play step by step. For the second option, co-leaders themselves role-play a scenario using multiple skills and have the group members write down every skill they observe. For skills such as considering other factors, challenging worry thoughts, or optional THINK skills, the actor in the role play can think aloud to demonstrate the thought process. Afterward, have a group discussion about the skills used and how they worked. A role-play scenario for using several skills at the same time follows.

Sample Role-Play Scenarios

A teen wants to ask a teacher for an extension on a paper deadline because she was out sick for a week. She is afraid the teacher might be annoyed with her and say "no" [*worry thought*], and then she tells herself, "If I don't ask, I will never know. And, asking for help skillfully can be a sign of strength" [*Wise Mind self-statements*]. She considers the teacher's capability to grant her request (she can), the relationship (seems appropriate for student–teacher relationship), and the give-and-take nature of their interaction (she's been a good student and always gets her assignments in on time) [*factors to consider*]. She then makes a clear, assertive request with a specific extended deadline [*DEAR*], but she also asks the teacher if she would prefer to set another extended deadline [*MAN*]. She is gentle and validates the teacher [*GIVE*], while being honest without overapologizing for or exaggerating her illness [*FAST*].

The teacher says "no" because it is right near the end of the semester, and she needs time to do all of her grading. The teen feels very angry and assumes that the teacher hates her and is out to get her. She then takes a moment to think about it differently, to have some empathy for the teacher (she has five classes of 30 students each), and generates a more benign interpretation: She is truly busy right now; she has been a supportive teacher through the year, always willing to tutor me when I came for extra help [*THINK*]. This wider understanding helps her use kindness in her approach, and she tells the teacher she understands, but since she expects this assignment not to be her best work, she offers to do an extra credit assignment, if the teacher will allow it.

Another option is to present a scenario and lead group members through a discussion of what could interfere with using skills, how to overcome those obstacles, and how to apply which skills.

Let's say you finally get invited to a sleepover with the "popular" kids and now they are playing "truth or dare." You and others are getting asked to do things that violate privacy (i.e., reveal highly personal information), are embarrassing (e.g., you are asked to demonstrate for everyone how you dance at parties, as they all look on mockingly), are mean to you (e.g., you are asked to swallow a teaspoonful of a strong spice from the pantry), or are mean to others (post something mean or embarrassing on somebody's Facebook wall). You feel "stuck" in this situation. What might be stopping you from asking for what you want (to play something else or "tone it down") or to say "no"?

- Lack of skill: You don't know what to say or how to ask.
- Worry thoughts: You think, "They won't like me"; "They won't invite me again"; "They'll think I'm a loser"; or "They'll make fun of me."
- Emotions: You feel a mix of strong emotions, including anger, loneliness, fear, and shame, with a lump in your throat and tears in your eyes when you get close to speaking up.
- Can't decide: You are not sure if you should speak up or if you should just relax, throw yourself in, and have fun—after all, this is what kids do, and you did want to be here.
- Environment: Maybe you do try speaking up and they ignore you or say flippantly, "Sorry, majority rules!" and continue with the same activities.

Discussing Obstacles to Skills Use

If worry thoughts get in the way, what might a Wise Mind statement be? [*Take one response from group. Responses should be along the lines of "Better to be true to myself than do something I'll really regret."*]

What if strong emotions get in your way? You might use a mindfulness skill, such as observing your emotions nonjudgmentally and staying focused. [*If emotion regulation skills have been taught:*] Or use an emotion regulation skill such as taking the opposite action.

What if you just can't decide? Use mindfulness skills to get into Wise Mind to help you decide on the response you want to make.

If you decide to not participate and then speak up but the environment ignores you, you can then decide whether to accept the situation or maybe to leave.

Discussing Which Skills to Use and How

If you decide that your goals are to try to maintain these relationships (or at least not make enemies), get what you want or say "no," and keep your self-respect, what might you say?

Ask for volunteers from the group to try to craft a skillful response. As one co-leader coaches them through this, the other can write the specific skills being demonstrated on the board (e.g., describe, be truthful, stick to values). The gist of the response should include GIVE, DEAR MAN, and FAST skills, and sound something like this: "I know you guys are just having fun. But some of what we're doing is making me uncomfortable. I'd rather not go any further with this, especially the dancing, eating spices, and the stuff we're doing online. I'm willing to watch a movie or see what else you guys might want to do."

Additional role-play scenarios for using multiple skills:

- Kid wants to stay out late whereas parent wants early curfew.
- Wanting to tell a family member "I can't come to your _____ [important event]."
- Asking to stay home from school for a "mental health" day, or parent saying "no" to this.

ASSIGNMENT OF HOMEWORK

Assign Interpersonal Effectiveness Handout 11, "Practice Exercise: Factors to Consider in Asking or Saying 'No.'" Group members complete this homework to practice considering various important factors when making a request or saying "no."

Assign Interpersonal Effectiveness Handout 12, "Practice Exercise: Using Skills at the Same Time." This worksheet provides a final and integrative practice for the main skills taught in this module. Since real-life situations often require combining the interpersonal effectiveness skills, this practice allows members to apply multiple skills to an interpersonal interaction.

Optional: If taught, leaders can assign Interpersonal Effectiveness Optional Handout 14, "Practice Exercise: THINK Skills." This worksheet reviews the THINK skills for perspective taking, reducing negative inferences about another's behavior, and considering more positive and gentler response options.

PART III

Skills Training Handouts

DISTRESS TOLERANCE HANDOUTS

WALKING THE MIDDLE PATH HANDOUTS

EMOTION REGULATION HANDOUTS

INTERPERSONAL EFFECTIVENESS HANDOUTS

ORIENTATION HANDOUTS

What Is Dialectical Behavior Therapy (DBT)?

- DBT is an effective treatment for people who have difficulty controlling their emotions and behaviors.

- DBT aims to replace problem behaviors with skillful behaviors.

- DBT skills help people experience a range of emotions without necessarily acting on those emotions.

- DBT skills help teens navigate relationships in their environment (family/school/peers).

- DBT helps people create a life worth living.

What Does "Dialectical" Mean?

Dialectical = two opposite ideas can be true at the same time, and when considered together, can create a new truth and a new way of viewing the situation. There is always more than one way to think about a situation.

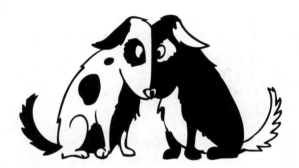

Goals of Skills Training

Problems to Decrease

1. **REDUCED AWARENESS AND FOCUS; CONFUSION ABOUT SELF**
   (Not always aware of what you are feeling, why you get upset, or what your goals are, and/or have trouble staying focused)

2. **EMOTIONAL DYSREGULATION**
   (Fast, intense mood changes with little control and/or steady negative emotional state; mood-dependent behaviors)

3. **IMPULSIVITY**
   (Acting without thinking it all through; escaping or avoiding emotional experiences)

4. **INTERPERSONAL PROBLEMS**
   (Pattern of difficulty keeping relationships steady, getting what you want, keeping self-respect; loneliness)

5. **TEENAGER AND FAMILY CHALLENGES**
   (Extreme thinking, feeling, and acting; absence of flexibility; difficulty navigating family conflict or effectively influencing others' behaviors)

Behaviors to Increase

1. **CORE MINDFULNESS SKILLS**

2. **EMOTION REGULATION SKILLS**

3. **DISTRESS TOLERANCE SKILLS**

4. **INTERPERSONAL EFFECTIVENESS**

5. **WALKING THE MIDDLE PATH SKILLS**

PERSONAL GOALS:

Behaviors to Decrease

1. _____
2. _____
3. _____
4. _____
5. _____

Behaviors to Increase

1. _____
2. _____
3. _____
4. _____
5. _____

DBT Skills Training Group Format

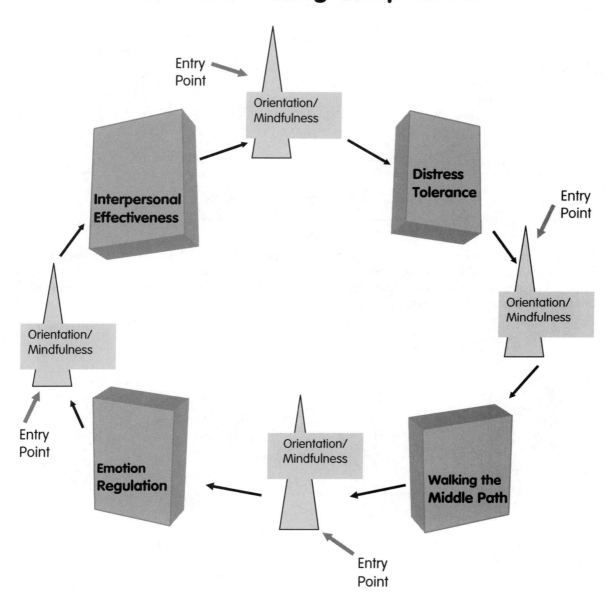

Biosocial Theory

BIO:

A. There is a biological vulnerability to emotions
   1. high sensitivity
   2. high reactivity
   3. slow return to baseline

plus

B. An inability to effectively regulate emotions.

TRANSACTING ⬇ ⬆ **WITH . . .**

SOCIAL:

An invalidating environment communicates that what you are feeling, thinking, or doing doesn't make sense or is considered inaccurate or an overreaction. Environments include parents, teachers, peers, therapists, coaches, and others. Sometimes there is a "poor fit" (e.g., temperament) between the person and the environment.

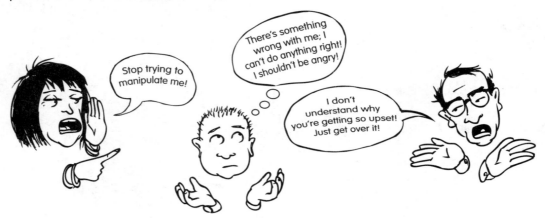

The invalidating environment punishes or sometimes reinforces emotional displays and contributes to the person's suppression or escalation of emotions, and sometimes leaves the person feeling confused and unable to trust one's own emotional experiences (**self-invalidation**).

OVER TIME LEADS TO . . .

**Multiple Problems
(Chronic Emotional Dysregulation)**

DBT Assumptions

1. People are doing the best they can.

2. People want to improve.

3. People need to do better, try harder, and be more motivated to change.

4. People may not have caused all of their own problems and they have to solve them anyway.

5. The lives of emotionally distressed teenagers and their families are painful as they are currently being lived.

6. Teens and families must learn and practice new behaviors in all the different situations in their lives (e.g., home, school, work, neighborhood).

7. There is no absolute truth.

8. Teens and their families cannot fail in DBT.

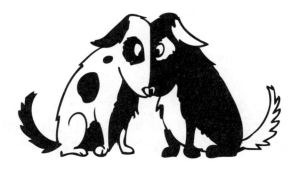

Adapted from *DBT® Skills Training Handouts and Worksheets, Second Edition.* Copyright 2015 by Marsha M. Linehan. Adapted by permission.

Guidelines for the Adolescent Skills Training Group

1. Information obtained during sessions (including the names of other group members) must remain confidential.

2. People are not to come to sessions under the influence of drugs or alcohol.

3. If you miss more than five group sessions (absences) in a 24-week program, you have dropped out of treatment. You can reapply one complete module after being out of the group. Attendance is kept on each family member individually.

4. If you are more than 15 minutes late, you will be allowed in but will be considered absent.

5. People are not to discuss any risk behaviors with other group members outside of sessions. Participants do not tempt others to engage in problem behaviors.

6. Group members may not contact one another when in crisis and instead should contact their skills coach or therapist.

7. People may not form private (cliques, dating) relationships with one another while they are in skills training together.

8. People may not act in a mean or disrespectful manner toward other group members or leaders.

9. *For teens in a comprehensive DBT program*, each adolescent must be in ongoing individual DBT therapy.

DBT Contract

 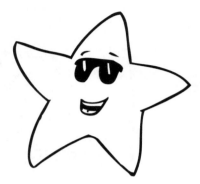

I am familiar with the theory, assumptions, and format of DBT Skills Training.

I agree to participate in DBT Skills Training and complete all of the modules.

I will come to group on time with my materials and practice exercises. If I don't do the practice, I agree to do a behavioral analysis (so we understand what got in the way and can problem-solve for next time).

I am fully aware of the attendance policy, and if I exceed the allotted amount of absences, I understand that I will have dropped out of DBT Skills Training. (As a caregiver, I am aware that the attendance policy applies to me as well.)

_____   _____
(Your signature)   **(date)**

_____   _____
(Skills trainer signature)   **(date)**

MINDFULNESS HANDOUTS

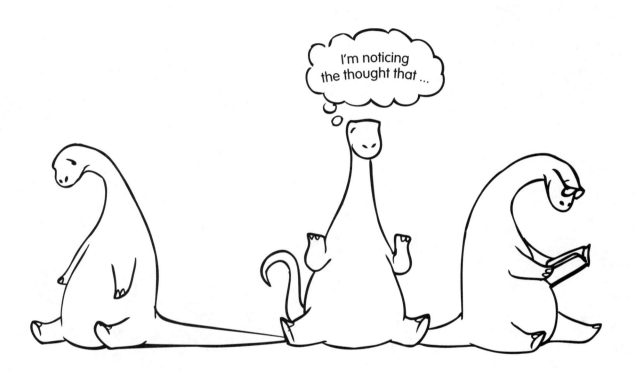

Mindfulness: Taking Hold of Your Mind

Being in control of your mind rather than letting your mind be in control of you.

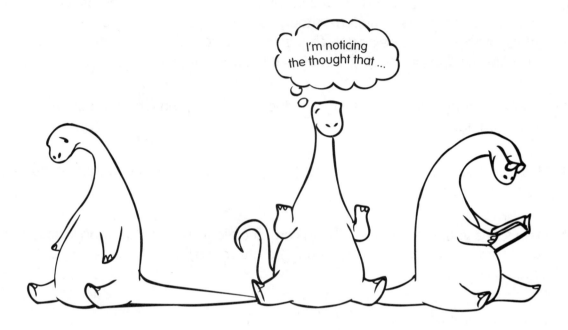

1. **FULL AWARENESS (Opened Mind):** Being aware of the present moment (e.g., thoughts, emotions, and physical sensations) without judgment and without trying to change it.

2. **ATTENTIONAL CONTROL (Focused Mind):** Staying focused on one thing at a time.

Mindfulness: Why Bother?

Being mindful can . . .

1. Give you more choices and more control over your behavior. It helps you slow down and notice emotions, thoughts, and urges (i.e., increases self-awareness), and helps you choose a behavior more thoughtfully, rather than act impulsively and make situations worse.

2. Reduce your emotional suffering and increase your pleasure and sense of well-being.

3. Help you make important decisions (and balance overly emotional or overly logical decisions).

4. Help focus your attention (i.e., be in control of your mind rather than letting your mind be in control of you) and therefore make you more effective and productive.

5. Increase compassion for self and others.

6. Lessen your pain, tension, and stress, and in turn can even improve your health.

Practice, practice, practice

Three States of Mind

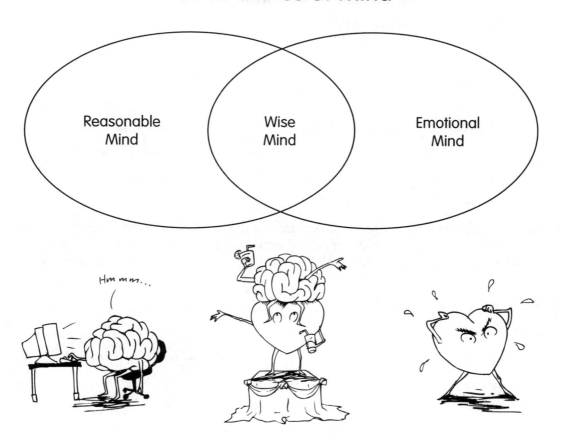

Emotional Mind is "hot," ruled by your feelings and urges.

When I am in Emotional Mind, I tend to: _____

_____

_____

_____

_____

_____

_____

(continued)

Reasonable Mind is "cool," ruled by thinking, facts, and logic.

When I am in Reasonable Mind, I tend to: _____

_____

_____

_____

_____

_____

_____

Wise Mind includes both reason and emotion; it is the wisdom within each person and the state of mind to access to avoid acting impulsively and when you need to make an important decision. *(Wise mind helps us think more clearly in the presence of strong emotions.)*

When I am in Wise Mind, I tend to: _____

_____

_____

_____

_____

_____

_____

_____

Practice Exercise:
Observing Yourself in Each State of Mind

Due Date: _____

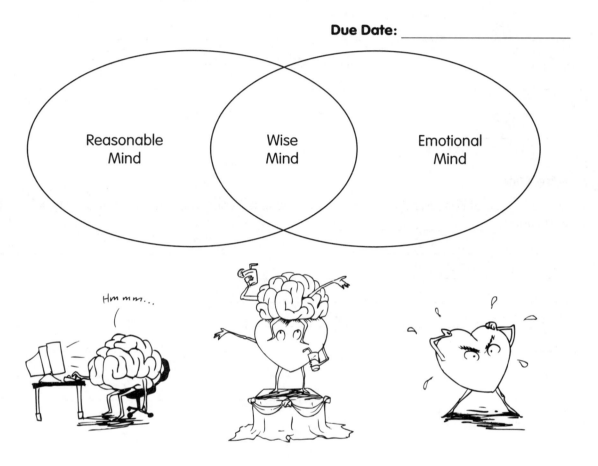

Emotional Mind

One example of Emotional Mind this week was (please describe your emotions, thoughts, behaviors): _____

_____

_____

_____

_____

(continued)

Reasonable Mind

One example of Reasonable Mind this week was (please describe your emotions, thoughts, behaviors): _____

_____

_____

_____

_____

_____

Wise Mind

One example of Wise Mind this week was (please describe your emotions, thoughts, behaviors): _____

_____

_____

_____

_____

_____

_____

_____

Mindfulness "What" Skills

Observe

- *Wordless watching*: Just notice the experience in the present moment.

- Observe both inside and outside yourself, using all of your five senses.

- Watch your thoughts and feelings come and go, as if they were on a conveyer belt.

- Have a "Teflon mind," letting experiences come into your mind and slip right out (not holding on).

- Don't push away your thoughts and feelings. Just let them happen, even when they're painful.

- Note: we cannot observe another's inner experience ("He's upset.")—only external features (e.g., a tear rolling down a cheek) or our thoughts about another's experience ("I observed the thought 'He's upset.' ").

Describe

- Put words on the experience: Label what you observe with words.

- For example: "I feel sad," "My face feels hot," "I feel my heart racing," "I'm having the thought that . . . ," "I'm having an urge to. . . ."

- Describe only what you observe *without* interpretations. Stick to the facts! Instead of "that person has an attitude," you could describe that person as "rolling her eyes, speaking with a loud voice."

Participate

- Throw yourself into the present moment fully (e.g., dancing, cleaning, taking a test, feeling sad in the moment). Try not to worry about tomorrow or focus on yesterday.

- Become one with whatever you're doing: *Get into the zone*.

- Fully experience the moment without being self-conscious.

- Experience even negative emotions fully to help your Wise Mind make a decision about what to do (instead of acting impulsively).

Mindfulness "How" Skills

Don't Judge

- Notice but don't evaluate as good or bad. Stick to the observable facts of the situation, using only what is observed with your senses.

- Acknowledge the harmful and the helpful, but don't judge it. For example, replace "He's a jerk" with "He walked away while we were talking."

- You can't go through life without making judgments; your goal is to catch and replace them with descriptions so you have more control over your emotions.

- When you find yourself judging, *don't judge your judging.*

Stay Focused

- One-mindfully: Focus your attention on *only* one thing in this moment. Slow yourself down to accomplish this.

- Stop doing two things at once (the opposite of multitasking).

- Concentrate your mind: Let go of distractions and refocus your attention when it drifts, again and again.

- Stay focused so that past, future, and current distractions don't get in your way.

Do What Works

- Be effective: Focus on what works to achieve your goal.

- Don't let emotions control your behavior; cut the cord between feeling and doing.

- Play by the rules (which may vary at home, school, work).

- Act as skillfully as you can to achieve your goals.

- Let go of negative feelings (e.g., vengeance and useless anger) and "shoulds" (e.g., "My teacher should have. . . .") that can hurt you and make things worse.

Mindfulness Cheat Sheet

1. Identify what you will focus on:

   Examples: Your breath

   An object (a picture, burning candle)

   An activity (brushing your hair, cleaning your room, reading)

2. Bring your attention to the object of focus.

3. When your attention wanders away from the object of focus (and sometimes it will, so don't judge yourself for it!) . . .

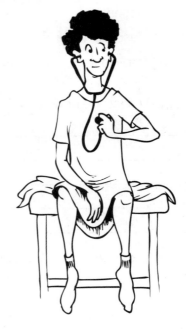

   - Notice that this has happened.
   - Gently bring your attention back to the object of focus.

To Get Started

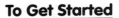

Begin practicing mindfulness by noticing your attention and how it wanders. Gradually work on doing this practice for 30 seconds, 1 minute and 2 minutes at a time. Practice *a lot*. No one will know you are doing it!

Your attention may wander to noises around you, worry thoughts, judgmental thoughts such as "this is stupid," body sensations, urges to talk, and so on). Notice them, let them go, and return your attention to the object of focus.

Practice Exercise:
Mindfulness "What" and "How" Skills

Due Date _____

Check off one **"what"** skill and one **"how"** skill to practice during the week.

"What" Skills	**"How" Skills**
____Observe	____Don't Judge
____Describe	____Stay Focused
____Participate	____Do What Works

Briefly describe how you used each skill during the week (include what, when, and where):

_____

_____

_____

_____

_____

Briefly describe how the skills affected your thoughts, feelings, or behaviors:

_____

_____

_____

_____

_____

_____ Were you able to get into Wise Mind?

_____ Were you able to better notice the present moment?

_____ Were you able to better focus your attention on just one thing at a time?

_____ Any other effects on thoughts, feelings, or behaviors? _____

_____

DISTRESS TOLERANCE HANDOUTS

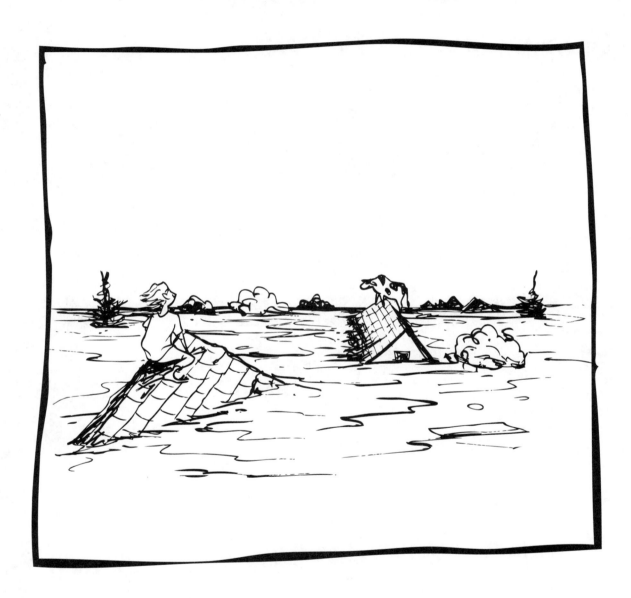

Why Bother Tolerating Painful Feelings and Urges?

Because . . .

> 1. Pain is part of life and can't always be avoided.

> 2. If you can't deal with your pain, you may act impulsively.

> 3. When you act impulsively, you may end up hurting yourself, hurting someone else, or not getting what you want.

Crisis Survival Skills Overview

Skills for tolerating painful events and emotions when you can't make things better right away and you don't want to make things worse!

Distract with "Wise Mind ACCEPTS"

Activities
Contributing
Comparisons
Emotions
Pushing Away
Thoughts
Sensations

SELF-SOOTHE with Six Senses

Vision
Hearing
Smell
Taste
Touch
Movement

IMPROVE the Moment

Imagery
Meaning
Prayer
Relaxation
One thing in the moment
Vacation
Encouragement

PROS AND CONS

TIPP

Temperature
Intense exercise
Paced breathing
Progressively relaxing your muscles

Adapted from *DBT® Skills Training Handouts and Worksheets, Second Edition.* Copyright 2015 by Marsha M. Linehan. Adapted by permission.

Crisis Survival Skills:
Distract with "Wise Mind ACCEPTS"

Activities   ***Do something.*** Call, e-mail, text, or visit a friend; watch a favorite movie or TV show; play your instrument or sing; play videogames; draw, cook, or bake; write in a journal; clean your room; go for a walk or exercise; read a book; listen to your iPod, go online and download music, apps; play a game with yourself or others.

Contributing   ***Contribute to (do something nice for) someone.*** Help a friend or sibling with homework; make something nice for someone else; donate things you don't need; surprise someone with a hug, a note, or a favor; volunteer.

Comparisons   ***Compare yourself*** to those less fortunate. Compare how you are feeling now to a time when you were doing worse. Think about others who are coping the same or less well than you.

Emotions   ***Create different emotions.*** Watch a funny TV show or emotional movie; listen to soothing or upbeat music; get active when you are sad; go to a store and read funny greeting cards or joke books.

Pushing away   ***Push the painful situation out of your mind temporarily.*** Leave the situation mentally by moving your attention and thoughts away; build an imaginary wall between you and the situation. Put the pain in a box and on a shelf for a while.

Thoughts   ***Replace your thoughts.*** Read; do word or number puzzles; count numbers, colors in a poster, tiles on a wall, anything; repeat the words to a song in your mind.

Sensations   ***Intensify other sensations.*** Hold or chew ice; listen to loud music; take a warm or cold shower; squeeze a stress ball; do sit-ups and push-ups; pet your dog or cat.

Adapted from *DBT® Skills Training Handouts and Worksheets, Second Edition.* Copyright 2015 by Marsha M. Linehan. Adapted by permission.

Practice Exercise:
Distract with "Wise Mind ACCEPTS"

Due Date _____

Write down at least two specific Distract skills to practice during the week when you feel upset (e.g., activity—play the guitar; contributing—bake cookies for my neighbor):

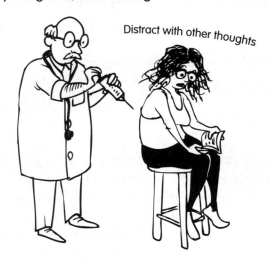

Distract with other thoughts

<u>Distract with "ACCEPTS"</u>

Activities _____

Contributing _____

Comparisons _____

Emotions _____

Pushing away _____

Thoughts _____

Sensations _____

(continued)

Briefly describe the stressful situations you were in and the specific skills you used: _____

_____

_____

_____

_____

_____

Did using the skills help you to (1) cope with uncomfortable feelings and urges and/or (2) avoid conflict of any kind?

Circle   Yes   or   No.

(Note: If the skill helped you to *not* do anything to make the situation worse, it worked!)

If YES, please describe how it helped: _____

_____

_____

_____

If NO, please describe why you believe it did not help: _____

_____

_____

_____

If you did not practice this skill, please explain why: _____

_____

_____

_____

_____

_____

_____

Crisis Survival Skills: Self-Soothe with Six Senses

VISION	**HEARING**
SMELL	**TASTE**
TOUCH	**MOVEMENT**

Vision   Go to your favorite place and take in all the sights; look at a photo album; zone out to a poster/picture; notice colors in a sunset; people watch.

Hearing   Listen to your favorite music and play it over and over again; pay attention to sounds in nature (birds, rain, thunder, traffic); play an instrument or sing; listen to a sound machine.

Smell   Put on your favorite lotion; use a scented aftershave or body wash; make cookies or popcorn; smell freshly brewed coffee; go to the park and "smell the roses."

Taste   Eat some of your favorite foods; drink your favorite nonalcoholic beverage; have your favorite flavor of ice cream; really notice the food you eat; eat one thing mindfully; don't overdo it!

Touch   Take a long bath or shower; pet your dog or cat; get a massage; brush your hair; hug or be hugged; put a cold cloth on your head; change into your most comfortable clothes.

Movement   Rock yourself gently; stretch; go for a run; do yoga; dance!

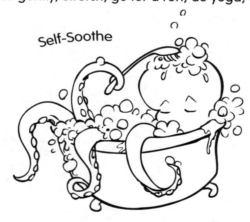

Self-Soothe

Adapted from *DBT® Skills Training Handouts and Worksheets, Second Edition.* Copyright 2015 by Marsha M. Linehan. Adapted by permission.

Practice Exercise: Self-Soothe Skills

Due Date _____

Write down at least two specific SELF-SOOTHE Skills to practice during the week when you feel upset:

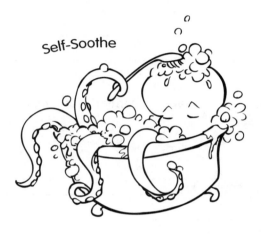

Self-Soothe

SELF-SOOTHE WITH SIX SENSES:

VISION _____

HEARING _____

SMELL _____

TASTE _____

TOUCH _____

MOVEMENT _____

(continued)

Briefly describe the stressful situations you were in and the specific skills you used:

1. _____

_____

_____

2. _____

_____

_____

Did using this skill help you to (1) cope with uncomfortable feelings and urges and/or (2) avoid conflict of any kind?

Circle   Yes   or   No.

If <u>YES</u>, please describe how it helped: _____

_____

_____

_____

_____

If <u>NO</u>, please describe why you believe it did not help: _____

_____

_____

_____

_____

If you did not practice this skill, please explain why: _____

_____

_____

_____

_____

_____

Crisis Survival Skills: IMPROVE the Moment

IMPROVE the Moment with:

Imagery   Imagine very relaxing scenes of a calming, safe place. Imagine things going well; imagine coping well. Imagine painful emotions draining out of you like water out of a pipe.

Meaning   Find or create some purpose, meaning, or value in the pain. Make lemonade out of lemons.

Prayer   Open your heart to a supreme being, greater wisdom, or your own Wise Mind. Ask for strength to bear the pain in this moment.

Relaxation   Try to relax your muscles by tensing and relaxing each large muscle group, starting with the forehead and working down. Download a relaxation audio or video; stretch; take a bath or get a massage.

One thing in the Moment   Focus your entire attention on what you are doing right now. Keep your mind in the present moment. Be aware of body movements or sensations while you're walking, cleaning, eating.

Vacation   Give yourself a brief vacation. Get outside, take a short walk, go get your favorite coffee drink or smoothie, read a magazine or newspaper; surf the web; take a 1-hour breather from hard work that must be done. Unplug from all electronic devices.

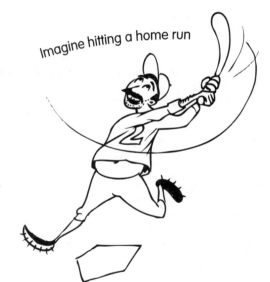

Imagine hitting a home run

Encouragement   Cheerlead yourself. Repeat over and over: "I can stand it," "It won't last forever," "I will make it out of this," "I'm doing the best I can."

Practice Exercise: IMPROVE the Moment

Due Date _____

Write down at least two specific IMPROVE Skills to practice during the week when you feel distressed:

Imagery _____

Meaning _____

Prayer _____

Relaxation _____

One Thing in the Moment _____

Vacation _____

Encouragement _____

Briefly describe the stressful situation(s) you were in and the specific skills you used: _____

_____

_____

_____

_____

_____

_____

_____

(continued)

Did using the skills help you to (1) cope with uncomfortable feelings and urges and/or (2) avoid conflict of any kind?

Circle   YES   or   NO

If <u>YES</u>, please describe how it helped: _____

_____

_____

_____

_____

If <u>NO</u>, please describe why you believe it did not help: _____

_____

_____

_____

_____

If you did not practice this skill, please explain why: _____

_____

_____

_____

_____

_____

_____

Crisis Survival Skills: Pros and Cons

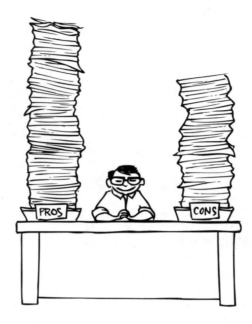

Select one crisis (emotionally upsetting situation) where you find it *really* hard to tolerate your distress, avoid destructive behavior, and not act impulsively.

Crisis I am faced with: _____

_____

Crisis urges: _____

_____

- An urge can intensify a crisis when it is intense and acting on the urge will make things worse in the long term.

- Make a list of the pros and cons of acting on your crisis urges. These might be to engage in addictive or harmful behavior or it might be to give in, give up, or avoid doing what is necessary to build a life you want to live.

- Make another list of the pros and cons of resisting crisis urges—that is, tolerating the distress skillfully and not giving into the urge.

(continued)

	PROS	CONS
Acting on Crisis Urges	Pros of acting on impulsive urges:	Cons of acting on impulsive urges:
Resisting Crisis Urges	Pros of resisting impulsive urges:	Cons of resisting impulsive urges:

1. Consider short-term and long-term PROS and CONS.

2. <u>Before</u> an overwhelming urge hits:

    Write out your PROS and CONS and carry them with you.

3. <u>When</u> an overwhelming urge hits:

    Review your PROS and CONS and imagine the positive consequences of resisting the urge.

    Imagine (and remember past) negative consequences of giving in to crisis urges.

Practice Exercise: Pros and Cons

Due Date _____

Select one crisis (emotionally upsetting situation) where you find it *really* hard to tolerate your distress, avoid destructive behavior, and not act on your urges.

Crisis I am faced with: _____

_____

Crisis urges: _____

_____

	PROS	**CONS**
Acting on Crisis Urges	Pros of acting on impulsive urges:	Cons of acting on impulsive urges:
Resisting Crisis Urges	Pros of resisting impulsive urges:	Cons of resisting impulsive urges:

1. Consider short-term and long-term PROS and CONS.

2. <u>Before</u> an overwhelming urge hits:

Write out your PROS and CONS and carry them with you.

3. <u>When</u> an overwhelming urge hits:

Review your PROS and CONS and imagine the positive consequences of resisting the urge.

Imagine (and remember past) negative consequences of giving in to crisis urges.

Crisis Survival Skills:
TIPP Skills for Managing Extreme Emotions

When emotional arousal is very HIGH!!!!!!!!!

- You are completely caught in Emotion Mind.
- Your brain is not processing information.
- You are emotionally overwhelmed.

"TIPP" your body chemistry to reduce extreme Emotion Mind quickly with:

Temperature

- **Tip the temperature of your face with cold water to calm down fast**. Holding your breath, put your face in a bowl of cold water; keep water above 50° F. Or, hold a cold pack or ziplock bag with ice water on your eyes and cheeks, or splash cold water on your face. Hold for 30 seconds.

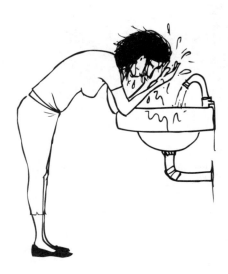

  Caution: Ice water decreases your heart rate rapidly. Intense exercise will increase heart rate. If you have a heart or medical condition, lowered base heart rate due to medications, take a beta blocker, or have an eating disorder, consult your health care provider before using these skills. Avoid ice water if allergic to the cold.

Intense Exercise

- **To calm down your body when it is revved up by emotion**. Engage in intense aerobic exercise, if only for a short while (10–15 minutes). Expend your body's stored-up physical energy by running, walking fast, jumping rope or jumping jacks, playing basketball, weight lifting, putting on music and dancing. *Don't overdo it!*

(continued)

Paced Breathing

- **Slow your pace of breathing way down** (to about 5–7 in and out breaths per minute). Breathe deeply from the abdomen. Breathe *out* more slowly than you breathe *in* (e.g., 4 seconds in and 6 seconds out). Do this for 1–2 minutes to bring down your arousal.

Progressive Muscle Relaxation

- **Tense and relax each muscle group**, head to toe, one muscle group at a time. *Tense* (5 seconds), then let go; *relax* each muscle all the way. *Notice* the tension; *notice* the difference when relaxed.

Practice Exercise: TIPP Skills

Due Date _____

Choose one TIPP skill to practice this week. Check it off now and prepare yourself to use this skill when emotional arousal gets very high.

Rate your emotional arousal before you use the skill: 1–100: _____

TIPP your body chemistry with:

____**T**emperature

Alter your body temperature by holding your breath and placing head in bowl of cold water. Or, splash cold water on your face or place a cold gel mask on your eyes or forehead. Hold for at least 30 seconds. Works best if bent over forward.

____**I**ntense exercise

Run in place, do a high-intensity weight circuit, jump, put on music and dance (10–15 minutes). *Don't* overdo it!

____**P**aced breathing

Slow down your breath so that you're breathing in for about 4 seconds and out for 5–8 seconds. Do this for 1–2 minutes to bring down your arousal.

____**P**rogressive muscle relaxation

Tense and relax each muscle group, head to toe, one muscle group at a time.

Rate your emotional arousal after using the skill: 1–100: _____

Adapted from *DBT® Skills Training Handouts and Worksheets, Second Edition.* Copyright 2015 by Marsha M. Linehan. Adapted by permission.

Create Your Crisis Survival Kit
for Home, School, or Work

List below 10 "tools" that go into your home crisis survival kit. Choose from your Distract with Wise Mind ACCEPTS skills, your Self-Soothe skills, your IMPROVE skills, and your TIPP skills. Take a shoebox, sturdy bag, or basket and place the relevant items inside: for example, your iPod, a stress ball, your favorite scented lotion or aftershave, picture of your favorite vacation spot, a favorite magazine, a crossword book, herbal tea bags, a favorite piece of candy, a relaxation CD or DVD.

1. _____
2. _____
3. _____
4. _____
5. _____
6. _____
7. _____
8. _____
9. _____
10. _____

Create a smaller version of your kit for school or work that fits in a pencil case or lunchbox. Consider items that can be used at your desk: for example, multicolored rubber bands to stretch; paper and pens for doodling; a mini-pack of playdough; a squeeze ball; silly putty; a list of visual stimuli in your class or office that can distract or soothe you; snacks to self-soothe; a list of friends, teachers, counselors, or colleagues you can approach when you have a break.

1. _____
2. _____
3. _____
4. _____
5. _____
6. _____

Accepting Reality: Choices We Can Make

Five optional ways of responding when a serious problem comes into your life:

1. Figure out how to solve the problem.
2. Change how you feel about the problem.
3. Accept it.
4. Stay miserable (no skill use).
5. Make things worse (act on your impulsive urges).

When you can't solve the problem or change your emotions about the problem, try acceptance as a way to reduce your suffering.

Why Bother Accepting Reality?

✓ Rejecting reality does not change reality.

✓ Changing reality requires first accepting reality.

✓ Rejecting reality turns pain into suffering.

✓ Refusing to accept reality can keep you stuck in unhappiness, anger, shame, sadness, bitterness, or other painful emotions.

Radical Acceptance

✓ RADICAL ACCEPTANCE is the skill of <u>accepting the things you can't change.</u>

✓ RADICAL = complete and total accepting in mind, heart, and body.

✓ ACCEPTANCE = seeing reality for what it is, even if you don't like it.

✓ ACCEPTANCE can mean to acknowledge, recognize, endure, not give up or give in.

✓ It's when you stop fighting reality, stop throwing tantrums about reality, and let go of bitterness. It is the opposite of "Why me?" It **is** "Things <u>are</u> as they <u>are</u>."

✓ Life can be worth living, even with painful events in it.

(continued)

Adapted from *DBT® Skills Training Handouts and Worksheets, Second Edition.* Copyright 2015 by Marsha M. Linehan. Adapted by permission.

List one important thing that you need to accept in your life *now*: _____

_____

_____

List one less important thing you need to accept *this week*: _____

_____

_____

Accepting Reality: Turning the Mind

✓ ACCEPTANCE is a choice. It is like coming to a "fork in the road." You may have to turn your mind toward the ACCEPTANCE road and away from the REJECTING "Reality Road."

✓ First notice you are not accepting reality (anger, bitterness, "Why me?")

✓ Second, make an inner commitment to ACCEPT.

✓ You may have to turn your mind over and over and over again.

Factors That Interfere with Acceptance

✓ Beliefs get in the way: You believe that if you accept your painful situation, you will become weak and just give up (or give in), approve of reality, or accept a life of pain.

✓ Emotions get in the way: Intense anger at the person or group that caused the painful event; unbearable sadness; guilt about your own behavior; shame regarding something about you; rage about the injustice of the world.

REMEMBER: ACCEPTANCE DOES NOT MEAN APPROVAL!

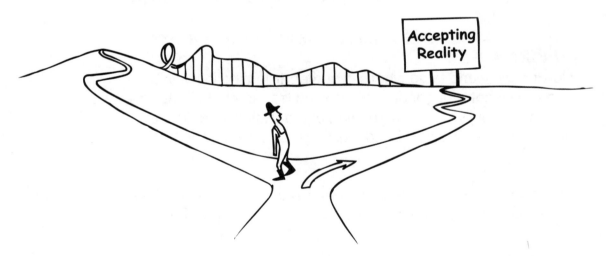

Adapted from *DBT® Skills Training Handouts and Worksheets, Second Edition.* Copyright 2015 by Marsha M. Linehan. Adapted by permission.

Willingness

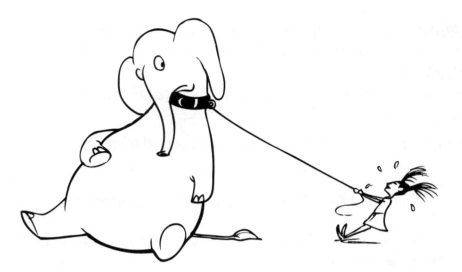

WILLFULNESS IS . . .
- Willfulness is refusing to tolerate a situation or giving up.
- Willfulness is trying to change a situation that cannot be changed, or refusing to change something that must be changed.
- Willfulness is "the terrible twos"—"no . . . no . . . no . . ."
- Willfulness is the opposite of "DOING WHAT WORKS"

REPLACE WILLFULNESS WITH *WILLINGNESS*.
WILLINGNESS IS . . .
- allowing the world to be what it is and participating in it fully.
- doing just what is needed—no more, no less. It is being effective.
- listening carefully to your Wise Mind and deciding what to do.
- When willfulness doesn't budge, ask: "What is the threat?"

How can you feel the difference between when you are *willing* and when you are *willful*? Clues that you are being willful: extreme thoughts like "No way!"; muscles tightening.

(continued)

Describe a situation when you noticed your **willingness**
and one in which you noticed your **willfulness:**

Where were you willful? _____

_____

_____

How were you willful (e.g., thoughts, feelings, body sensations)? _____

_____

_____

_____

What happened? _____

_____

_____

_____

Where were you willing? _____

_____

_____

How were you willing (e.g., thoughts, feelings, body sensations)? _____

_____

_____

_____

What happened? _____

_____

_____

_____

Ways to Practice Accepting Reality

1. Acceptance of reality <u>as it is</u> sometimes requires an act of CHOICE.

2. Breathe mindfully to be in the moment and to help develop a more accepting mindset.

3. Accept reality with your face: half-smile.

4. Rehearse in your mind those things that you would do if you really did accept reality *as it is*.

5. Practice willingness.

6. Remember to turn the mind back to accepting Reality Road.

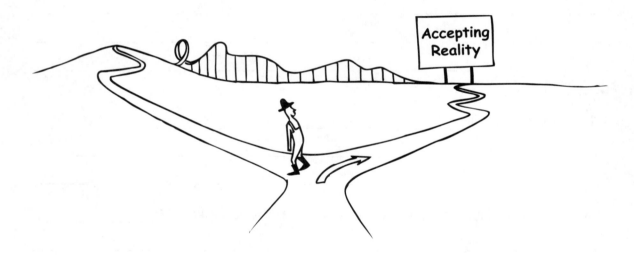

Adapted from *DBT® Skills Training Handouts and Worksheets, Second Edition*. Copyright 2015 by Marsha M. Linehan. Adapted by permission.

Practice Exercise: Accepting Reality

Due Date _____

Describe a situation during the week in which you were distressed and there was no way to change the situation right away: _____

_____

_____

_____

Rate your distress from 1 to 10 (with 10 being the worst): _____

If you couldn't solve the problem right away or change how you felt about it, what did you choose to do (circle one of the remaining three possibilities)?:

1. ~~Solve the problem.~~
2. ~~Change how you feel about the problem.~~
3. ACCEPT the situation.
4. Stay miserable (refuse to accept situation).
5. Make the situation worse.

If you tried to radically accept the situation, what exactly did you do or say to yourself? _____

_____

_____

_____

Did you notice that you had to "turn your mind" back to radical acceptance? If yes, how? _____

_____

_____

_____

If you chose to stay miserable or make things worse, what did you do? _____

_____

_____

_____

Rate your distress after you turned your mind toward acceptance (rate 0–10, with 10 being the worst distress): _____

WALKING THE MIDDLE PATH HANDOUTS

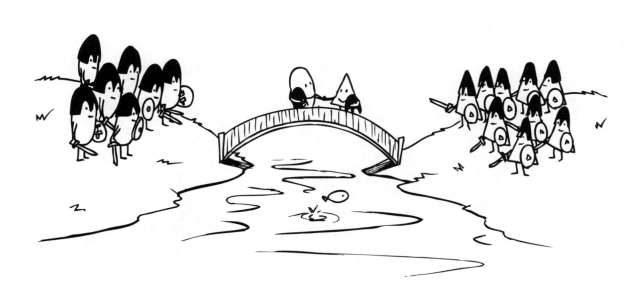

Dialectics: What Is It?

Dialectics teach us that:

- There is always more than one way to see a situation and more than one way to solve a problem.
- All people have unique qualities and different points of view.
- Change is the only constant.
- Two things that seem like (or are) opposites can both be true.
- *Honor* the truth on both sides of a conflict. This does not mean giving up your values or selling out. Avoid seeing the world in "black-and-white," "all-or-nothing" ways.

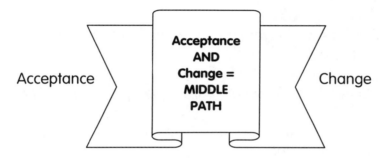

Acceptance

Acceptance AND Change = MIDDLE PATH

Change

Examples:

I am doing the best I can **AND** I need to do better, try harder, and be more motivated to change.

I can do this **AND** it's going to be hard. My mom is really strict **AND** she really cares about me. I've got big problems **AND** I can try to solve them. You are tough **AND** you are gentle.

This perspective helps pave the way toward the middle path by helping you:

- Expand your thoughts and ways of considering life situations.
- "Unstick" standoffs and conflicts.
- Be more flexible and approachable.
- Avoid assumptions and blaming.

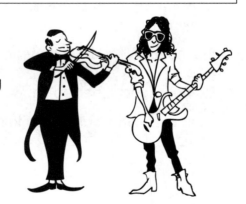

Dialectics "How-to" Guide

Hints for Thinking and Acting Dialectically:

1. Move to "both–and" thinking and away from "either/or" thinking. Avoid extreme words: *always, never, you make me*. Be descriptive.

   Example: Instead of saying "Everyone *always* treats me unfairly," say "*Sometimes* I am treated fairly *and* at other times, I am treated unfairly."

2. Practice looking at all sides of a situation and all points of view. Be generous and dig deep. Find the kernel of truth in every side by asking "What is being left out?"

   Example: "Why does Mom want me to be home at 10:00 P.M.?" "Why does my daughter want to stay out until 2:00 A.M.?

3. Remember: No one has the absolute truth. Be open to alternatives.

4. Use "I feel . . ." statements, instead of "You are . . .," "You should . . .," or "That's just the way it is" statements.

   Example: Say "I feel angry when you say I can't stay out later just because you said so" instead of, "You never listen and you are always unfair to me."

5. Accept that different opinions can be valid, even if you do not agree with them.

   Example: "I can see your point of view even though I do not agree with it."

6. Check your assumptions. Do not assume that you know what others are thinking.

   Example: "What did you mean when you said . . .?"

7. Do not expect others to know what you are thinking.

   Example: "What I am trying to say is. . . ."

(continued)

Practice:

Circle the dialectical statements:

1. a. "It is hopeless. I just cannot do it."

    b. "This is easy . . . I've got no problems."

    c. "This is really hard for me and I am going to keep trying."

2. a. "I know I am right about this."

    b. "You are totally wrong about that and I am right."

    c. "I can understand why you feel this way, and I feel different about it."

Thinking Mistakes

1. **ALL-OR-NOTHING, BLACK-AND-WHITE THINKING:** If you're not perfect, you're a total loser. If you don't get everything you want, it feels like you got nothing. If you're having a good day, the whole rest of your life is perfect and you don't need therapy anymore.

2. **CATASTROPHIZING (FORTUNETELLING ERROR):** You predict the future negatively without considering other, more likely outcomes. "I'm definitely going to fail my test," or "If I tell her that, she'll hate me forever."

3. **MIND READING:** You believe you know what other people are thinking even without asking. "He clearly doesn't think I will do a good job."

4. **OVERGENERALIZATION:** You make a sweeping, negative conclusion that goes far beyond the current situation. "Since I felt uncomfortable in my first day of class, I know that I won't be able to enjoy the rest of the year."

5. **MENTAL FILTER:** You develop selective hearing and vision and only hear and see the one negative thing and ignore the many positive things. "Because my supervisor gave me one low rating on my evaluation (that also had many higher ratings), it means I'm doing a terrible job."

6. **DISQUALIFYING THE POSITIVE:** You tell yourself that the positive experiences, actions, or qualities do not count. "I did well in that one basketball game because I just got lucky."

7. **EMOTIONAL REASONING:** You start thinking your emotions are fact. "I feel . . .; therefore, it is. I feel like she hates me; therefore, she does." "I feel stupid; therefore I am stupid." "I dread school, so it's a bad idea to go."

8. **"SHOULD" STATEMENTS:** You "should" on yourself or someone else by having a fixed idea of how you or others should behave, and you overestimate how bad it will be if these expectations are not met. "It's terrible that I made a mistake; I should always do my best." "You shouldn't be so upset."

9. **LABELING:** Overgeneralization is taken a step further by the use of extreme language to describe things. "I spilled my milk. I am SUCH A LOSER!" "My therapist didn't call me right back; she is the most uncaring, heartless therapist ever!"

10. **PERSONALIZATION:** You see yourself as the cause for things you have absolutely no control over or the target of stuff that may have absolutely nothing to do with you. "My parents divorced because of me." "The receptionist was short with me because I did something wrong."

From *Cognitive Behavior Therapy: Basics and Beyond, Second Edition*, by Judith S. Beck. Copyright 2011 by Judith S. Beck. Adapted by permission.

Dialectical Dilemmas

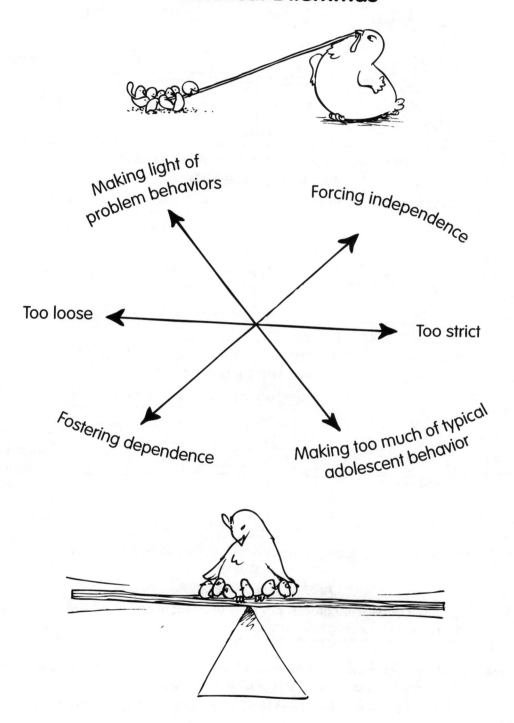

Making light of
problem behaviors

Forcing independence

Too loose

Too strict

Fostering dependence

Making too much of typical
adolescent behavior

Dialectical Dilemmas:
How Does the Dilemma Apply to You?

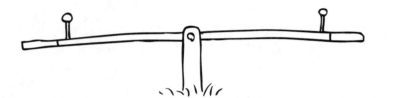

Too loose   Too strict

> Have clear rules and enforce them consistently
> **AND AT THE SAME TIME**
> Be willing to negotiate on some issues and don't overuse consequences

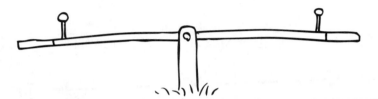

Making light of problem behaviors   Making too much of typical adolescent behavior

> Recognize when a behavior "crosses the line" and get help for that behavior
> **AND AT THE SAME TIME**
> Recognize which behaviors are part of typical adolescent development

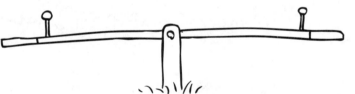

Forcing independence   Fostering dependence

> Give your adolescent guidance, support, and coaching to help figure out how to be responsible
> **AND AT THE SAME TIME**
> SLOWLY give your adolescent greater amounts of freedom and independence while continuing to encourage an appropriate amount of reliance on others

Place an "X" on each continuum to note where you are, a "Y" where your family member is, and a "Z" for a second family member.

What do you need to do to think and act more dialectically?

What's Typical for Adolescents and What's Cause for Concern?

Typical	Not Typical: Cause for Concern
1. Increased moodiness	Intense, painful, long-lasting moods; risky mood-dependent behavior, major depression, or panic attacks; self-injury or suicidal thinking
2. Increased self-consciousness, of feeling "on stage," increased focus on body image	Social phobia or withdrawal; perfectionism and unrealistic standards; bingeing, purging, or restricted eating; obsessive about or neglectful of hygiene
3. Increased dawdling	Multiple distractions to point of not being able to complete homework or projects, lack of focus that interferes with daily work or tasks, regularly late for appointments
4. Increased parent–adolescent conflict	Verbal or physical aggression, running away
5. Experimentation with drugs, alcohol, or cigarettes	Substance abuse, selling drugs, substance-using peer group
6. Increased sense of invulnerability (may lead to increased sensation seeking or risk taking)	Multiple accidents; encounters with firearms; excessive risk taking (e.g., subway surfing, driving drunk or texting while driving), getting arrested
7. Stressful transitions to middle and high school	School refusal; bullying or being bullied; lack of connection to school or peers; school truancy, failure, or dropout
8. Increased argumentativeness, idealism, and criticism; being opinionated	Rebellious questioning of social rules and conventions; causing trouble with family members, teachers, or others who attempt to assert authority over the adolescent

(continued)

Typical	**Not Typical: Cause for Concern**
9. Increased sexual maturation; sexual interest or experimentation	Sexual promiscuity, multiple partners, unsafe sexual practices, pregnancy
10. Becoming stressed by everyday decision making	Becoming paralyzed with indecision
11. Increased desire for privacy	Isolation from family; breakdown of communication, routine lying, and hiding things
12. Strong interest in technology; social media	Many hours per day spent on computer, on high-risk or triggering websites; casually meeting partners online; revealing too much (e.g., "sexting," overly personal posts on Facebook, Tumblr, Instagram, in blog)
13. Messy room	Old, rotting food; teen not able to find basic necessities; dirty clothes covering floor chronically
14. Sleep cycle shifts later (urge to be a "night owl" and to sleep late on weekends)	Often up nearly all night; sleeps almost all day on weekends; routinely late (or missing school) because of sleep schedule

Practice Exercise: Thinking and Acting Dialectically

Due Date _____

Identify a time this week when you did *not* think or act dialectically.

Example 1: Briefly describe the situation (who, what, when) _____

_____

_____

How did you think or act in this situation? _____

_____

_____

Are you thinking in extremes (e.g., all or nothing or catastrophizing)? Examples: _____

_____

_____

What is a more dialectical thought (or action) about the situation? _____

_____

_____

What was the outcome? _____

_____

_____

Identify a time this week when you *did* think or act dialectically.

Example 2: Briefly describe the situation (who, what, when) _____

_____

How did you think or act in this situation? _____

_____

What was the outcome? _____

_____

_____

Validation

VALIDATION communicates to another person that his or her feelings, thoughts, and actions **make sense** and are understandable to you in a particular situation.

SELF-VALIDATION involves perceiving your *own* feelings, thoughts, and actions as making sense, accurate, and acceptable in a particular situation.

INVALIDATION communicates (intentionally or not, through words or actions) that another person's feelings, thoughts, and actions in a particular situation make no sense, are "manipulative," or "stupid," or an "overreaction," or not worthy of your time, interest, or respect.

Remember: Validation ≠ Agreement

Validation *does not* necessarily mean that you like or agree with what the other person is doing, saying, or feeling. It means that you understand where they are coming from.

WHY VALIDATE?

- Validation improves relationships!!!!
- It can deescalate conflict and intense emotions.
- Validation can show that:
  - We are listening.
  - We understand.
  - We are being nonjudgmental.
  - We care about the relationship.
  - We can disagree without having a big conflict.

WHAT TO VALIDATE?

- Feelings, thoughts, and behaviors in ourselves or others

Validate the valid, not the invalid. You can still validate the feeling *without* validating the behavior. For example: Validate someone feeling upset about a low test grade even though you know he or she didn't study, but *don't* validate the lack of studying that led to the low grade.

How Can We Validate Others?

1. Actively listen. Make eye contact and stay focused.

2. Be mindful of your verbal and nonverbal reactions in order to avoid invalidation (e.g., rolling eyes, sucking teeth, heavy sighing, walking away, making light of serious things, or saying, for example, "That's stupid, don't be sad," "I don't care what you say," "Whatever!").

3. Observe what the other person is feeling in the moment. Look for a word that describes the feeling.

4. Reflect the feeling back without judgment. The goal is to communicate that you *understand* how the other person feels (e.g., "It makes sense that you're angry"; "I understand that you are having a tough time right now").

   For *self-validation*: "I have a right to feel sad." Avoid "Yes, but . . ." thinking. Instead, think about what your best friend in Wise Mind would say to you.

5. Show tolerance! Look for how the feelings, thoughts, or actions make sense given the other's (or your own) history and current situation, even if you don't approve of the behavior, emotion, or action itself.

6. Respond in a way that shows that you are taking the person seriously (with or without words); for example, "That sounds awful." If someone is crying, give a tissue or a hug. You may ask, "What do you need right now? For me to just listen or to help you problem-solve?"

How Can We Validate Ourselves?

How can I validate myself?

1. Actively listen and pay attention to yourself: Be mindful of your thoughts, feelings, and behaviors.

2. Describe your feelings without passing judgment: "Wow, I'm really angry right now!" or "It makes sense that I'm a little nervous."

3. Respond in a way that shows that you take yourself seriously: Accept that it is OK to have your emotion(s) (e.g., "It's OK to feel sad sometimes").

4. Acknowledge that the emotion may make sense in the situation. Show tolerance for yourself and your emotions (e.g., "It makes sense that I'm not able to focus very well with all of the stress I am under").

5. Do not judge your own emotion (or yourself).

6. Use interpersonal effectiveness skills for self-respect to be fair to yourself, not apologize for feeling how you feel, stick up for yourself, and stay true to your values (FAST).

Practice Exercise: Validation of Self and Others

Due Date _____

List *one* self-invalidating statement and *two* self-validating statements:

1. _____

2. _____

3. _____

List *one* invalidating statement to others and *two* validating statements to others:

1. _____

2. _____

3. _____

Choose a situation during the week in which you used validation skills with someone else or yourself.

Situation: _____

_____

Who did you validate? _____

What *exactly* did you do or say to validate yourself or that person? _____

_____

What was the outcome? _____

_____

_____

How did you feel afterward? _____

_____

Would you say or do something differently next time? What? _____

_____

_____

Behavior Change

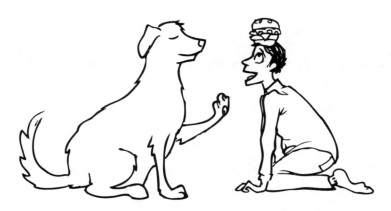

Behavior change skills are strategies used to *increase* behaviors we want and to *reduce* behaviors we don't want (in ourselves and others).

BEHAVIORS TO INCREASE

Remember to be specific and measurable.

SELF:

What behaviors would you like to increase in yourself (e.g., exercising, saving money, going to school, doing homework)? _____

_____

_____

_____

_____

OTHERS:

What behaviors would you like to increase in someone else (e.g., spending more time with you, listening to you, making eye contact, putting dirty dishes in the sink)? _____

_____

_____

_____

_____

(continued)

BEHAVIORS TO DECREASE

SELF:

What behaviors would you like to decrease in yourself (e.g., overeating, cigarette smoking, cutting, blurting out impulsively, arguing back, running away, fighting, skipping classes, lying in bed during the day)? _____

_____

_____

_____

_____

OTHERS:

What behaviors would you like to decrease in someone else (e.g., nagging, breaking curfew, running away, yelling, avoiding school, invalidation, playing videogames, staying up past bedtime)? _____

_____

_____

_____

_____

Ways to Increase Behaviors

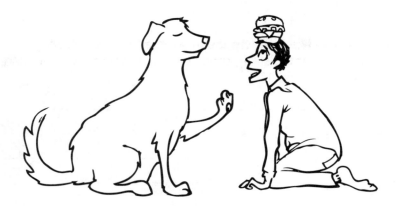

Reinforcers are *consequences* that result in an *increase* in a behavior. They provide information to a person about what you want them to do.

- **Positive reinforcement:** Increases the frequency of a behavior by providing a "rewarding" consequence.(e.g., labeled praise; a genuine compliment; an A on an exam).

   HINT: Timing is very important. Give the reward immediately and choose motivating reinforcers! Don't forget to reinforce yourself!

   Examples: _____

   _____

   _____

- **Negative reinforcement:** Increases the frequency of a behavior by removing something negative; it's *relief* from something unpleasant.

   Examples: Why take an aspirin when you have a headache? It *relieves* the headache and that makes you more likely to take aspirin next time you have a headache (aversive stimulus). Aspirin taking is negatively reinforced.

   If your mom is nagging you, you are more likely to clean your room in order to stop the nagging. If you have intense negative emotions, and a harmful behavior provides temporary relief, you are more likely to repeat the harmful behavior. Remember, you are learning skills to manage this better!

   (continued)

Examples of negative reinforcements that are *not* harmful (e.g., positive ways to soothe yourself, leaving painful situations): _____

_____

_____

- **Shaping:** Reinforcing small steps that lead toward the ultimate goal (e.g., going from *A* to *Z* in 26 steps, each step rewarded).

  Example: A teenager is anxious about going to school and doesn't usually go. She might be encouraged to go for 1 hour on Monday, 2 hours on Tuesday, and so on, until she's able to stay for a whole day, ultimately leading up to staying every day, all week long. Reinforce each step!

Practice Exercise: Positive Reinforcement

Due Date _____

1. Look for opportunities (since they are occurring all of the time) to positively reinforce yourself and someone else. First, simply notice or acknowledge something positive that occurred (positive tracking).

   What is something positive that *you* did this week? _____

   What is something positive that your *family member* did this week? _____

   _____

2. Using a different example, identify a specific behavior you wanted to increase and the reinforcer you used to help increase it. Remember, you can reinforce even a small step in the right direction (shaping)!

   A. For yourself:

      Behavior: _____

      Reinforcer: _____

   B. Someone else: _____

      Behavior: _____

      Reinforcer: _____

3. Describe the situation(s) when you used reinforcement:

   A. For yourself: _____

   B. Someone else: _____

4. What was the outcome? What did you observe?

   A. For yourself: _____

   _____

   _____

   B. Someone else: _____

   _____

   _____

Ways to Decrease or Stop Behaviors

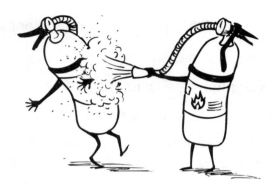

Extinction: Reduces a behavior by *withholding* previous reinforcement. When attention is reinforcing, ignore the unwanted behavior. Make sure you reinforce a desirable replacement behavior.

- If a parent ignores a child's tantrum, the child will eventually stop tantruming.

- Beware of the **behavioral burst,** a temporary increase in the behavior you are trying to extinguish. DON'T GIVE UP or forget to orient the person in whom you are beginning to extinguish a particular behavior!

- Beware of **intermittent reinforcement**: Behavior that is reinforced only occasionally is the hardest behavior to extinguish (e.g., never give candy to stop a tantrum after you've ignored episodes).

Punishment: A *consequence* that results in a *decrease* in behavior. It tells another person what you don't want him or her to do. **Use sparingly because:**

- Punishment does not teach new behavior.

- Punishment can lead to resentment and a feeling of demoralization.

- Punishment may lead to self-punishment.

(continued)

To use punishment effectively:

- First, reinforce desired behaviors to **prevent** undesired ones.

- Communicate **clear rules and expectations.**

- Have a menu of possible punishments ready in advance.

- Pair a negative consequence with **reinforcement of desired behavior**.

- Be specific, time limited, and make the punishment fit the crime (e.g., if you're out past curfew 1 hour, your curfew is 1 hour earlier next time).

- Ask yourself, is **Wise Mind** dictating the consequence?

- Apply the punishing consequence immediately or . . .

- Allow natural consequences (e.g., you failed the test because you stayed up all night and were too tired to focus in school).

Practice Exercise: Extinction and Punishment

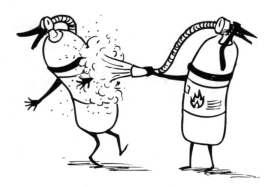

Extinction

Practice ignoring what peers or family members do that is annoying or provocative.

Important Note 1: Don't use with behaviors that are dangerous!

Important Note 2: If provocative behaviors include bullying or pressuring you to do something that goes against your values, ignoring (extinction) might not be enough. You may need to tell a trusted authority figure and ask for help!

Briefly describe the situation and what you ignored. How did it work out? _____

_____

_____

_____

_____

_____

_____

Punishing Consequences: Use Sparingly or as Last Resort

Parents:

List three Wise Mind–based short-term consequences you can apply when other methods of behavior change haven't worked:

1. _____

2. _____

3. _____

EMOTION REGULATION HANDOUTS

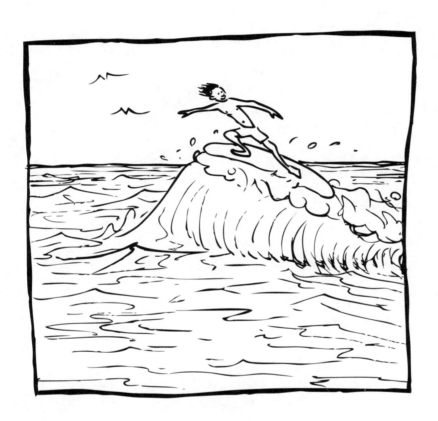

Taking Charge of Your Emotions: Why Bother?

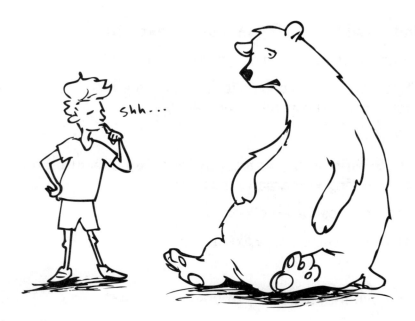

Taking charge of your emotions is important because:

Adolescents often have intense emotions that are difficult to manage, such as anger, shame, depression, or anxiety.

Difficulties controlling these emotions often lead to problematic behaviors that affect you and those around you.

Problematic behaviors are often ineffective solutions to intensely painful emotions.

Goals of Emotion Regulation Skills Training

I. **Understand the emotions that you experience.**

- Identify (observe and describe/name) emotions.
- Know what emotions do for you (are your emotions working for or against you in this moment?).

II. **Reduce emotional vulnerability and stop unwanted emotions from starting in the first place.**

- Increase positive emotions.
- Decrease vulnerability to Emotion Mind.

III. **Decrease the frequency of unwanted emotions.**

IV. **Decrease emotional suffering; stop or reduce unwanted emotions once they start.**

- Let go of painful emotions using *mindfulness*.
- Change emotions through *opposite action*.

Short List of Emotions

LOVE **HATE** *FEAR* **JOY** shame Guilt ANXIETY
loneliness

ANGER Excited FRUSTRATION *sadness* shyness envy
BOREDOM SURPRISE! embarrassed

CONFUSED CURIOUS PRIDE SUSPICIOUS HAPPY

Rage INTEREST DEPRESSED **WORRY** IRRITABLE PANIC

Jealous optimistic hopeless Disgust *hurt*
sympathy DISAPPOINTED Content Calm

Other names for emotions I frequently have:

_____   _____
_____   _____
_____   _____
_____   _____
_____   _____
_____   _____
_____   _____
_____   _____

What Good Are Emotions?

Emotions Give Us Information.

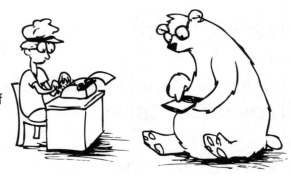

- Emotions provide us with a signal that something is happening (e.g., "I feel nervous standing alone in this dark alley").

- Sometimes our emotions communicate by "gut feeling" or intuition. This can be helpful if our emotions get us to check out the facts.

- It's a problem when we treat emotions as if they are facts about the world. For example: "If I am afraid, there must be a threat," or "I love him, so he must be good for me."

- We need to be mindful that emotions are *not* facts. Therefore, it is important to check the facts about the situation.

Emotions Communicate to, and Influence, Others.

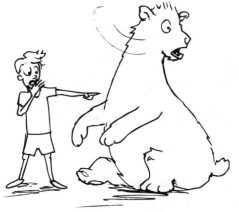

- Facial expressions, body posture, and voice tone say a lot about how you're feeling. They communicate emotions to others (e.g., your sad face may cause someone to ask you if you are OK and to give you support).

- Whether you realize it or not, your emotions—expressed by words, face, or body language—influence how other people respond to you.

Emotions Motivate and Prepare Us for Action.

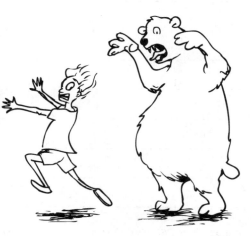

- The action urge connected to specific emotions is often "hardwired." For example, when we hear a loud horn beep suddenly, we startle.

- Emotions save time in getting us to act in important situations. Our nervous system activates us (e.g., we instantly jump out of the way of an oncoming car). We don't have to think everything through.

- Strong emotions can help us overcome obstacles—in our mind and in the environment.

A Model of Emotions

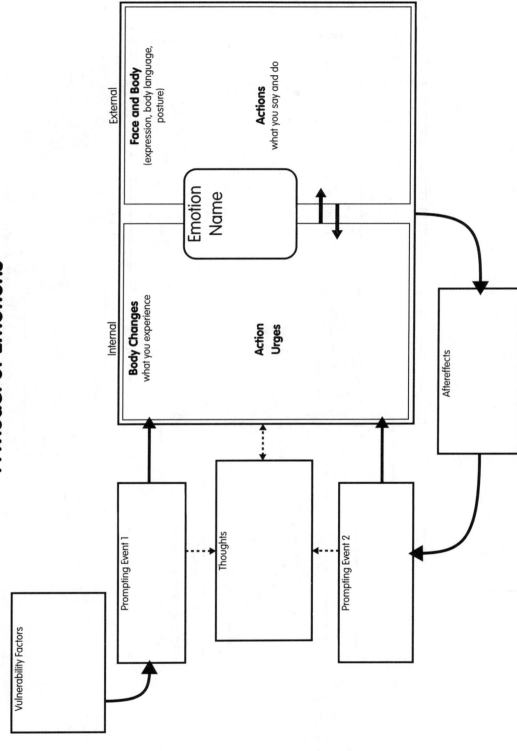

Adapted from *DBT® Skills Training Handouts and Worksheets, Second Edition*. Copyright 2015 by Marsha M. Linehan. Adapted by permission.

A Model of Emotions with Skills

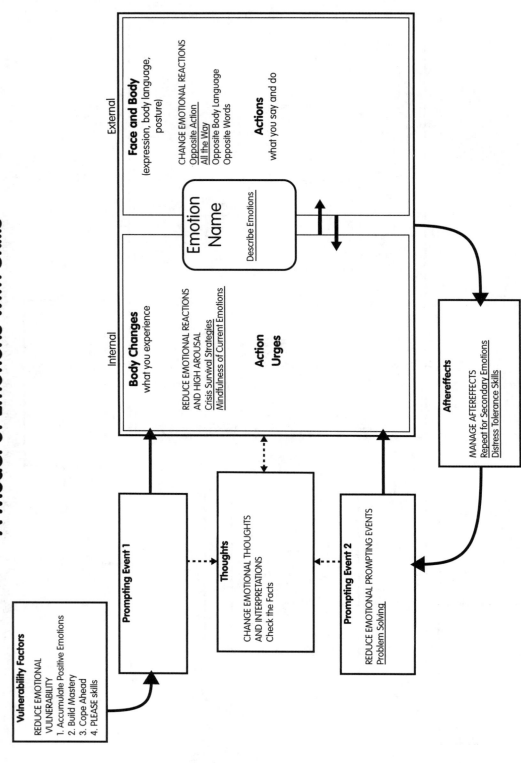

Practice Exercise: Observe and Describe an Emotion

Due Date _____

External

Face and Body Language
What is my facial expression?
Posture? Gestures?

Actions and Words
What I said and did:

Emotion Name
_____
_____
_____
Intensity (0–100)

Internal

Face and Body Change/Sensing
What am I feeling in my body?

Action Urge
What do I feel like doing?
What do I want to say?

Aftereffects (secondary emotions, behavior, thoughts, etc.)

Vulnerability Factors:
What happened before to make me more vulnerable to the prompting event?

Prompting Event:
What triggered the emotion? What happened in the minutes right before the emotion fired? Just the facts!

Thoughts (thoughts, beliefs, assumptions):

Prompting Event 2
What happened next to trigger more emotion firing?

Adapted from *DBT® Skills Training Handouts and Worksheets, Second Edition.* Copyright 2015 by Marsha M. Linehan. Adapted by permission.

ABC PLEASE Overview

How to **increase** positive emotions

and

reduce vulnerability to Emotional Mind

Accumulating positive experiences

Build mastery

Cope ahead of time with emotional situations

Treat **P**hysica**L** illness

Balance **E**ating

Avoid mood-altering drugs

Balance **S**leep

Get **E**xercise

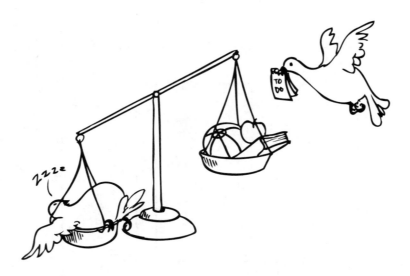

Adapted from *DBT® Skills Training Handouts and Worksheets, Second Edition.* Copyright 2015 by Marsha M. Linehan. Adapted by permission.

ACCUMULATING Positive Experiences—Short Term
(To Build a Dam between You and the Sea of Emotional Dyscontrol)

In the Short Term:

Do pleasant things that are possible right now.

- Increase pleasant activities that lead to positive emotions.

- Do one thing each day from the Pleasant Activities List. Also consider the Parent-Teen Shared Pleasant Activities List.

- Be mindful of positive experiences.

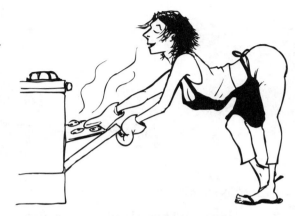

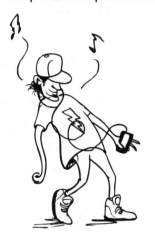

Be Mindful of Positive Experiences:

- Focus your attention on positive events while they are happening.

- Refocus your attention when your mind wanders to the negative.

- Participate fully in the experience.

Be Unmindful of Worries:

- Don't destroy positive experiences by thinking about when they will end.

- Don't think about whether you deserve this positive experience.

- Don't think about how much more might be expected of you now.

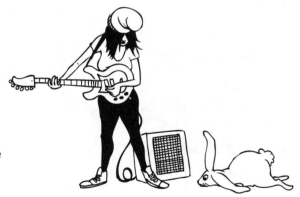

Pleasant Activities List

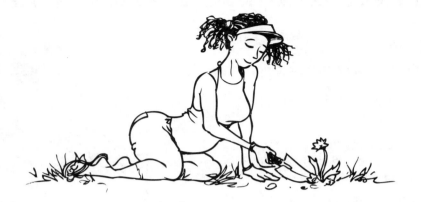

1. Soaking in the bathtub
2. Thinking about how it will be when school ends
3. Going out with friends
4. Relaxing
5. Going to a movie
6. Going running
7. Listening to music
8. Lying in the sun (with sunscreen)
9. Reading
10. Saving money
11. Planning the future
12. Dancing
13. Fixing or cleaning things around the house
14. Having a quiet night
15. Cooking good food
16. Taking care of your pets

17. Going swimming
18. Writing
19. Drawing or doodling
20. Playing sports (list: _____)
21. Going to a party
22. Talking with friends
23. Working out
24. Singing
25. Going ice skating
26. Going to a beach
27. Playing a musical instrument
28. Traveling
29. Making a gift for someone
30. Downloading music or new apps
31. Watching sports on TV

32. Going out to dinner
33. Baking
34. Planning a party for someone
35. Buying clothes
36. Getting a haircut or styling your hair
37. Enjoying a cup of hot chocolate, coffee, or tea
38. Kissing
39. Going to hear live music
40. Getting a manicure or pedicure
41. Spending some time with little kids
42. Going for a bike ride
43. Going sledding in a snowstorm
44. Getting a massage

(continued)

45. E-mailing or texting friends

46. Writing in a diary or journal

47. Looking at photos

48. Dressing up however you like

49. Playing videogames

50. Walking around where you live

51. Noticing birds or trees (something in nature)

52. Surfing the Internet

53. Surprising someone with a favor

54. Completing something you will feel great about

55. Shooting pool or playing ping-pong

56. Contacting a relative with whom you have been out of touch

57. Tweeting, posting online

58. Thinking about taking lessons (sports, dance, music, martial arts)

59. Bowling

60. Fantasizing about life getting better

61. Saying "I love you"

62. Writing a poem, song, or rap

63. Thinking about a friend's good qualities

64. Putting on makeup

65. Making a smoothie and drinking it slowly

66. Putting on your favorite piece of clothing

67. Playing a game

68. Writing a story

69. Instant messaging someone

70. Watching reruns on TV

71. Making a card and giving it to someone you care about

72. Figuring out your favorite scent

73. Buying yourself a little treat

74. Noticing a storm coming

75. Building furniture or carpentry

Add Your Own!

76. _____

_____

77. _____

_____

78. _____

_____

79. _____

_____

80. _____

_____

Parent–Teen Shared Pleasant Activities List

Instructions: Check off the activities on this list that you would enjoy doing with your parent/teen. Then compare lists (or fill this out together) and select a few activities that you can enjoy together—aim for at least 3 per week.

*Also, remember to respect each other's need for privacy and alone time.

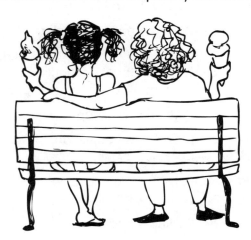

1. Going bicycling

2. Going for coffee

3. Going out for ice cream/yogurt

4. Cooking or baking

5. Getting a manicure

6. Going for a massage

7. Walking by the beach

8. Planning a vacation

9. Going shopping

10. Watching a ballgame

11. Doing yard work/gardening

12. Playing with pets, walking the dog

13. Bowling

14. Playing golf

15. Going for a drive

16. Fixing up part of your home

17. Doing a crossword puzzle

18. Skiing, ice skating

19. Having some quiet reading time together

20. Going to a café/out to eat

21. Going to an amusement park

22. Going to a museum

23. Playing catch

24. Having a barbecue

25. Going camping

26. Listening to music you both like

27. Going to a show, game, or concert

28. Watching a favorite TV show or movie together

29. Going for a walk/run

30. Getting your hair or makeup done together

31. Talking about when you were little

32. Visiting relatives or friends together

(continued)

33. Doing community service/volunteer work

34. Shopping for a gift

35. Talking about your day

36. Playing videogames

37. Playing board games or cards

38. Looking thru photos

39. Going to a park

40. Working out/going to the gym

41. Take a yoga/exercise class

42. Playing music/jamming together

43. Talking about future plans together

44. Planning a surprise for someone

45. Joking around/being silly

46. Doing a creative hobby together (e.g., painting, drawing, knitting, scrapbooking, model building)

47. Taking an art class

48. Looking at/showing your favorite website

49. Teaching the other one something new (e.g., in technology, photography)

50. Telling family stories

Add Your Own!

51. _____

_____

52. _____

_____

53. _____

_____

54. _____

_____

55. _____

_____

ACCUMULATING Positive Experiences—Long Term
(To Build a Life Worth Living)

In the Long Term:

Make changes in your life so that positive events will occur more often. Build a life worth living. Check "Wise Mind" Values and Priorities List.

Work toward goals based on your values:
- Identify *one* goal (e.g., graduate from high school).
- List small steps toward goals (e.g., get out of bed, go to first class).
- Take first step (e.g., buy an alarm clock or set cell phone alarm).

1. Goal: _____

   _____

2. Some steps toward my goal: _____

   _____

   _____

   _____

3. What's a simple first step I can take? _____

   _____

Pay attention to relationships:
- Repair old, create new, work on current relationships, and end destructive relationships.

What can I do this week to work on a relationship? _____

_____

Avoid avoiding:
- Avoiding makes problems build up and increases vulnerability to Emotion Mind. Return that call, schedule that doctor's appointment, face that work, discuss that problem.
- Avoid giving up.

What have I been avoiding? _____

_____

Wise Mind Values and Priorities List

Mark the items that are important to you:

- **Contribute** (e.g., be generous, help people in need, make sacrifices for others, volunteer, service to society).

- **Attend to relationships** (e.g., build new relationships, work on current relationships, repair old relationships, end destructive relationships, treat others well).

- **Be part of a group** (e.g., be social, have close friends, have people to do things with, feel sense of belonging).

- **Build character** (e.g., have integrity, be honest, be loyal, stand up for my beliefs, keep my word, be respectful, be courageous in facing and living life, keep growing as a human being).

- **Be responsible** (e.g., get my work done, earn money, take care of myself more and more, be reliable).

- **Achieve things** (e.g., get good grades, work hard, be financially secure).

- **Learn** (e.g., seek knowledge and information, read, study).

- **Have fun** (e.g., enjoy what I do, laugh, go out and have a good time, relax).

- **Focus on family** (e.g., see family often, keep family relationships strong, do things for family, respect family traditions).

- **Be a leader** (e.g., be seen by others as successful; be in charge of something like a club, team, or committee; be respected by others; be accepted).

- **Be healthy** (e.g., be physically fit, exercise, eat and sleep well, see my doctors when needed, practice yoga).

- **Strive for moderation** (e.g., avoid excesses and achieve balance).

- Other _____

  _____

Practice Exercise: ACCUMULATING Positive Experiences in the Short and Long Term

Due Date _____

In the short term:

1. Engage in at least one activity from your list each day. Also consider the Parent–Teen Shared Pleasant Activities List. Please write down each activity on the list below. Add more rows if you need them.

2. Rate your mood *before* you start the activity and then *after.* Use rating scale below.

3. Remember to try to *stay mindful* of activity and unmindful of worries.

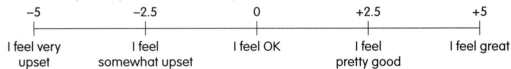

–5	–2.5	0	+2.5	+5
I feel very upset	I feel somewhat upset	I feel OK	I feel pretty good	I feel great

Date:						
Monday	Tuesday	Wednesday	Thursday	Friday	Saturday	Sunday
/	/	/	/	/	/	/
/	/	/	/	/	/	/

4. Were you mindfully participating in each activity? If yes, describe the effect on your emotional state. If no, what happened?

_____

_____

In the long term:

1. List your **goal** and a **value** with which it is associated: _____

_____

2. What is the first step in achieving your goal? _____

_____

3. Take the first step. Describe how taking the first step made you feel? _____

_____

Building Mastery and Coping Ahead

Build Mastery

1. Do at least one thing each day to feel competent and in control of your life. The idea is to challenge yourself a little, get better at something, or cross something off your "to-do" list. Examples: Put together a piece of furniture, practice your instrument, get one HW assignment done, start a project.

   Example: _____

2. Plan for success, not failure.
   - Do something difficult, *but* possible.

3. Gradually increase the difficulty over time.
   - If the first task is too difficult, do something a little easier next time.

Cope Ahead of Time with Emotional Situations
Rehearse a plan ahead of time so that you are prepared when there is a threat.

1. **Describe** a situation that is likely to create negative emotions.
   - Be specific in describing the situation. **Check the facts!**
   - Name the emotions you are likely to experience in the situation.

2. **Decide** what DBT skills (including **problem-solving)** you want to use in the situation.
   - Be specific. Write them out: _____

3. **Imagine the situation** in your mind as vividly as possible.
   - Imagine yourself *in* the situation *now*.

4. **Rehearse coping effectively in your mind**.
   - Rehearse exactly what you could do to cope effectively in your mind.
   - Rehearse your actions, your thoughts, what you say, and how to say it.
   - *Troubleshoot*: Rehearse coping with problems that might arise.

PLEASE Skills

Treat **P**hysica**L** illness: Take care of your body. See a doctor when necessary. Take medications as prescribed.

Balance **E**ating: Don't eat too much or too little. Stay away from foods that may make you overly emotional.

Avoid mood-altering drugs: Stay off nonprescribed drugs such as marijuana, other street drugs, and alcohol.

Balance **S**leep: Try to get the amount of sleep that helps you feel rested. Stay on a regular schedule in order to develop good sleep habits.

Get **E**xercise: Do some sort of exercise every day, including walking. Start small and build on it!

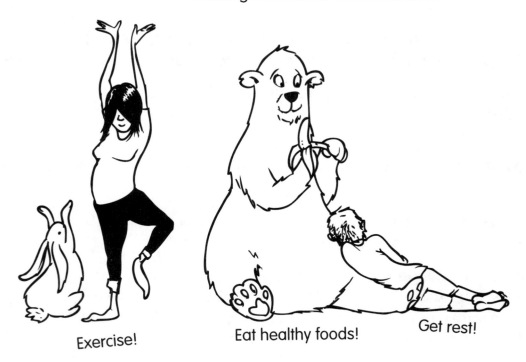

Exercise!   Eat healthy foods!   Get rest!

FOOD and Your MOOD

Step 1: Observe how certain foods affect your mood (both negatively and positively).

Negative examples:

- Soda and sugary snacks might make you feel tired and irritable.
- Heavy, fatty foods (e.g., french fries, potato chips, fried chicken, greasy foods) might make you feel sluggish.
- Caffeine might make you feel jittery and more anxious and interfere with your sleep.

Positive examples:

- Complex carbohydrates and fiber (e.g., sweet potatoes, whole wheat pasta, oatmeal, whole-grain cereals, salads) give you slow and steady energy.
- Proteins (e.g., lean meats and poultry, beans, nuts, fish, eggs) also provide your body with steady energy that helps you stay active and strong both physically and mentally.
- Dairy foods (e.g., low-fat milks, cheeses, yogurts) have protein and calcium, which help with energy and bone strength.
- Fruits and vegetables provide you energy, boost your health, and give you a sweet or crunchy treat without zapping your energy or making you feel guilty.
- Once you know what foods make up a balanced diet, you can determine what changes might be needed.

Step 2: Notice whether you are eating too much or too little.

Step 3: Start thinking about changes.

How can you begin to increase the amount of healthy foods you eat? Keep track of your food choices in a food diary every day so you see your progress!

(continued)

Step 4: Start small.

Don't try to make dramatic changes to your diet all at once. You may feel overwhelmed, which might set yourself up to fail. Start slowly and gradually to change your habits.

For example:

- Cut down on processed foods and add more fresh foods.
- Add more fruits and vegetables to meals and have them for snacks.
- Add lettuce, tomato, cucumber, and onion to sandwiches.
- Add fruit to cereal.

Step 5: Notice the effects of eating well on your mood.

BEST Ways to Get REST: 12 Tips for Better Sleep

Maintaining a balanced sleep pattern will decrease your emotional vulnerability.

1. **Stick to a schedule** and don't sleep late on weekends. If you sleep late on Saturday and Sunday morning, you will disrupt your sleep pattern. Instead, go to bed and get up at about the same time every day.

2. **Establish a bedtime routine**. This might include shutting off screens (TV, computer, cell phone), changing into comfy PJs, sipping herbal tea, lowering bright lights and reducing noise, and reading.

3. **Don't eat or drink a lot before bed**. Eat a light dinner at least 2 hours before sleeping. If you drink too many liquids before bed, you'll wake up repeatedly for trips to the bathroom. Watch out for spicy foods, which may cause heartburn and interfere with sleep.

4. **Avoid caffeine and nicotine**. Both are stimulants and can keep you awake. Caffeine should be avoided for 8 hours before your desired bedtime.

5. **Exercise**. If you're trying to sleep better, the best time to exercise is in the morning or afternoon. A program of regular physical activity enhances the quality of your sleep.

6. **Keep your room cool**. Turn the temperature in the room down, as this mimics the natural drop in your body's temperature during sleep. Use an air conditioner or a fan to keep the room cool. If you get cold, add more layers. If you are hot, remove some layers.

7. **Sleep primarily at night**. Daytime naps steal hours from your nighttime sleep. Limit daytime sleep to less than 1 hour, no later than 3:00 P.M.

8. **Keep it dark, quiet, and NO SCREENS**. Use shades, blinds, and turn off lights. Silence helps you sleep better. Turn off the radio and TV. Use earplugs. Use a fan, a white noise machine, or some other source of constant, soothing, background noise to mask sounds you can't control. No laptops, iPads, phones, or screens for at least 1 hour before bedtime.

(continued)

9. **Use your bed only for sleep**. Make your bed comfortable and appealing. Use only for sleep—not for studying or watching TV. Go to bed when you feel tired and turn out the lights. If you don't fall asleep in 30 minutes, get up and do something else relaxing like reading books or magazines—NO SCREENS! Go back to bed when you are tired. Don't stress out! This will make it harder to fall asleep.

10. **Soak and sack out**. Taking a hot shower or bath before bed helps relax tense muscles.

11. **Don't rely on sleeping pills**. If they are prescribed to you, use them only under a doctor's close supervision. Make sure the pills won't interact with other medications!

12. **Don't catastrophize.** Tell yourself "It's OK; I'll fall asleep eventually."

Practice Exercise:
Build Mastery, Cope Ahead, and PLEASE Skills

Due Date _____

Building Mastery:

List two ways that you built mastery this week.

1. _____

2. _____

Coping Ahead of Time with Emotional Situations:

Describe your plan to effectively manage a future emotional situation. Include skills you will use.

_____

_____

_____

_____

Check off two PLEASE Skills to practice during the week:

_____ Treat **P**hysica**L** illness

_____ Balance **E**ating

_____ **A**void mood-altering drugs

_____ Balance **S**leep

_____ Get **E**xercise

Describe specifically what you did to practice your PLEASE Skills. _____

_____

_____

_____

Did you notice a difference in your mood? _____

_____

_____

The Wave Skill: Mindfulness of Current Emotions

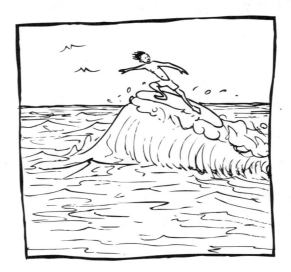

EXPERIENCE YOUR EMOTION

- Observe your feeling.
- Step back and just notice it.
- Get unstuck.
- Experience it as a WAVE, coming and going.
- Don't try to GET RID of it or PUSH it away.
- And don't try to HOLD ON to it.

PRACTICE MINDFULNESS OF EMOTIONAL BODY SENSATIONS

- Notice WHERE in your body you are feeling emotional sensations.
- Experience the SENSATIONS as fully as you can.

REMEMBER: YOU ARE NOT YOUR EMOTION

- You don't need to ACT on the feeling.
- Remember times when you have felt differently.

DON'T JUDGE YOUR EMOTION

- Radically accept it as part of you.
- Invite it home for dinner; name the emotion.
- Practice *willingness* to experience the emotion.

Check the Facts and Problem Solving

These two skills can be used as part of Cope Ahead, or as independent emotion regulation skills to help reduce/change intense emotions regarding situations that have already occurred or are ongoing.

1. DESCRIBE the problem situation.

2. CHECK THE FACTS! (Check all the facts; sort them from interpretations.)
   a. Are you interpreting the situation correctly? Are there other possible interpretations?
   b. Are you thinking in extremes (all-or-nothing, catastrophic thinking?)
   c. What is the probability of the worst happening?
   d. Even if the worst were to happen, could you imagine coping well with it?
   e. If you are still faced with a big problem, then start the steps below.

3. IDENTIFY your GOAL in solving the problem.
   a. Identify what needs to happen or change for you to feel OK.
   b. Keep it simple; keep it something that can actually happen.

4. BRAINSTORM lots of solutions.
   a. Think of as many solutions as you can. Ask for suggestions from people you trust.
   b. Do not be critical of any ideas at first (wait for Step 5 to evaluate ideas).

5. CHOOSE a solution that is likely to work.
   a. If unsure, choose two or three solutions that look good.
   b. Do pros and cons to compare the solutions. Choose the best to try first.

6. Put the solution into ACTION.
   a. ACT: Try out the solution.
   b. Take the first step, and then the second . . .

7. EVALUATE outcomes.
   a. Did it work? YEAH! Reward yourself!
   b. It didn't work? Reward yourself for trying and DON'T GIVE UP!
   c. Try a new solution.

Adapted from *DBT® Skills Training Handouts and Worksheets, Second Edition.* Copyright 2015 by Marsha M. Linehan. Adapted by permission.

Opposite Action to Change Emotions

Emotions come with specific ACTION URGES that push us to act in certain ways.

Often we escape the pain of the emotion in harmful ways.

These are common URGES associated with a sample of emotions:

FEAR   → Escaping or avoiding

ANGER   → Attacking

SADNESS   → Withdrawing, becoming passive, isolating

SHAME   → Hiding, avoiding, withdrawing, saving face by attacking others

GUILT   → Overpromise that you will not commit the offense again, disclaim all responsibility, hiding, lowering head, begging forgiveness

JEALOUSY → Verbal accusations, attempt to control, acting suspicious

LOVE   → Saying "I love you," making effort to spend time with the person, doing what the other person wants and needs, and giving affection

ACTING OPPOSITE = act opposite to the action urge when the emotion is doing more harm than good (see Emotion Regulation Handout 4, "What Good Are Emotions?").

EMOTION---------**OPPOSITE ACTION**

Fear/Anxiety------APPROACH
- Approach events, places, tasks, activities, people you are afraid of, over and over; confront.
- Do things to increase a sense of control and mastery over fears.

Anger-----------GENTLY AVOID
- Gently avoid the person you are angry with (rather than attacking).
- Take a time out and breathe in and out deeply and slowly.
- Be kind rather than mean or attacking. (Try to have sympathy or empathy for the other person.)

Sadness---------GET ACTIVE
- Approach, don't avoid.
- Build mastery and increase pleasant activities.

(continued)

EMOTION- - - - - - - - -**OPPOSITE ACTION**

Shame- - - - - - - - - -**FACE THE MUSIC** (when your behavior violates your moral values or something shameful has been revealed about you and the shame fits the facts):

- Apologize and repair the harm when possible.
- Try to avoid making same mistake in the future and accept consequences.
- Forgive yourself and let it go.

GO PUBLIC (when your behavior DOES NOT violate your moral values and the shame does NOT fit the facts):

- You continue to participate fully in social interactions, hold your head high, keep your voice steady, and make eye contact.
- Go public with your personal characteristics or your behavior (with people who won't reject you).
- Repeat the behavior that sets off shame over and over (without hiding it from those who won't reject you).

Guilt- - - - - - - - - - - -**FACE THE MUSIC** (when your behavior violates your moral values, hurts feelings of significant others, and the guilt fits the facts):

- Experience the guilt.
- You ask, but don't beg, for forgiveness and accept the consequences.
- You repair the transgression and work to prevent it from happening again.

DON'T APOLOGIZE OR TRY TO MAKE UP FOR IT (when your behavior DOES NOT violate your moral values and the guilt does NOT fit the facts):

- Change your body posture, look innocent and proud, head up, puff up your chest, maintain eye contact, keep voice steady and clear.

Jealousy- - - - - - - - -**LET GO OF CONTROLLING OTHERS' ACTIONS** (when it does not fit the facts or is not effective):

- Stop spying or snooping.
- Relax your face and body.

Love- - - - - - - - - - - - -**STOP EXPRESSING LOVE** (when it does not fit the facts or is not effective, e.g., the relationship is truly over, not accessible, or abusive):

- Avoid the person and distract yourself from thoughts of the person.
- Remind yourself of why love is not justified and rehearse the "cons" of loving this person.
- Avoid contact with things that remind you of the person (e.g., pictures).

(continued)

OPPOSITE ACTION WORKS BEST WHEN:

1. **The emotion does NOT FIT THE FACTS.**
   - An emotion does ***not fit the facts*** when:
     o The emotion does *not fit the facts* of the actual situation (e.g., terror in response to speaking in public)

or

     o The emotion, its intensity, or its duration are *not effective* for your goals in the situation (e.g., you feel angry at your math teacher, but three periods later you're still fuming and can't focus on science).

2. **The opposite action is done ALL THE WAY.**
   - Opposite behavior
   - Opposite words and thinking
   - Opposite facial expression, voice tone, and posture

OPPOSITE ACTION REQUIRES THESE seven STEPS:

1. Figure out the emotion you are feeling.

2. What is the action URGE that goes with the emotion?

3. Ask yourself: Does the emotion fit the facts in the situation? If yes, will acting on the emotion's urge be effective?

4. Ask yourself: Do I want to change the emotion?

5. If yes, figure out the OPPOSITE ACTION.

6. Do the opposite action—ALL THE WAY!

7. Repeat acting in the opposite way until the emotion goes down enough for you to notice.

Practice Exercise: Opposite Action

Due Date _____

Ask yourself the following questions as a guide to OPPOSITE ACTION:

Observe and **Describe** the emotion.

What is the current emotion you want to change?

What is your action urge?

Do the opposite action ALL THE WAY.

How did you feel after acting opposite to your emotion?

Adapted from *DBT® Skills Training Handouts and Worksheets, Second Edition.* Copyright 2015 by Marsha M. Linehan. Adapted by permission.

INTERPERSONAL EFFECTIVENESS HANDOUTS

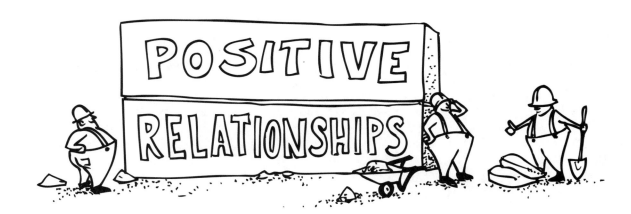

What Is Your Goal and Priority?

Keeping and maintaining healthy relationships (GIVE Skills)

Question: How do I want the other person to feel about me?

Example: If I care about the person or if the person has authority over me, act in a way that keeps the person respecting and liking me.

Getting somebody to do what you want (DEAR MAN Skills)

Question: What do I want? What do I need? How do I get it? How do I effectively say "no"?

Example: How do I ask for something, resolve a problem, or have people take me seriously?

Maintaining Your Self-Respect (FAST Skills)

Question: How do I want to feel about myself after the interaction?

Example: What are my values? Act in a way that makes me feel positive about myself.

What Stops You from Achieving Your Goals?

I. Lack of skill

You actually *don't know* what to say or how to act.

II. Worry thoughts

You have the skill, but your worry thoughts interfere with your doing or saying what you want.

- Worries about bad consequences:
  - "They won't like me"; "He will break up with me."
- Worries about whether you deserve to get what you want:
  - "I'm such a bad person, I don't deserve this."
- Worries about being ineffective and calling yourself names:
  - "I won't do it right"; "I'm such a loser."

III. Emotions

You have the skill, but your emotions (anger, fear, shame, sadness) make you unable to do or say what you want. Emotion Mind, instead of skills, controls what you say and do.

IV. Can't decide

You have the skills, but you *can't decide* what you really want: asking for too much versus not asking for anything; saying "no" to everything versus giving in to everything.

V. Environment

You have the skill, but the environment gets in the way:

- Other people are too powerful (sometimes despite your best efforts).
- Other people may have some reason for not liking you if you get what you want.
- Other people won't give you what you need unless you sacrifice your self-respect.

Building and Maintaining Positive Relationships: GIVE Skills

Remember **GIVE**:

(be) **G**entle

(act) **I**nterested

Validate

(use an) **E**asy manner

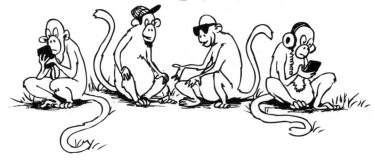

(be) **G**entle:	Be nice and respectful! Don't attack, use threats, or cast judgments. Be aware of your tone of voice.
(act) **I**nterested:	LISTEN and act interested in what the other person is saying. Don't interrupt or talk over him or her. Don't make faces. Maintain good eye contact.

Validate:	Show that you understand the other person's feelings or opinions.
	Be nonjudgmental out loud.
	    "I can understand how you feel *and* . . ."
	    "I realize this is hard . . ."
	    "I see you are busy, *and* . . ."
	    "That must have felt . . ."

(use an) **E**asy manner:	SMILE. Use humor. Use nonthreatening body language. Leave your attitude at the door.

Practice Exercise: GIVE Skills

Due Date _____

Choose two situations during the week in which you used your GIVE skills and describe how.

Remember **GIVE . . .**

(be) **G**entle

(act) **I**nterested

Validate

(use an) **E**asy manner

SITUATION 1:

With whom are you trying to keep a good relationship? _____

What was the situation in which you chose to use your GIVE skills? _____

_____

_____

What was the outcome? _____

_____

How did you feel after using your skills? _____

_____

SITUATION 2:

With whom are you trying to keep a good relationship? _____

What was the situation in which you chose to use your GIVE skills? _____

_____

_____

What was the outcome? _____

_____

How did you feel after using your skills? _____

_____

Getting Someone to Do What You Want: DEAR MAN Skills

Remember **DEAR MAN:**

Describe	**M**indful
Express	**A**ppear Confident
Assert	**N**egotiate
Reinforce	

Describe: Describe the situation. Stick to the facts. "The last three weekends, I have noticed you coming home after curfew."

Express: Express your feelings using "I" statements ("I feel . . .," "I would like . . ."). Stay away from "you should . . ."; instead, say, "When you come home late, *I feel* worried about you."

Assert: Ask for what you want or say "no" clearly. Remember, the other person cannot read your mind. "*I would like* you to come home by curfew."

Reinforce: Reward (reinforce) the person ahead of time by explaining the positive effects of getting what you want. "I would be able to trust you more and give you more privileges if you stuck to our curfew agreement."

Mindful: Keep your focus on what you want, avoiding distractions. Come back to your assertion over and over, like a "broken record." Ignore attacks. "I know the other kids stay out later than you, *and* I would still like you to do your best to meet your curfew."

Appear Confident: Make (and maintain) eye contact. Use a confident tone of voice—do not whisper, mumble, or give up and say "Whatever."

Negotiate: Be willing to **GIVE TO GET**. Ask for the other person's input. Offer alternative solutions to the problem. Know when to "agree to disagree" and walk away. "If you can do this for the next 2 weeks, then I will feel comfortable letting you stay out later for the party."

Adapted from *DBT® Skills Training Handouts and Worksheets, Second Edition.* Copyright 2015 by Marsha M. Linehan. Adapted by permission.

Practice Exercise: DEAR MAN Skills

Due Date _____

Choose one situation during the week in which you used your DEAR MAN skills and describe below.

What happened? (Who did what? What led up to what? What is the problem?) _____

_____

_____

_____

What did you want (e.g., asking for something, saying "no," being taken seriously)?

Be specific: _____

_____

_____

DEAR MAN Skills used (write down _exactly_ how you used each one):

<u>D</u>escribe (describe the situation; just the facts): _____

_____

<u>E</u>xpress (feelings): _____

<u>A</u>ssert: _____

<u>R</u>eward: _____

<u>M</u>indful: _____

<u>A</u>ppear confident: _____

<u>N</u>egotiate: _____

What was the result of using your DEAR MAN skills? _____

_____

_____

_____

Maintaining Your Self-Respect: FAST Skills

Remember **FAST:**

(be) **F**air
(no) **A**pologies
    Stick to values
(be) **T**ruthful

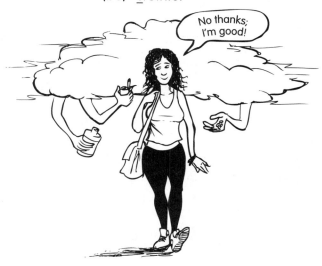

(be)	**F**air:	Be fair to *yourself* and to the *other* person.
(no)	**A**pologies:	Don't *over*apologize for your behavior, for making a request, or for being you.
		(If you wronged someone, don't underapologize.)
	Stick to values:	Stick to your own values and opinions.
		Don't sell out to get what you want, to fit in, or to avoid saying "no."
		(Refer to Emotion Regulation Handout 13, "Wise Mind Values and Priorities List.")
(be)	**T**ruthful:	Don't lie.
		Don't act helpless when you are not.
		Don't make up excuses or exaggerate.

Worry Thoughts and Wise Mind Self-Statements

Turn negative thoughts into realistic ones.

1. Why bother asking? It won't make a difference anyway.

   WISE MIND STATEMENT: _____

2. If I ask for something, she'll think I'm stupid.

   WISE MIND STATEMENT: _____

3. I can't take it if he's [she's] upset with me.

   WISE MIND STATEMENT: _____

4. If I say "no," they won't like me or want to hang out with me anymore.

   WISE MIND STATEMENT: _____

5. If I say "no," they'll be really angry at me.

   WISE MIND STATEMENT: _____

6. If I make a request or ask for help, I will look weak.

   WISE MIND STATEMENT: _____

Examples of Wise Mind Self-Statements:

1. "Just because I didn't get what I wanted last time does not mean that if I ask skillfully this time that I won't get it."
2. "I can handle it if I don't get what I want or need."
3. "It takes a strong person to admit that he [she] needs help from someone else and then ask for it."
4. "If I say 'no' to people and they get angry, it doesn't mean I should have said 'yes.'"
5. "I can deal with it if he [she] is annoyed with me."

Others? _____

_____

_____

_____

Practice Exercise: FAST Skills

Due Date _____

Choose two situations during the week in which you used your FAST skills and describe below.

Remember **FAST** . . .

        (be) **F**air
        (no) **A**pologies
              Stick to values
        (be) **T**ruthful

SITUATION 1:

In what way are you trying to maintain your self-respect? _____

_____

What was the situation in which you chose to use your FAST skills and how did you use them? _____

_____

What was the outcome? _____

_____

How did you feel after you used your skills? _____

SITUATION 2:

In what way are you trying to maintain your self-respect? _____

_____

What was the situation in which you chose to use your FAST skills and how did you use them? _____

_____

What was the outcome? _____

_____

How did you feel after you used your skills? _____

Factors to Consider in Asking for What You Want
(or Saying "No" to an Unwanted Request)

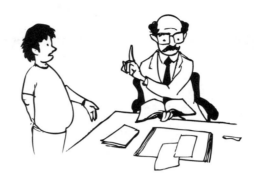

1. Priorities: Objectives very important? (Is it important to get what I want?)

Relationship shaky? On good terms?

Self-respect on the line?

2. Capability: Is the person able to give me what I want? (Or do I have what the person wants?)

3. Timeliness: Is this a good time to ask? Is the person in the mood to listen or able to pay attention to me? (Is this a bad time to say "no"?)

4. Preparation: Do I know all the facts I need to know? Am I clear about what I want? (Am I clear on the facts that I am using to explain why I am saying "no"?)

5. Relationship: Is what I want appropriate to the current relationship? (Is what the person is asking me appropriate to our current relationship?)

6. Give and take: Has the other person helped me in the past? Have I overused his [her] help? (Have I helped the other person in the past? Has he [she] overused my help?)

Which of the above do you need to pay more attention to? _____

_____

_____

Practice Exercise:
Factors to Consider in Asking or Saying "No"

Due Date _____

Choose a situation during the week in which it was hard to determine whether to ask for something or to say "no," or how *strong* your request or your "no" should be.

Did you consider each of the factors below? Check off which ones applied. If the factor applied, what was the circumstance, and did considering it lead you to still ask for what you wanted or say "no" to what someone else wanted? Did it make your request or your "no" stronger or weaker?

✓		**Describe Circumstance**
_____	**Priorities**	_____
		_____
_____	**Capability**	_____
		_____
_____	**Timeliness**	_____
		_____
_____	**Preparation**	_____
		_____
_____	**Relationship**	_____
		_____
_____	**Give and take**	_____
		_____

So, what did you decide to do, and how did it work out? _____

_____

_____

_____

Practice Exercise: Using Skills at the Same Time

Due Date _____

Choose a situation during the week that required more than one interpersonal effectiveness skill.

Describe situation: _____

_____

_____

What were my priorities? (Check all that apply.)

_____ Build/maintain relationship

_____ Get what I want, say "no," or be taken seriously

_____ Build/maintain self-respect

What I said or did and how I did so (check and describe):

_____Gentle	_____Describe	_____Fair
_____Interested	_____Express	_____No apologies
_____Validate	_____Assert	_____Stick to values
_____Easy manner	_____Reinforce	_____Truthful
	_____Mindful	
	_____Appear confident	
	_____Negotiate	

_____

_____

_____

_____

THINK Skills

When you want to make peace, reduce conflict, and reduce anger, **THINK** about it differently.

We often make interpretations or assumptions about others that fuel our Emotion Minds and can make the situation worse. So . . .

What's the situation? _____

_____

_____

How are your interpretations about the other person fueling your Emotion Mind? __

_____

_____

Now try these steps to THINK about it differently:

Think . . .   about it from the other person's perspective.

Have empathy   What might he or she be feeling or thinking?

Interpretations Can you think of more than one possible interpretation or explanation for the other's behavior? List other possible reasons for the behavior; come up with at least *one benign reason*:

        _____   _____

        _____   _____

        _____   _____

Notice . . .   ways the other person has been trying to make things better, to help, or to show he or she cares. Or, notice how the other person may be struggling with his or her own stress or problems.

Use **K**indness   Can you use kindness and be gentle when you approach the other person?

Practice Exercise: THINK Skills

THINK about it differently:

With whom did you want to make peace/reduce conflict/reduce anger? _____

Briefly, what was the situation? _____

_____

How were your interpretations or assumptions about the other person fueling your Emotion Mind or making things worse? _____

Indicate which steps you used and HOW you used them to THINK about it differently:

<u>T</u>hink about it from the other person's perspective—what was his or her perspective?

_____

_____

<u>H</u>ave empathy—what might he or she have been feeling or thinking? _____

_____

<u>I</u>nterpretations—were you able to think of more than one possible interpretation or explanation for the other's behavior? List other possible reasons for the behavior; did you come up with at least *one benign reason*?

_____   _____

_____   _____

_____   _____

<u>N</u>otice: What are ways the other person had been trying to make things better, to help, or to show he or she cared? _____

_____

Or, how was the other person struggling with his or her own stress or problems? _____

_____

Did you use <u>**K**indness</u> and were you gentle when you approached the other person? _____

_____

What was the outcome? _____

_____

_____

References

Albers, S. (2003). *Eating mindfully: How to end mindless eating and enjoy a balanced relationship with food*. Oakland, CA: New Harbinger.

Arnett, J. J. (1999). Adolescent storm and stress, reconsidered. *American Psychologist, 54*(5), 317–326.

Barkley, R. A., Edwards, G. H., & Robins, A. L. (1999). *Defiant teens: A clinician's manual for assessment and family intervention*. New York: Guilford Press.

Barley, W. D., Buie, S. E., Peterson, E. W., Hollingsworth, A. S., Griva, M., Hickerson, S. C., et al. (1993). Development of an inpatient cognitive-behavioral treatment program for borderline personality disorder. *Journal of Personality Disorders, 7*(3), 232–240.

Baumrind, D. (1991). The influence of parenting style on adolescent competence and substance use. *Journal of Early Adolescence, 11*(1), 56–95.

Berk, L. E. (2000). *Child development* (5th ed.). Boston: Allyn & Bacon.

Berzins, L. G., & Trestman, R. L. (2004). The development and implementation of dialectical behavior therapy in forensic settings. *International Journal of Forensic Mental Health, 3*(1), 93–103.

Birmaher, B., Brent, D. A., Kolko, D., Baugher, M., Bridge, J., Holder, D., et al. (2000). Clinical outcome after short-term psychotherapy for adolescents with major depressive disorder. *Archives of General Psychiatry, 57*(1), 29.

Bohus, M., Haaf, B., & Simms, T. (2004). Effectiveness of inpatient dialectical behavior therapy for borderline personality disorder: A controlled trial. *Behaviour Research and Therapy, 42*, 487–499.

Bohus, M., Haaf, B., Stiglmayr, C., Pohl, U., Bohme, R., & Linehan, M. (2000). Evaluation of inpatient dialectical-behavioral therapy for borderline personality disorder: A prospective study. *Behaviour Research and Therapy, 38*, 875–887.

Bradley, R. G., & Follingstad, D. R. (2003). Group therapy for incarcerated women who experienced interpersonal violence: A pilot study. *Journal of Traumatic Stress, 16*(4), 337–340.

Brent, D. A., Baugher, M., Bridge, J., Chen, T., & Chiappetta, L. (1999). Age- and sex-related risk factors for adolescent suicide. *Journal of the American Academy of Child and Adolescent Psychiatry, 38*(12), 1497–1505.

Brown, B. B. (1990). Peer groups and peer cultures. In S. S. Feldman & G. R. Elliott (Eds.), *At the threshold* (pp. 171–196). Cambridge, MA: Harvard University Press.

Brown, M. (2012, November). *Enhancing emotional regulation with resonance frequency paced breathing training.* Paper presented at the annual meeting of the International Society for the Improvement and Training of DBT, National Harbor, MD.

Cooney, E., Davis, K., Thompson, P., Wharewera-Mika, J., Stewart, J., & Miller, A. L. (2012, November). *Feasibility of comparing dialectical behavior therapy with treatment as usual for suicidal & self-injuring adolescents: Follow-up data from a small randomized controlled trial.* Paper presented at the annual meeting of the Association of Behavioral and Cognitive Therapies, National Harbor, MD.

Crick, N. R., & Dodge, K. A. (1994). A review and reformulation of social information-processing mechanisms in children's social adjustment. *Psychological Bulletin, 115,* 74–101.

Dishion, T. J., McCord, J., & Poulin, F. (1999). When interventions harm: Peer groups and problem behavior. *American Psychologist, 54,* 755–764.

Epstein, L. J., & Mardon, S. (2006). *The Harvard Medical School guide to a good night's sleep.* New York: McGraw-Hill.

Evershed, S., Tennant, A., Boomer, D., Rees, A., Barkham, M., & Watson, A. (2003). Practice-based outcomes of dialectical behaviour therapy (DBT) targeting anger and violence, with male forensic patients: A pragmatic and non-contemporaneous comparison. *Criminal Behaviour and Mental Health, 13*(3), 198–213.

Fleischhaker, C., Munz, M., Böhme, R., Sixt, B., & Schulz, E. (2006). Dialectical behaviour therapy for adolescents (DBT-A): A pilot study on the therapy of suicidal, parasuicidal, and self-injurious behaviour in female patients with a borderline disorder. *Zeitschrift fur Kinder-und Jugendpsychiatrie und Psychotherapie, 34*(1), 15–25.

Fleischhaker, C., Böhme, R., Sixt, B., Brück, C., Schneider, C., & Schulz, E. (2011). Dialectical behavior therapy for adolescent (DBT-A): A clinical trial for patients with suicidal and self-injurious behavior and borderline symptoms with a one-year follow-up. *Child and Adolescent Psychiatry and Mental Health, 5*(3). Retrieved from *www.capmh.com/content/5/1/3.*

Fruzzetti, A. (2006). *The high conflict couple.* Oakland, CA: New Harbinger.

Garber, J., Clarke, G. N., Weersing, V. R., Beardslee, W. R., Brent, D. A., Gladstone, T. R., et al. (2009). Prevention of depression in at-risk adolescents: A randomized controlled trial. *Journal of the American Medical Association, 301*(21), 2215–2224.

Goldstein, T., Axelson, D. A., Birmaher, B., & Brent, D. A. (2007). Dialectical behavior therapy for adolescents with bipolar disorder: A 1-year open trial. *Journal of the American Academy of Child and Adolescent Psychiatry, 46,* 820–830.

Goldstein, T., Fersch-Podrat, R., Rivera, M., Axelson, D., Brent, D. A., & Birmaher, B. (2012, November). *Is DBT effective with multi-problem adolescents?: Show me the data!* Paper presented at the annual meeting of the Association of Behavioral and Cognitive Therapies, National Harbor, MD.

Groves, S., Backer, H. S., van den Bosch, W., & Miller, A. (2012). Dialectical behaviour therapy with adolescents. *Child and Adolescent Mental Health, 17,* 65–75.

Halaby, K. S. (2004). Variables predicting noncompliance with short-term dialectical behavior therapy for suicidal and parasuicidal adolescents. *Dissertation Abstracts International: Section B: The Sciences and Engineering, 65*(6), 3160B.

Hashim, R., Vadnais, M., & Miller, A. L. (2013). Improving adherence in adolescent chronic kidney disease: A DBT feasibility trial. *Clinical Practice in Pediatric Psychology, 1,* 369–379.

Hoffman, P. D., & Steiner-Grossman, P. (Eds.). (2008). *Borderline personality disorder: Meeting the challenges to successful treatment.* New York: Routledge.

Hope, D. A., Heimberg, R. G., Juster, H. R., & Turk, C. L. (2000). *Managing social anxiety client workbook: A CBT approach.* Boulder, CO: TherapyWorks, Graywind.

James, A. C., Taylor, A., Winmill, L., & Alfoadari, K. (2008). A preliminary community study of dialectical behaviour therapy (DBT) with adolescent females demonstrating persistent, deliberate self-harm (DSH). *Child and Adolescent Mental Health, 13*(3), 148–152.

Kabat-Zinn, J. (1990). *Full catastrophe living.* New York: Delacorte Press.

Katz, L. Y., Cox, B. J., Gunasekara, S., & Miller, A. L. (2004). Feasibility of dialectical behavior therapy for suicidal adolescent inpatients. *Journal of the American Academy of Child and Adolescent Psychiatry, 43*(3), 276–282.

Kaufman, J., Birmaher, B., Brent, D., Rao, U., Flynn, C., Moreci, P., et al. (1997). Schedule for affective disorders and schizophrenia for school-age children present and lifetime version (K-SADS-PL): Initial reliability and validity data. *Journal of the American Academy of Child and Adolescent Psychiatry, 36*, 980–988.

Keuthen, N. J., Rothbaum, B. O., Welch, S. S., Taylor, C., Falkenstein, M., Heekin, M., et al. (2010). Pilot trial of dialectical behavior therapy-enhanced habit reversal for trichotillomania. *Depression and Anxiety, 27*(10), 953–959.

Koons, C. R., Robins, C. J., Tweed, J. L., Lynch, T. R., Gonzalez, A. M., Morse, J. Q., et al. (2001). Efficacy of dialectical behavior therapy in women veterans with borderline personality disorder. *Behavior Therapy, 32*, 371–390.

Linehan, M. M. (1993a). *Cognitive-behavioral treatment of borderline personality disorder.* New York: Guilford Press.

Linehan, M. M. (1993b). *Skills training manual for treating borderline personality disorder.* New York: Guilford Press.

Linehan, M. M. (1997). Validation and psychotherapy. In A. Bohart & L. Greenberg (Eds.), *Empathy reconsidered: New directions in psychotherapy* (pp. 353–392). Washington, DC: American Psychological Association.

Linehan, M. M. (1999). Standard protocol for assessing and treating suicidal behaviors for patients in treatment. In D. G. Jacobs (Ed.), *The Harvard Medical School guide to suicide assessment and intervention* (pp. 146–187). San Francisco: Jossey-Bass.

Linehan, M. M. (2015a). *DBT skills training handouts and worksheets* (2nd ed.). New York: Guilford Press.

Linehan, M. M. (2015b). *DBT skills training manual* (2nd ed.). New York: Guilford Press.

Linehan, M. M., Armstrong, H. E., Suarez, A., Allmon, D., & Heard, H. L. (1991). Cognitive-behavioral treatment of chronically parasuicidal borderline patients. *Archives of General Psychiatry, 48*(12), 1060–1064.

Linehan, M. M., Comtois, K. A., Murray, A. M., Brown, M. Z., Gallop, R. J., Heard, H. L., et al. (2006). Two-year randomized controlled trial and follow-up of dialectical behavior therapy vs. therapy by experts for suicidal behaviors and borderline personality disorder. *Archives of General Psychiatry, 63*(7), 757–767.

Linehan, M. M., Comtois, K. A., & Ward-Ciesielski, E. (2012). Assessing and managing risk with suicidal individuals. *Cognitive and Behavioral Practice, 19*(2), 218–232.

Linehan, M. M., Dimeff, L. A., Reynolds, S. K., Comtois, K. A., Welch, S. S., Heagerty, P., et al. (2002). Dialectical behavior therapy versus comprehensive validation therapy plus 12-step for the treatment of opioid dependent women meeting criteria for borderline personality disorder. *Drug and Alcohol Dependence, 67*(1), 13–26.

Linehan, M. M., Heard, H. L., & Armstrong, H. E. (1993). Naturalistic follow-up of a behavioral treatment for chronically parasuicidal borderline patients. *Archives of General Psychiatry, 50*(12), 971–974.

Linehan, M. M., Schmidt, H., Dimeff, L. A., Craft, J. C., Kanter, J., & Comtois, K. A. (1999). Dialectical behavior therapy for patients with borderline personality disorder and drug-dependence. *American Journal on Addictions, 8*(4), 279–292.

Lynch, T. R. (2000). Treatment of elderly depression with personality disorder comorbidity using dialectical behavior therapy. *Cognitive and Behavioral Practice, 7*(4), 468–477.

Lynch, T. R., Morse, J. Q., Mendelson, T., & Robins, C. J. (2003). Dialectical behavior therapy for depressed older adults: A randomized pilot study. *American Journal of Geriatric Psychiatry, 11*(1), 33–45.

Lynch, T. R., Trost, W. T., Salsman, N., & Linehan, M. M. (2007). Dialectical behavior therapy for borderline personality disorder. *Annual Review of Clinical Psychology, 3*, 181–205.

Mason, P., Catucci, D., Lusk, V., & Johnson, M. (2009, November). *An overview of a modified dialectical behavioral therapy adolescent skills training program in a school setting.* Poster presented at the Child and School-Related Issues SIG at ABCT Convention, New York.

Mazza, J. J., Dexter-Mazza, E. T., Murphy, H. E., Miller, A. L., & Rathus, J. H. (in press). *Skills training for emotional problem solving for adolescents (STEPS-A): Implementing DBT skills training in schools.* New York: Guilford Press.

McDonell, M. G., Tarantino, J., Dubose, A. P., Matestic, P., Steinmetz, K., Galbreath, H., et al. (2010). A pilot evaluation of dialectical behavioral therapy in adolescent long-term inpatient care. *Child and Adolescent Mental Health, 15*(4), 193–196.

McKnight-Eily, L. R., Eaton, D. K., Lowry, R., Croft, J. B., Presley-Cantrell, L., & Perry, G. S. (2011). Relationships between hours of sleep and health-risk behaviors in adolescent students. *Preventive Medicine, 53,* 271–273.

Mehlum, L., Ramberg, M., Tørmoen, A., Haga, E., Larsson, B., Stanley, B., et al. (2012, November). *Dialectical behavior therapy for adolescents with recent and repeated suicidal and self-harm behavior: A randomized controlled trial.* Paper presented at the annual meeting of the Association of Behavioral and Cognitive Therapies, National Harbor, MD.

Mehlum, L., Tørmoen, A., Ramberg, M., Haga, E., Diep, L., Laberg, S., et al. (2014). Dialectical behavior therapy for adolescents with recent and repeated self-harming behavior: First randomized controlled trial. *Journal of the American Academy of Child and Adolescent Psychiatry, 53,* 1082–1091.

Miller, A. L., & Rathus, J. H. (2000). Dialectical behavior therapy: Adaptations and new applications. *Cognitive and Behavioral Practice, 7,* 420–425.

Miller, A. L., Rathus, J. H., & Linehan, M. M. (2007). *Dialectical behavior therapy with suicidal adolescents.* New York: Guilford Press.

Miller, A. L., Rathus, J. H., Linehan, M. M., Wetzler, S., & Leigh, E. (1997). Dialectical behavior therapy adapted for suicidal adolescents. *Journal of Psychiatric Practice, 3*(2), 78.

Morin, C. M. (1993). *Insomnia: Psychological assessment and management.* New York: Guilford Press.

Moss, M. (2013). *Salt, sugar, fat.* New York: Random House.

Nelson-Gray, R. O., Keane, S. P., Hurst, R. M., Mitchell, J. T., Warburton, J. B., Chok, J. T., et al. (2006). A modified DBT skills training program for oppositional defiant adolescents: Promising preliminary findings. *Behaviour Research and Therapy, 44*(12), 1811–1820.

Nock, M. K., & Kazdin, A. E. (2005). Randomized controlled trial of a brief intervention for increasing participation in parent management training. *Journal of Consulting and Clinical Psychology, 73,* 872–879.

Otto, M. W., & Smits, J. A. J. (2011). *Exercise for mood and anxiety: Proven strategies for overcoming depression and enhancing well-being.* New York: Oxford University Press.

Palmer, R. L., Birchall, H., Damani, S., Gatward, N., McGrain, L., & Parker, L. (2003). A dialectical behavior therapy program for people with an eating disorder and borderline personality disorder: Description and outcome. *International Journal of Eating Disorders, 33*(3), 281–286.

Parker-Pope, T. (2010, June 7). An ugly toll of technology: Impatience and forgetfulness. *New York Times,* p. A13.

Perepletchikova, F., Axelrod, S. R., Kaufman, J., Rounsaville, B. J., Douglas-Palumberi, H., & Miller, A. L. (2011). Adapting dialectical behaviour therapy for children: Towards a new research agenda for pediatric suicidal and non-suicidal self-injurious behaviours. *Child and Adolescent Mental Health, 16*(2), 116–121.

Phelan, T. W. (1998). *Surviving your adolescents: How to manage—and let go of—your 13–18 year olds.* Glen Ellyn, IL: Independent Publishers Group.

Pollan, M. (2009). *In defense of food.* New York: Penguin Press.

Porr, V. (2010). *Overcoming borderline personality disorder: A family guide for healing and change.* New York: Oxford University Press.

Pryor, K. (2002). *Don't shoot the dog!: The new art of teaching and training.* Lydney, UK: Ringpress Books.

Rathus, J. H., Campbell, B., & Miller, A. (in press). Feasibility of Walking the Middle Path: A new DBT skills module. *American Journal of Psychotherapy.*

Rathus, J. H., & Feindler, E. L. (2004). *Assessment of partner violence: A handbook for researchers and practitioners*. Washington, DC: American Psychological Association.

Rathus, J. H., & Miller, A. L. (2000). DBT for adolescents: Dialectical dilemmas and secondary treatment targets. *Cognitive and Behavioral Practice, 7*, 425–434.

Rathus, J. H., & Miller, A. L. (2002). Dialectical behavior therapy adapted for suicidal adolescents. *Suicide and Life-Threatening Behavior, 32*, 146–157.

Rathus, J. H., Wagner, D., & Miller, A. L. (2013). *Self-report assessment of emotion dysregulation, impulsivity, interpersonal chaos, and confusion about self: Development and psychometric evaluation of the Life Problems Inventory*. Manuscript submitted for publication.

Ritschel, L. A., Cheavens, J. S., & Nelson, J. (2012). Dialectical behavior therapy in an intensive outpatient program with a mixed-diagnostic sample. *Journal of Clinical Psychology, 68*, 221–235.

Robins, C. J., & Chapman, A. L. (2004). Dialectical behavior therapy: Current status, recent developments, and future directions. *Journal of Personality Disorders, 18*(1), 73–89.

Safer, D. L., Lock, J., & Couturier, J. L. (2007). Dialectical behavior therapy modified for adolescent binge eating disorder: A case report. *Cognitive and Behavioral Practice, 14*, 157–167.

Safer, D. L., Telch, C. F., & Agras, W. S. (2001). Dialectical behavior therapy for bulimia nervosa. *American Journal of Psychiatry, 158*, 632–634.

Safer, D. L., Telch, C. F., & Chen, E. Y. (2009). *Dialectical behavior therapy for binge eating and bulimia*. New York: Guilford Press.

Salbach-Andrae, H., Bohnekamp, I., Pfeiffer, E., Lehmkuhl, U., & Miller, A. L. (2008). Dialectical behavior therapy of anorexia and bulimia nervosa among adolescents: A case series. *Cognitive and Behavioral Practice, 15*, 415–425.

Salbach, H., Klinkowski, N., Pfeiffer, E., Lehmkuhl, U., & Korte, A. (2007). Dialectical behavior therapy for adolescents with anorexia and bulimia nervosa (DBT-AN/BN): A pilot study. *Praxis der Kinderpsychologie und Kinderpsychiatrie, 56*(2), 91–108.

Sally, M., Jackson, L., Carney, J., Kevelson, J., & Miller, A. L. (2002, November). *Implementing DBT skills training groups in an underperforming high school*. Poster session presented at the annual meeting of the International Society for the Improvement and Training of DBT, Reno, NV.

Scheel, K. R. (2000). The empirical basis of dialectical behaviour therapy: Summary, critique, and implications. *Clinical Psychology: Science and Practice, 7*(1), 68–86.

Simpson, E. B., Pistorello, J., Begin, A., Costello, E., Levinson, J., Mulberry, S., et al. (1998). Use of dialectical behavior therapy in a partial hospital program for women with borderline personality disorder. *Psychiatric Services, 49*, 669–673.

Springer, T., Lohr, N. E., Buchtel, H. A., & Silk, K. R. (1996). A preliminary report of short-term cognitive-behavioral group therapy for inpatients with personality disorders. *Journal of Psychotherapy Practice and Research, 5*(1), 57–71.

Sunseri, P. A. (2004). Preliminary outcomes on the use of dialectical behavior therapy to reduce hospitalization among adolescents in residential care. *Residential Treatment for Children and Youth, 21*(4), 59–76.

Telch, C. F., Agras, W. S., & Linehan, M. M. (2000). Group dialectical behavior therapy for binge-eating disorder: A preliminary uncontrolled trial. *Behavior Therapy, 31*, 569–582.

Thakkar, V. G. (2013, April 28). Diagnosing the wrong deficit. *New York Times*, Week in Review, p. SR1.

Trautman, P. D., Stewart, N., & Morishima, A. (1993). Are adolescent suicide attempters noncompliant with outpatient care? *Journal of the American Academy of Child and Adolescent Psychiatry, 32*(1), 89–94.

Trupin, E. W., Stewart, D. G., Beach, B., & Boesky, L. (2002). Effectiveness of a dialectical behavior therapy program for incarcerated juvenile offenders. *Child and Adolescent Mental Health, 7*, 121–127.

van den Bosch, L. M. C., Koeter, M., Stijnen, T., Verheul, R., & van den Brink, W. (2005). Sustained efficacy of dialectical behaviour therapy for borderline personality disorder. *Behaviour Research and Therapy, 43*, 1231–1241.

Velting, D. M., & Miller, A. L. (1999, April). *Diagnostic risk factors for adolescent parasuicidal behavior*.

Paper presented at the 9th annual conference of the American Association of Suicidology, Houston, TX.

Verheul, R., van den Bosch, L. M., Koeter, M. W., de Ridder, M. A., Stijnen, T., & van den Brink, W. (2003). Dialectical behaviour therapy for women with borderline personality disorder: 12-month, randomised clinical trial in the Netherlands. *British Journal of Psychiatry, 182,* 135–140.

Walsh, R. (2011). Lifestyle and mental health. *American Psychologist, 66,* 579–592.

Wansink, B. (2006). *Mindless eating: Why we eat more than we think.* New York: Bantam.

Woodberry, K. A., & Popenoe, E. J. (2008). Implementing dialectical behavior therapy with adolescents and their families in a community outpatient clinic. *Cognitive and Behavioral Practice, 15*(3), 277–286.

Index

Page numbers followed by *f* indicate a figure; *t* indicate a table.